Jay A. Goldstein, MD

Betrayal by the Brain
The Neurologic Basis
of Chronic Fatigue Syndrome,
Fibromyalgia Syndrome,
and Related Neural Network Disorders

Pre-pu   , and an
REVIE   compre-
COMM   eview of
EVALU   ire."

"An
   th
rochemis   into
lems of   brain in
myalgia.   body. I
sight wit   book to
gram for   ues as a
                                          read."

Richard
Clinical I   **1PH**
Departme
UNDNJ-R
Medical S   *na*

"**T**his book bridges the chasm of molecular biology and clinical practice. Dr. Goldstein utilizes a wide range of resources from the basic sciences to form the foundation for clinical research and effective treatments for what were, until recently, considered vague syndromes, including fibromyalgia, chronic fatigue, and irritable bowel. . . . Like many others who have discovered new treatments, his work chronicles the very tight reasoning and sequential clinical trials that systematically led him to his conclusions."

Robert H. Gerner, MD
Department of Veterans Affairs,
Medical Center, West Los Angeles;
Associate Research Psychiatrist,
UCLA

"**T**his is the first truly scholarly, erudite, and definitive work on several complex but related entities. I was most impressed with the neuropharmacology and Goldstein's perception as to its place in his evolving therapeutic pharmacologic armamentarium. All of us in clinical practice have been frustrated with the illusory and transitory treatment regimens heretofore offered. This work offers new and exciting dynamism in the treatment of these most difficult and refractory disorders."

Melvin J. Tonkon, MD
Cardiology Associates Medical Group,
Anaheim, California;
Clinical Professor,
University of California, Irvine

"**I** find reading this book such an education in basic neuroscience, let alone its implications for CFS. . . . We need more of such efforts, no matter how offensive they may be to mainstream scientists and medical school-based academic clinicians. . . . The potential contribution of this book to CFS in particular and the whole array of neurosomatic patients in general is immense, and if carefully read, it will offer any dedicated researcher a whole slew of potentially experimental, testable hypotheses regarding etiology, neuropathology, and treatment."

Peter V. Madill, MD
Sebastopol, California

More pre-publication
REVIEWS, COMMENTARIES, EVALUATIONS . . .

"**J** udged from the vantage point of a pharmaceutical company, this book is an important and challenging synthesis. . . . In my view, CFS is an illness that investigators and clinicians alike wish would go away until such time as we know enough to deal with it more effectively. It represents a lesion that is probably too complex for our current state of knowledge in neurobiology. . . . Into this confusion, Dr. Goldstein launches this book, claiming that he is able to supply most of the missing answers. . . . Most importantly, he offers his program of pharmacological interventions. The success he has reported and the ambitiousness of the undertaking make this book well worth the careful study it requires."

Paul Gladstone, PhD
Senior Research Investigator,
Pharmaceutical Research Institute,
Bristol Myers Squibb,
Seattle, Washington

"**I** am very impressed by his encyclopedic knowledge and his unconventional and daring conclusions and share most of his views."

Robert Olin, PhD
Professor, Huddinge Hospital,
Karolinska Institute,
Stockholm, Sweden

"**T** his book is a primer on neurosomatic medicine. In it, Dr. Goldstein dissects the brain's neurochemical pathways leading to and from the limbic system in order to explain a number of disease states. He has incorporated an incomparable breadth of detail from existing studies to which he has added his own analytic thinking and broad neurochemical perspective to come to the conclusions presented here. . . . Presenting a blueprint for those altered neural pathways, Dr. Goldstein provides a useful guide for research and, at the same time, provides insights that have implications for treatment."

Herbert P. Gordon, DDS, PhD
Associate Clinical Professor,
School of Medicine and Dentistry,
University of Washington

"**R** evolutionary and fascinating. Cuts through established boundaries with an intense intuition to connect relationships [one] never would have thought of."

Mike Paul, PhD
Senior Training Analyst,
Los Angeles Psychoanalytic Society
and Institute

More pre-publication
REVIEWS, COMMENTARIES, EVALUATIONS . . .

"**D**r. Goldstein provides the reader with valuable insights into the complex neural networks that regulate human brain function. He explores, in a scholarly fashion, how disruptions of these networks result in neurosomatic illnesses. . . . This pioneering effort has resulted in an integrated, cohesive model of neural disease. Goldstein's profound understanding of the dysfunctional brain has led to the application of novel therapeutic regimens of proven efficacy. . . . This book makes a very important contribution and should be widely read by practicing clinicians and basic neuroscientists."

W. John Martin, MD, PhD
Professor of Pathology,
USC School of Medicine

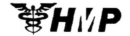

The Haworth Medical Press
An Imprint of The Haworth Press, Inc.

Betrayal by the Brain
*The Neurologic Basis
of Chronic Fatigue Syndrome,
Fibromyalgia Syndrome,
and Related Neural
Network Disorders*

The Haworth Library of the
Medical Neurobiology of Somatic Disorders
Neuroimmunoendocrine Networks
in Health & Illness

Volume I: *Chronic Fatigue Syndromes: The Limbic Hypothesis*

Volume II: *Betrayal by the Brain: The Neurologic Basis of Chronic Fatigue Syndrome, Fibromyalgia Syndrome, and Related Neural Network Disorders*

Editor-in-Chief

Jay A. Goldstein, MD, Director
Chronic Fatigue Syndrome Institute, Anaheim, California

Betrayal by the Brain

The Neurologic Basis
of Chronic Fatigue Syndrome,
Fibromyalgia Syndrome,
and Related Neural
Network Disorders

Jay A. Goldstein, MD

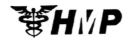

The Haworth Medical Press
An Imprint of The Haworth Press, Inc.
New York • London

Published by

The Haworth Medical Press, an imprint of The Haworth Press, Inc., 10 Alice Street, Binghamton, NY 13904-1580

DISCLAIMER
Medicine is an ever-changing science. As new research and clinical experience broaden our knowledge, changes in treatment and drug therapy are required. While many suggestions for drug usages are made herein, the book is intended for educational purposes only, and the author, editor, and publisher do not accept liability in the event of negative consequences incurred as a result of information presented in this book. We do not claim that this information is necessarily accurate by the rigid, scientific standard applied for medical proof, and therefore make no warranty, expressed or implied, with respect to the material herein contained. Therefore the patient is urged to consult his or her own physician prior to following a course of treatment. The physician is urged to check the product information sheet included in the package of each drug he or she plans to administer to be certain the protocol followed is not in conflict with the manufacturer's inserts. When a discrepancy arises between these inserts and information in this book, the physician is encouraged to use his or her best professional judgement.

Cover designed by Marylouise Doyle.

Library of Congress Cataloging-in-Publication Data

Goldstein, Jay A.
    Betrayal by the brain : the neurologic basis of chronic fatigue syndrome, fibromyalgia syndrome, and related neural network disorders / Jay A. Goldstein.
        p.   cm.
    Companion v. to: Chronic fatigue syndromes : the limbic hypothesis / Jay A. Goldstein. ©1993.
    Includes bibliographical references and index.
    ISBN 1-56024-981-1 (alk. paper).
    1. Chronic fatigue syndrome. 2. Fibromyalgia. 3. Psychoneuroimmunology. 4. Neural networks (Neurobiology). 5. Limbic system. I. Goldstein, Jay A. Chronic fatigue syndromes. II. Title.
    [DNLM: 1. Nervous System Diseases. 2. Nerve Net–physiopathology. 3. Fatigue Syndrome, Chronic–physiopathology. 4. Fatigue Syndrome, Chronic–drug therapy. 5. Fibromyalgia–physiopathology. 6. Fibromyalgia–drug therapy. WL 300 G624b 1994]
    RB 150.F37G649 1994
    616.8'4–dc20
    DNLM/DLC
    for Library of Congress   95-51124
                                                                                                        CIP

This book is dedicated to the two most important people in my life—my wife, Gail, and our six-year-old son, Jordan. For 17 years she has been my partner, inspiration, and cheerleader. She has never flagged in her belief in me and the importance of my work. Gail's dogged persistence, hard work, and sacrifices enable me to plan and chair conferences and lectures about CFS/FMS in the United States and abroad, write books and articles, and still continue to treat my patients. She organizes, listens, edits, administrates, and advises. She suggests that I deflect the brickbats hurled at me, but learn from the intelligent critiques of my colleagues. She urges me not to be dissuaded by the ill-informed and biased opinions of those who have not read my work or do not seem to comprehend it. Jordan is the star atop the Christmas tree, the sparkle in our hearts, and reminds us by his very existence that my work must continue so that his generation will be healthier and wiser than ours. I give thanks every day for my wonderful, supportive family.

ABOUT THE AUTHOR

Jay A. Goldstein, MD, has specialized in Chronic Fatigue Syndrome and related disorders for the past nine years, and has been interested in the illness since 1985. He has written two books on the topic, *Chronic Fatigue Syndromes: The Limbic Hypothesis*, in 1993, and *Chronic Fatigue Syndrome: The Struggle for Health*, in 1990. He is also the author of *Symptoms and Solutions*, published by Berkeley Press. He was a contributing editor to the CFS encyclopedia, *The Clinical and Scientific Basis of Myalgic Encephalomyelitis/Chronic Fatigue Syndrome*, published in 1992. In 1994, a textbook entitled *Myofascial Pain Syndrome and Fibromyalgia*, edited by A. Masi, MD, was published. Dr. Goldstein has written a chapter for this book entitled "Fibromyalgia Syndrome: A Pain Modulation Disorder Related to Altered Limbic Function?" Since 1988, he has been a regular contributor of articles to the *CFIDS Chronicle*, the leading physician/patient publication dealing with Chronic Fatigue Syndrome, and has had over fifty publications in peer-reviewed journals.

Dr. Goldstein organizes annual international conferences about the neurobiology of Chronic Fatigue Syndrome and recently has broadened the scope of these meetings to include other disorders of regulatory physiology caused by dysfunction of brain neural networks. Referring to these illnesses as "neurosomatic," he includes fibromyalgia, irritable bowel syndrome, migraine headaches, interstitial cystitis, sleep disorders, and premenstrual syndrome in this category.

Having training in psychiatry and being board certified in family practice, Dr. Goldstein has taught in residency programs in both specialties. During the 1980s he gave an elective, "Internal Medicine of the Brain," in the UC Irvine Department of Psychiatry and Human Behavior. He was also a co-leader of a seminar there on advanced psychopharmacology. He currently coordinates a team of researchers from several southern California universities who are investigating Chronic Fatigue Syndrome. Dr. Goldstein has offices in Anaheim Hills and Santa Monica.

CONTENTS

Treatments   129

List of Abbreviations

^{133}Xe:	^{133}Xenon (a radioactive isotope)
5-HIAA:	5 hydroxyindoleacetic acid
5-HT:	serotonin
ACE:	angiotensin-converting enzyme
Ach:	acetylcholine
ACTH:	adrenocorticotropic hormone
ADH:	antidiuretic hormone
ADP:	adenosine diphosphate
AED:	antiepileptic drug
AMP:	adenosine monophosphate
ATP:	adenosine triphosphate
BEAM:	brain electrical activity mapping
BNST:	bed nucleus of the stria terminalis
Ca:	calcium
CA1:	cornu ammonis, area 1 (part of the hippocampus)
CCK:	cholecystokinin
CE:	central nucleus of the amygdala
CFS:	chronic fatigue syndrome
CGRP:	calcitonin gene-related peptide
CMV:	cytomegalovirus
CNS:	central nervous system
CO:	carbon monoxide
CO_2:	carbon dioxide
CPK:	creatinine phosphokinase
CRH:	corticotropin-releasing hormone
CSF:	cerebrospinal fluid
CSTC:	cortico-striatal-thalamo-cortical
CT:	computerized tomography
DA:	dopamine
DAG:	diacylglycerol
DDAVP:	desamino-D-arginine vasopressin

DLPFC:	dorsolateral prefrontal cortex
dynA:	dynorphin A
EAA:	excitatory amino acid
EBV:	Epstein-Barr virus
ECT:	electroconvulsive therapy
EDTA:	ethylenediaminetetraacetic acid
EEG:	electroencephalogram
EMG:	electromyogram
ET:	endothelin
FMS:	fibromyalgia syndrome
FPDD:	familial pure depressive disorder
GABA:	gamma-aminobutyric acid
GABA-T:	gamma-aminobutyric acid transaminase
GBP:	gabapentin
GH:	growth hormone
GHRH:	growth hormone releasing hormone
GMP:	guanosine monophosphate
GP:	globus pallidus
gp120:	glycoprotein 120
GR:	glucocorticoid receptor
GSH:	glutathione
HCTZ:	hydrochlorothiazide
HD:	Huntington's disease
HIS:	histamine
HIV:	human immunodeficiency virus
HLA:	human leukocyte antigen
HMPAO:	technetium hexamethyl propyleneamine oxime
HPA:	hypothalamic-pituitary-adrenal
HSV:	herpes simplex virus
HTLV:	human T-cell lymphotropic virus
HVA:	homovanillic acid
I.C.V.:	intracerebroventricular
IBS:	irritable bowel syndrome
IC:	interstitial cystitis
IEG:	immediate early gene
IGF:	insulin-like growth factor
IL-1:	interleukin-1
IP$_3$:	inositol triphosphate

IM:	intramuscular
IPSP:	inhibitory post-synaptic potential
IV:	intravenous
K:	potassium
LA:	lateral amygdala
LC:	locus ceruleus
LTG:	lamotrigine
LTP:	long-term potentiation
MAO:	monoamine oxidase
MAOI:	monoamine oxidase inhibitor
Mg:	magnesium
MHPG:	3-methoxy-4-hydroxyphenylglycol
MR:	mineralocorticoid receptor
MRI:	magnetic resonance imaging
mRNA:	messenger ribonucleic acid
MRS:	magnetic resonance spectroscopy
MSH:	melanocyte-stimulating hormone
N-100:	negative wave at 100 milliseconds after a stimulus, seen on computerized measures of electrical brain activity
Na:	sodium
NE:	norepinephrine
NGF:	nerve growth factor
NK:	natural killer cell
NMDA:	N-methyl-D-aspartate
NO:	nitric oxide
NPY:	neuropeptide Y
NREM:	non-rapid eye movement
NTG:	nitroglycerine
OCD:	obsessive-compulsive disorder
OFC:	orbitofrontal cortex
OXT:	oxytocin
P-300:	positive brain wave deflection seen at 300 milliseconds
PAG:	periaqueductal gray
PD:	Parkinson's disease
PET:	positron emission tomography
PFC:	prefrontal cortex
PG:	prostaglandin
PGD_2:	prostaglandin D_2

PKA:	protein Kinase A
PKC:	protein Kinase C
PMS:	premenstrual syndrome
PPI:	prepulse inhibition
PRL:	prolactin
PTSD:	posttraumatic stress disorder
PVN:	paraventricular nucleus
QD:	per day
rCBF:	regional cerebral blood flow
REM:	rapid eye movement
RSD:	reflex sympathetic dystrophy
RT:	reticular nucleus
SAH:	S-adenosylhomocysteine
SCG:	superior cervical ganglion
SLE:	systemic lupus erythematosus
SN:	substantia nigra
SNS:	sympathetic nervous system
SOM:	somatostatin
SP:	substance P
SPECT:	single photon emission computerized tomography
SRI:	serotonin reuptake inhibitor
STN:	signal-to-noise
SWS:	slow-wave sleep
TGF-beta:	transforming growth factor beta
TH:	tyrosine hydroxylase
THC:	tetrahydrocannabinol
TNF:	tumor necrosis factor
TRH:	thyrotropin-releasing hormone
TS:	Tourette's syndrome
VIG:	vigabatrin
VIP:	vasoactive intestinal peptide
VLM:	ventrolateral medulla
VMH:	ventromedial hypothalamus
VP:	vasopressin
VTA:	ventral tegmental area

Foreword

The book *Betrayal by the Brain: The Neurologic Basis of Chronic Fatigue Syndrome, Fibromyalgia Syndrome, and Related Neural Network Disorders* is a work of major importance. It is a culmination of at least ten years of indefatigable, fully dedicated clinical work limited to chronic fatigue syndrome patients. Five years ago Jay Goldstein, MD, summarized his experience in the book *Chronic Fatigue Syndromes: The Struggle for Health* and two years ago published his monograph entitled *Chronic Fatigue Syndromes: The Limbic Hypothesis.* In this later contribution he gives arguments that point to the limbic origin of the apparently diverse symptomatology exhibited by these patients. On one hand, symptomatology clearly related to the central nervous system, e.g., depression, cognitive impairment, and sleep disorders are accompanied by other symptoms of apparently different nature. These include fatigue, allergy, and immunological disorders (e.g., asthma, rhinitis, chemical sensitivity) and cardiac, dermatologic, endocrine, gastroenterologic syndromes as well. The challenge to trace the diverse origin of these symptoms had contributions from many disciplines: neuropsychiatry, immunology, pharmacology, functional neuroimaging, etcetera.

The contribution of neuroimaging, and in particular, Neuro-SPECT, to the unraveling of the etiopathogenic mechanism of this disorder began in 1988 when I had the opportunity to collaborate with Dr. Goldstein to apply the first brain SPECT functional imaging to patients with CFS. It became apparent that these patients were different from normal controls determined by age-matched data bases. They presented with diminished rCBF (regional cerebral blood flow) in the frontal and temporal lobes, while global assessment of CBF, measured with ^{133}XE imaging, was also reduced. The patterns of cerebral regional perfusion appeared significantly different in patients suffering with depression of onset after 50 years of age, while patients suffering with CFS and developing depression afterward were indistinguishable from the pure CFS patients. These observations were later confirmed by investigators in the USA, Canada, and Europe with additional information on the participation of the basal ganglia and brainstem.

Jay Goldstein's insight into the physiopathology of CFS led him to explore brain function after stress exercise, based on the well-known exacerbation of fatigue and cognitive impairment after physical and sometimes mental activity. Brain SPECT demonstrated marked impairment of brain function persisting in many patients 24 hours after a bicycle stress test. Thus, in the same individual there was a direct correlation between brain function and brain perfusion. This concept holds in the basal state and during activation studies. However, there are pharmacological responses that appear paradoxical in their manifestations. This book has an in-depth analysis of the functional neuroanatomy which unravels the incognita of relationships of limbic system, frontal and temporal cortex, diaschitic phenomena and other manifestations of the complexities of these systems.

My collaboration with Jay Goldstein, MD, has been fruitful and challenging and I recommend this book to the readers as an up-to-date essay on the physiopathology of chronic fatigue syndrome and its presentation as a disorder of brain neural networks. Pharmacological interventions are extensively discussed and justified in their rationale, thus leading to treatment or amelioration of the crippling symptoms of this disorder, only recently fully defined.

Ismael Mena, MD
Emeritus Distinguished Professor
Radiological Sciences
UCLA School of Medicine

Introduction

There will come a time when our descendants will be amazed that we did not know things that are so plain to them.

–Seneca (first century)
Natural Questions, Book Seven

Most patients with chronic fatigue syndrome and fibromyalgia, as well as other disorders of central information processing, which I term "neurosomatic," are not difficult to treat applying the neurosomatic paradigm. About 50 percent of my new patients feel dramatically improved after the first office visit; 25 percent more are better after the second. Twenty percent more eventually respond to treatment, leaving about 5 percent that I cannot help very much. This rate of improvement is tremendously higher than six years ago, when I wrote *Chronic Fatigue Syndrome, The Struggle for Health,* and much better than even three years ago, when I wrote the companion volume to this book, *Chronic Fatigue Syndromes: The Limbic Hypothesis.*

This rapid rate of advance is related to (1) an explosion of knowledge in neuroscience, virtually none of which has filtered down to clinical practice; (2) a few new medications; and (3) attaining a "critical mass" in my data base, so that integrating new research and clinical findings into the neurosomatic paradigm is much easier.

Many of the illnesses treated using this model are still termed "psychosomatic" by the medical community and are treated psychodynamically by psychiatrists, neurologists, and general physicians. Social anthropologists also have their theories, describing chronic fatigue syndrome as the "neurasthenia" of the 1990s, and a "culture bound syndrome" that displaces the repressed conflicts of patients unable to feel or express their emotions ("alexithymics") into a culturally acceptable viral illness or immune dysfunction. Cognitive-behavioral therapy is perhaps more appropriate, since

1

coping with the vicissitudes of these illnesses, which wax and wane unpredictably, is a major problem for most of those afflicted.

Few investigators in psychosomatic illness (except those researching panic disorder) have concerned themselves about the pathophysiology of the patients they study, seeming content to define this population in psychosocial phenomenological terms. This position becomes increasingly untenable as the mind-body duality disappears. This book has been written to explain the neurology of "psychosomatic" disorders, and to propose exciting new therapeutic interventions based on these insights that essentially constitute a new neuropsychopharmacology, one for *neurosomatic* disorders.

I treat my patients pharmacologically. Referrals to psychotherapists are made primarily for patients who are suicidally depressed about their illness, who have relationship problems as a result of it, who have difficulty coping with an altered lifestyle, or who have psychosocial problems such as addictions or sociopathies. I now make these referrals rather infrequently. My wife, Gail, a psychologist, educator, and nurse, has helped me integrate medicine and principles of psychodynamics into the present paradigm and is quite comfortable using this neurosomatic model as a format for her therapeutic interactions with clients.

The legions of paramedical personnel in my office of five to ten years ago are gone. Massage therapists, chiropractors, acupuncturists, nutritional specialists, biofeedback specialists, sleep disorder experts, and physical therapists all helped patients in a palliative manner, but could not remediate the medical concerns of my patients. I make referrals for neuropsychological testing fairly frequently to define the nature and extent of cognitive impairment, but do not do cognitive rehabilitation. It does not work very well in this patient group, since the problems are caused by a biochemical neural network dysfunction, rather than by maladaptive or deficient learning strategies. Memory deficits are usually remedied in short order. We commonly observe patients doubling or tripling their scores on the Irvine Memory Battery one hour after taking the appropriate individualized regimen of medication (Sandman et al., 1993). This response is not transitory, but one that has a lasting effect as long as therapy is continued.

In order to make the diagnostic and therapeutic process cost-effective, I administer multiple medications sequentially in the same office visit, waiting until one has had time to exert its effect before trying the next. The medications do not interact appreciably. When a patient feels almost normal, he or she leaves with samples of and/or prescriptions for the medications that seemed effective, and then reports back to me or returns to the office in one to seven days. This novel therapeutic "immersion" process is disturbing to an occasional patient who may question this approach. Patients who travel long distances to see me usually come to the office for three or four days in a row and then are followed up by telephone. I work in conjunction with their local primary care physicians whenever possible.

The population that consults me is, in general, the more severely impaired, having been helped little by other treatment modalities. Although I still perform a focused physical exam, it is usually superfluous (Deale and David, 1994), except checking for fibromyalgia tender points, the elimination of which I use as the main in-office physical sign of therapeutic efficacy, aside from an alteration in the patient's demeanor and self-report. Sometimes I ask previously fatigued patients to run up and down the stairs, or use the treadmill. I have patients who complain of attentional or developmental learning disorders read a magazine article and then tell me what it was about. There are more precise techniques to assess cognition and endurance, but they are expensive and not necessary at the initial office visit. The amount of money many of these individuals have spent searching for relief is staggering and unnecessary.

Neurosomatic disorders are the most common group of illnesses for which patients consult physicians (Yunus, 1994). Fatigue, depression, anxiety, diffuse pain, cognitive dysfunction, and other neurosomatic disorders present to different specialists in different ways and the final diagnosis often depends on the orientation and specialty of the doctor.

TABLE 1:
EXAMPLES OF NEUROSOMATIC DISORDERS

Allergy and Immunology: allergic rhinitis, asthma, food intolerance, chemical sensitivity, environmental illness, IgG (Immunoglobulin G) subclass deficiency, Gulf War syndrome.

Cardiology: chest pain of unknown etiology, microvascular angina, palpitations, mitral valve prolapse, supraventricular tachycardia.

Dermatology: atopy, psoriasis, lichen simplex chronicus, urticaria, pruritus, diffuse alopecia, granuloma annulare, seborrheic dermatitis, recurrent herpes simplex, hand dermatitis.

Endocrinology: heat and cold intolerance, fatigue, hypothyroidism, autoimmune thyroiditis, adrenal insufficiency, hypercholesterolemia, rapid weight gain or loss, pituitary disorders, nausea.

Gastroenterology: proctalgia fugax, non-ulcer dyspepsia, abdominal pain and bloating, constipation, diarrhea, heartburn, belching, irritable bowel syndrome, intestinal pseudo-obstruction.

Hematology-Oncology: exhaustion, lymphadenopathy, rule out occult neoplastic process, spontaneous ecchymoses.

Infectious disease: chronic viral illness, chronic Lyme disease, chronic mononucleosis.

Neurology: paresthesias, dysesthesias, weakness, numbness, pseudoseizures, blackouts, near-syncope, headaches, cognitive dysfunction, sleep disorders, dysarthria, photophobia, phonophobia, fasciculations, nocturnal myoclonus, paroxysmal movements of limbs during sleep, autonomic episodes during sleep (R/O [rule out] seizures), atypical multiple sclerosis, atypical myasthenia gravis, atypical amyotrophic lateral sclerosis, atypical transient ischemic attacks, atypical migraine, atypical trigeminal neuralgia, atypical gait disturbances, atypical dystonias, disorders of initiating and maintaining sleep, possible narcolepsy, disorders of excessive sleepiness, atypical sensory neuropathy.

Obstetrics and Gynecology: pelvic pain, dyspareunia, endometriosis, ovarian cysts, dysfunctional uterine bleeding, anorgasmia, postpartum mood disorders, hot flashes, premenstrual syndromes, dysmenorrhea.

Ophthalmology: blurred vision, oscillopsia, dim vision, rapid changes in prescription, constriction of visual fields, pupillary abnormalities, "accommodative inertia," ocular pain of unknown etiology.

Oral Surgery/Orthodontia/Periodontia: possible multiple root canal disease, temporomandibular dysfunction, periodontal disease, bruxism.

Orthopedic Surgery: chronic low back and neck pain, sciatic pain due to pyriform muscle syndrome, carpal tunnel syndromes, phantom limb pain, reflex sympathetic dystrophy, repetitive strain injury.

Otolaryngology: nasal congestion, recurrent sinusitis (or what appears to be sinusitis), some cases of hearing loss, tinnitus, recurrent hoarseness, atypical facial pain, dizziness, vertigo, chronic sore throat, aphthous stomatitis, idiopathic parotid enlargement, atypical facial pain.

Pediatrics: attention deficit disorder with and without hyperactivity, "growing pains," polyarthralgias misdiagnosed as rheumatic fever or juvenile rheumatoid arthritis, exertional intolerance, some cases of developmental learning disorders.

Psychiatry: virtually all psychiatric conditions except schizophrenia, pervasive developmental disorder, situational depression and anxiety, personality disorders, mental retardation, and mental disorders due to medical conditions could be subsumed under neurosomatic disorders, as could most of pain and sleep disorder medicine.

Pulmonary Medicine: shortness of breath, sleep apnea, dyspnea on exertion, recurrent cough, asthmatic patients with co-morbid neurosomatic disorders causing shortness of breath.

Rheumatology: fibromyalgia (surprisingly often misdiagnosed by rheumatologists), sicca syndrome (possible Sjögren's syndrome), immune complex disorder (Raji cell assay often elevated), atypical systemic lupus erythematosus (the ANA [antinuclear antibody] is often quite elevated) or mixed connective tissue disorder, atypical Behcet's syndrome, atypical Reiter's syndrome, atypical ankylosing spondylitis.

Urology: prostatodynia, irritable bladder, interstitial cystitis, decreased libido, some cases of incontinence, some cases of erectile or ejaculatory dysfunction.

What is important to understand is that the above conditions do exist, are most often appropriately diagnosed by the respective specialists, and are adequately treated. There is, however, the significant subset of patients with neurosomatic disorders who are misdiagnosed or ignored. It is this population that can most be helped by the neurosomatic paradigm.

Explanations that neurosomatic illnesses have their bases in dysregulated brain mechanisms were popular around the turn of the last century and have been termed "pseudo-neurophysiology" by Edward Shorter, a historian (Shorter, 1992). I can think of no other unifying hypothesis, however, to explain the manifold presentations of neurosomatic disorders.

Essentially, neurosomatic disorders are neurologic illnesses. They are caused by a complex interaction of genetic, developmental, and environmental factors. The mechanism of symptom production may be conceptualized as impaired sensory information processing in a neural network. If extero- and interoceptive sensory input is not distributed and processed properly, an individual may have sensations that would not be appropriate to the context of an experience. Light touch would be painful, mild odors could produce malaise and nausea, walking across the room could be exhausting, and reading a magazine article could cause cognitive impairment. If input processing is not properly controlled, output will not be correct. Thus, a patient may exhibit signs and symptoms of neuroimmunoendocrine dysregulation, feeling in general that "my body doesn't work right," a perception that might be appropriate.

I have written this book as a companion volume to *Chronic Fatigue Syndromes: The Limbic Hypothesis,* published in 1993. Using my model of neural dysregulation, I have been able to incorporate basic neuroscience research into pathophysiology and treatment at an increasingly rapid rate. Thus, I have added layers of regulation to the limbic system, primarily from the prefrontal cortex, but also from the basal ganglia, thalamus, and heteromodal association areas, that help to further explain limbic dysfunction in neurosomatic disorders and suggest novel methods of remediation. As a result, most of my patients feel significantly improved in one or two office visits. Other physicians in the United States and elsewhere have been adapting the treatments discussed in this book to their own patient populations and tell me they are surprised and pleased with the results.

My patients frequently ask me, "Why aren't more doctors following this protocol?" I have pondered the same question for many years, and have several explanations:

1. Most new thinking about pathophysiology and treatment emanates from medical research scientists. The typical scope of interest of such workers is quite narrow and very data-driven. Integrative thinking, which I hope my body of work represents, is mistrusted. Indeed, certain other researchers have sympathetically (I think) warned me that the most direct pathway to academic oblivion is to publish any manuscript that attempts a synthesis of apparently disparate information.

2. The data base necessary to propose an integrative hypothesis is very large. Many physicians feel quite uncomfortable reading work that they lack the expertise to understand or critique. Since neurosomatic medicine is a novel paradigm, few reviewers feel competent to offer substantive suggestions, and many researchers feel quite put off by the whole idea. "I don't have time for speculation," said one senior CFS (chronic fatigue syndrome) researcher whom I met at a conference. He forbade his entire research group to read my work.

3. Since the data base grows so rapidly, the knowledge of neuropsychopharmacology among any neurosomatic researchers becomes rapidly outdated. Since all my therapies attempt to modulate brain function, many of these scientists are poorly equipped to evaluate them, and often dismiss each treatment out of hand. If antidepressants and cognitive-behavioral therapy were the sole answers for most of my patients, it would not be necessary for me to be writing books and articles about how to treat them.

4. There is a widely held view in academia that any treatment not yet proven valid by double-blind, placebo-controlled experiments should not be prescribed unless it is part of an experiment approved by an institutional review board; some think it is actually unethical to do so. I believe it is unethical to withhold a treatment program that

may be efficacious. When I see a patient, I believe it is my obligation to help him/her in any way possible if the risk/benefit ratio is good. For both medicolegal and efficacy considerations, my treatment program uses FDA-approved medications for off-label indications. Forty percent of all drugs are prescribed this way. My therapies are pharmacologically driven, not symptom driven. In 1993 I was invited to a meeting about the management of CFS at the National Institutes of Health. I stated to a group of about 70 researchers that I had developed a paradigm that explained most of the findings of the illness, and treatments based on this paradigm improved most of my patients in very short order. Those in the assemblage who wished to discuss my work with me could do so after the meeting. Guess how many did? If you guessed *two,* you would be high, although one psychiatrist took the time to hiss at me: "All your patients are placebo reactors!" "If so," I replied, "then I've learned a lot about placebo pharmacology!" Since treatment response to agents on my neurosomatic profile is highly variable, double-blind studies would be difficult to perform and would be complex and expensive. Nevertheless, I have applied for grants to do such experiments several times, but the applications have always been rejected. It may be sufficient at the current stage of investigation to demonstrate that all successful neurosomatic treatments act through a common neurophysiologic mechanism, cerebral vasoconstriction, which reflects a basic pathophysiology, noradrenergic denervation hypersensitivity. I discuss the research that has elucidated this principle in subsequent chapters.

> As the Nobel Laureate, Sir Peter Medawar, so well pointed out in his book, *The Art of the Soluble,* no scientist is admired for failing in the attempt to solve problems that are beyond his competence. All successful scientists pick problems they can solve, avoiding the very, very difficult ones. Clinicians by contrast can never avoid the very, very difficult problems in their practice. They must often practice "The Art of the Insoluble." (Shelley and Shelley, 1994)

5. "You need to do double-blind, placebo-controlled experiments, or else no one will believe you," I have been told more than once. I am certainly in favor of this research method. When in solo, fee-for-ser-

vice practice in an era of managed care, it is difficult to do this sort of research without financial support. My grant applications, which are laborious to complete, have all been refused as being "premature." I have published controlled experiments about CFS/FMS (fibromyalgia syndrome) pathophysiology with my colleagues, and would do much more of this sort of thing if funds were available. In the meantime, it is up to the readers of this book to judge for themselves whether these postulates are reasonable, and whether these treatments have a good risk/benefit ratio.

6. It is increasingly difficult to practice non-"cookbook" medicine in an era of cost containment, gatekeepers, formularies, and patient management algorithms. I spend much of my time trying to explain what I want to do for a patient to clerks at insurance companies. Fortunately, much of the past menu of expensive tests and treatments is no longer necessary. Either the tests have been performed in so many previous patients that I generally can project what patterns will occur in most current patients, or I have devised inexpensive therapies (e.g., eyedrops, nitroglycerin, oxytocin) that can supplant costly ones such as intravenous immunoglobulin. Actually, the type of neurosomatic medicine I practice now is extremely cost-effective, requiring a records review, questionnaire analysis, history taking, focused physical exam, treatment trials, and patient education. Usually the appropriate screening evaluations have been done by previous physicians, and I order few tests if any. A neurosomatic symptom profile is very characteristic. If such patients could consult a neurosomatic specialist (or a generalist who had learned about this discipline), much time, money, and suffering possibly could be spared. Such a physician should be more attuned to diagnose unusual medical problems that may simulate neurosomatic disorders and to distinguish a primary illness from secondary symptomatology. A recent study showed that $26,000 was an average medical expenditure prior to consulting a "neurosomaticist" (Lapp, Cheney, and Ouyang, 1994).

Sometimes, when patients have an atypical presentation, or do not respond to treatment, CFS and fibromyalgia syndrome are less likely diagnoses. Sophisticated testing is then necessary.

Case Report

A 46-year-old married Caucasian female MBA consulted me in 1991 with a ten-year history of fatigue and myalgias following viral meningitis. She had seen psychiatrists and other medical specialists and had been treated unsuccessfully with a variety of psychotropic medications. Three years prior to seeing me she had been diagnosed as having CFS on the basis of elevated EBV (Epstein-Barr virus) and CMV (cytomegalovirus) titers. She developed weakness in her right arm, difficulty walking, and cramps in her feet. Shortly before seeing me, she had visited a well-known multispecialty clinic with complaints of myalgias, fasciculations, and paresthesias. CPK (creatinine phosphokinase) was elevated but no diagnosis was made. A neuropathy workup at a leading university including lab tests and EMGs (electromyograms) was normal. A nerve conduction study was "borderline." A mild sensory neuropathy was considered.

On her first visit with me she complained of cognitive dysfunction, which was progressive. A BEAM (brain electrical activity mapping) scan showed left temporal dysfunction. Neuropsychological testing was indicative of diffuse organic involvement and did not show the typical CFS profile of short-term memory deficit. A PET (positron emission tomography) scan was diffusely abnormal. Two brothers had similar symptoms but to a much milder degree. One brother had diabetes mellitus. Two uncles died of heart disease at an early age but were confined to wheelchairs with "arthritis" prior to their deaths. I referred her back to the university medical center to the neurology group who specialized in muscle disorders, because the only disease I knew that could present in this manner was a mitochondrial encephalomyopathy. In this disorder, the mitochondria, the energy-producing organelles of muscle and nerve cells, are structurally damaged and do not function properly. This provisional diagnosis was disregarded, but the patient did respond when I prescribed co-enzyme Q10, a suggested treatment for mitochondrial myopathies. She went on to have three unsuccessful cervical fusions for disc disease, the last in 1994. Three muscle biopsies were done. One taken from the biceps area was normal. The next two from the iliacus and splenius cervicis were done during the second cervical surgery and were placed in the chart. A third operation was performed.

When her local neurologist requested a copy of her university hospital medical records, the final diagnosis was "evidence of denervation atrophy; myopathic change with mitochondrial abnormalities and core-targetoid change," i.e., a mitochondrial myopathy. Her neurologist began to cry because she knew this diagnosis on her patient and friend was tantamount to a death sentence, and could also have explained why three cervical fusions were unsuccessful; the neck muscles could not heal enough to hold up the head.

The patient and her brother returned to the university neurologists for a consultation. She mentioned that three years ago she had been referred by me and that I had given a provisional diagnosis of muscle disease and abnormal brain function.

She related that one neurologist told her, "Dr. Goldstein is a jerk, always doing those scans that show holes in people's brains."

Then she showed him the cervical and iliacus muscle biopsy results. His eyes widened but he said nothing. "Why didn't you tell me I had this three years ago?" she asked.

"We couldn't have known," he replied.

"Dr. Goldstein knew," she said, displaying my referral letter, which ended "R/O mitochondrial myopathy."

"I'll give him that one," the neurologist said.

She is now being considered for a halo, a procedure that would put tongs in her skull to hold up her head. She is very weak. "I'm going down like a stone," she said during our last telephone conversation.

7. "If the only tool you have is a hammer, everything looks like a nail." This aphorism is appropriate to the psychologizing of neurosomatic disorders, especially by the British. There are four major journals concerned with psychosomatic medicine: *Journal of Psychosomatic Research, Psychological Medicine*, *Psychosomatic Medicine*, and *Psychosomatics*. One rarely finds articles discussing neurobiology in any of these journals, most of which appear to apply the concept of somatization to virtually every topic between their covers. Thus neurosomatic disorders have been shoehorned into existing psychodynamic or cognitive-behavioral models, with mostly unsatisfactory results for doctors and patients alike.

8. For the last several years most articles in high-circulation psychiatry journals have been in large part repetitive. Authors seem to be continually reinventing the wheel. Some of my colleagues in biological psychiatry have expressed the same opinion to me. I refer primarily to *The American Journal of Psychiatry, The Archives of General Psychiatry, The Journal of Clinical Psychiatry*, and *The Journal of Clinical Psychopharmacology*. Psychiatry journals that I much enjoy are *Biological Psychiatry, Journal of Neuropsychiatry and Clinical Neuroscience, Neuropsychopharmacology*, and *Psychopharmacology* (Berlin).

Most of my neurosomatic study is in neurobiology and neuroscience. My colleagues and I think that most academic and clinical psychiatrists are generally unaware of this literature. We find that reading basic neuroscience generates many more insights and testable hypotheses than going over the same territory with the same classes of medication. There is still a gap between the basic researchers and the clinicians, one that I am trying to bridge. *Brain Research, Trends in Neuroscience*, several pharmacology journals (especially *Trends in Pharmacology*), *NeuroReport*, various neuroendocrinology and psychoneuroimmunology journals, *Endocrinology, Journal of Clinical Endocrinology* and *Metabolism, Neuroscience, Journal of Neuroscience, Neuroscience Letters, Seminars in Neuroscience*, and *Current Opinion in Neurobiology* round out my "must read" publications. I also like to scan rheumatology, gastroenterology, and pain journals (*Pain* is my favorite), as well as headache and sleep periodicals. I do not like to miss an issue of the *Journal of Neurochemistry*, and skim the neurology journals for articles on behavioral neurology and neuropharmacology. I subscribe to general medical and science journals and read them at home rather than at the library. I listen to medical cassette tapes in the car, and have done so for decades.

I do not list these journals to proclaim how informed I am. Rather, I cite them to illustrate the breadth of interest that I believe a neurosomatic investigator must have. Since neurosomatic disorders involve every medical specialty and every organ system, maintaining an ongoing foundation in basic research and clinical medicine is vitally necessary so that important connections can be made. Scarcely an evening at the biomedical library reading specialty journals passes for me without an "Aha!" moment, relating an esoteric research finding to my clinical experiences.

9. It is important to have capable and curious collaborators. I have been fortunate to work with leading researchers in functional brain imaging, neuropsychology, neuropeptides, immunopathology, virology, psychoimmunology, and rheumatology. I believe that the investigation by this group of scientists into the pathophysiology of neurosomatic disorders is five to ten years ahead of the rest of the world. I attend conferences as frequently as my clinical responsibilities and budget allow, but commonly hear presentations of "new" research that rehash seminal work we did five years ago. Since other meetings in chronic fatigue syndrome and fibromyalgia were infrequently held and, to my way of thinking, almost totally unproductive, I organized a succession of symposia in Los Angeles that were quite successful and informative, primarily concerning the neurobiology of these disorders, integrating disparate research endeavors, and pointing the way for future study. Partly as a result of conferences such as these, neuroscience has gained a firm foothold in neurosomatic research, which no longer is solely concerned with investigation of multiple end-organs or "psychiatrization."

10. I have devoted 12 years of my life to studying chronic fatigue syndrome and neurosomatic disorders. I never imagined at the beginning that this work would lead me to a new conceptualization of mechanisms of health and illness, and what amounts to a superimposition of a dozen or more novel drug therapies onto the neuropsychopharmacologic armamentarium already in place. Having been able to help so many treatment-resistant patients so rapidly and efficiently has been tremendously rewarding. The path has been a lonely one, however, beset with skeptics and financial sacrifices. The unwavering assistance and unconditional support of my devoted wife, Gail, has made this journey possible. As one reviewer wrote, "He has connected all the dots" (Thorson, 1993). I cannot see how the basic principles discussed in this volume and the previous one can be wrong (they seem so obvious), and look forward to my paradigm increasingly being adopted by researchers and clinicians.

PATHOPHYSIOLOGY OF NEUROSOMATIC DISORDERS: A SUMMARY

Chronic Fatigue Syndrome is a disorder of the management of sensory input by the brain. Information from inside and outside the body is misperceived, resulting in inappropriate sensations. Touch can be painful, odors can cause illness, climbing a flight of stairs can be like climbing a mountain. If input is dysregulated, output will be also, because the brain will make regulatory decisions based on improper "data processing." Actually, processing occurs properly, but "gating," the control of data input and output from processing centers, is dysfunctional. Thus, patients frequently complain, "my body doesn't work right."

The basic problem is the misperception of the saliency of sensory information by the prefrontal cortex, which regulates sensory gating as well as neurotransmitter secretion by neurons which secrete the excitatory amino acid glutamate. There appears to be insufficient glutamate secretion resulting in decreased levels of several neurotransmitters, especially norepinephrine (NE). The cause of prefrontal cortex dysfunction is an interaction of genetic, developmental, and environmental factors.

Norepinephrine enhances the "signal-to-noise (STN) ratio" in the processing of sensory input by the brain. If there is a high STN ratio, important information will be extracted from a welter of sensory input. If STN ratio is low, much more sensory input will reach the cerebral cortex, some of it irrelevant. STN ratio is low in neurosomatic patients, accounting for misperception of sensory information, as well as distractibility in stimulus situations where cues are increased, environments as disparate as malls and short-term memory testing.

Substance P (SP) lowers STN ratio. There is a "Yin-Yang" relationship between NE and SP—when one is high, the other is low. NE metabolites are low in neurosomatic disorders and SP levels are quite elevated. Reasons for these abnormalities will be discussed later in the book.

There are four influences on the development of a neurosomatic illness in an individual:

1. *Genetic susceptibility.* This tendency can be strong, weak, or anywhere in between. If it is strong, the patient will develop a neurosomatic illness no matter what, often beginning in childhood. Otherwise, expression of the trait is influenced by other factors.

2. *Developmental issues.* If a child feels unsafe for a period of time from birth through puberty, he may become hypervigilant and interpret the saliency of sensory input differently than a child who feels secure. The neurochemical expression of this experience might be elevated levels of SP enabling him to attend to a wide range of stimuli, as well as transiently elevated cortisol with subsequent downregulation of the HPA axis. Central NE levels would also be low, contributing to dysautonomia as well as abnormalities in sensory processing in the circuit between the dorsolateral prefrontal cortex, thalamus, and the hippocampus.

3. *Viral encephalopathy.* Individuals may be exposed to microbes that produce a persistent infection in neurons and glia without being lytic or initiating an immune response. Susceptibility to such infections would be largely genetically predetermined, but could also be influenced by situational perturbations of the immune response. Persistent CNS viral infections could alter production of transmitters and receptors as well as cellular mechanisms.

4. *Increased susceptibility to environmental stressors due to a reduction in neural plasticity.* The summation of causes 1-3 results in an impaired flexibility of the brain to alter the function of its neural networks to deal with changing internal or external circumstances. An example of this deficit may be encountered in the well-known problem that many neurosomatic patients have in making new memories. In order to encode a memory, a fragile neural network must be strengthened. This process may occur by augmenting secretion of glutamate from firing presynaptic neurons by secretion of a retrograde messenger, such as nitric oxide (NO) by the post-synaptic neuron. NO diffuses in a paracrine manner into firing neurons in the locality, enhancing glutamate secretion. If insufficient glutamate or NO is secreted, neural networks will not be appropriately reorganized (strengthened) and encoding will be fragile. Neurosomatic patients have an impairment in neural plasticity. Deficiency in the neurobiology of encoding is one example of this pervasive disorder. Thus the individual who is predisposed to develop

a neurosomatic disorder may have neural network function dysregulated by overtaxing his capacity for neural plasticity. This concept relates to that of "allostatic load" to be discussed in Chapter 3, and explains why most neurosomatic patients develop their illness in a milieu of increased environmental stressors of various types. An example of this propensity may be seen in the predilection of neurosomatic patients to develop their illness after an acute infection, which produces an increase in hypothalamic activity and a decrease in NE (Dunn, 1993) (Watkins, Maier, and Goehler, 1995b), as do sustained attention, exercise, ejaculation, immunization, emergence from inhalation anesthesia (Chave et al., 1993) or other activities which may produce or exacerbate symptomatology (see Chapter 3).

A Typical Neurosomatic New Patient Treatment Protocol

Agents, tried sequentially	Onset of action	Duration of action
1. Naphazoline HCL 0.1% gtt ⊤ OU	2 - 3 seconds	3 - 6 hours
2. Nitroglycerin 0.04 mg sublingual	2 - 3 minutes	3 - 6 hours
3. Nimodipine 30 mg po	20 - 40 minutes	4 - 8 hours
4. Gabapentin 100-300 mg	30 minutes	8 hours
5. Baclofen 10 mg	30 minutes	8 hours
6. Oxytocin 5 - 10 U IM QD or BID or Syntocinon 1 - 2 puffs TID	15 minutes - 72 hours	12 - 24 hours
7. Pyridostigmine 30 - 60 mg po	30 minutes	4 - 6 hours
8. Hydralazine 10 - 25 mg po	30 - 60 minutes	6 - 12 hours
9. Mexiletine 150 mg po	30 - 45 minutes	6 - 8 hours
10. Tacrine 10 mg	30 minutes	4 - 6 hours
11. Risperidone 0.25 - 0.5 mg	45 - 60 minutes	8 - 12 hours
12. Pindolol 5 mg BID	15 minutes - 7 days	12 hours
13. Lamotrigine 25 - 50 mg QD	30 - 45 minutes	24 hours
14. Sumatriptan 3 - 6 mg SQ	15 - 30 minutes	16 hours
15. Ranitidine 150 mg BID	1 hour - 1 week	12 - 24 hours
16. Doxepin HCL elixir 2 - 20 mg HS	1 hour	variable
17. Sertraline 25 - 50 mg QAM or Paroxetine 10 - 20 mg QAM	1 hour - 8 weeks	1 - 2 days
18. Bupropion 100 mg TID	30 minutes - 8 weeks	8 - 24 hours
19. Nefazodone 100 - 300 mg BID	2 - 8 weeks	24 hours
20. Venlafaxine 37.5 - 75 mg BID	1 - 4 weeks	24 hours
21. Glycine powder 0.4 Gm/Kg/day in juice or Cycloserine 15 - 50 mg QD	1 hour	24 hours
22. Felbamate 400 mg	30 minutes	6 - 8 hours
23. Lidocaine 200 - 300 mg in 500 ml normal saline infused over 2 hours	2 hours - 2 weeks	

I halt sequential trials when the patient is virtually asymptomatic, using other medications if tolerance should develop. These drugs are all relatively free of adverse reactions and do not appreciably interact with one another. Two selective serotonin reuptake inhibitors (SSRIs) should not be given conjointly. I prefer sertraline (Zoloft) because it does not inhibit hepatic cytochrome P_{450}, and thus does not increase serum levels of other agents metabolized by the liver. Paroxetine, however, is less likely to cause agitation and GI (gastrointestinal) side effects. SSRI's do not have as effective an analgesic effect as these other agents. A patient taking tacrine requires regular liver function tests, and felbamate therapy must include routine hematologic and hepatic monitoring. Using this protocol, most patients are dramatically improved in one or two office visits.

Fibromyalgia Syndrome:
A Pain Modulation Disorder
Related to Altered Limbic Function?

Louis Pasteur's theory of germs is a ridiculous fiction. How do you think that these germs in the air can be numerous enough to develop into all these organic infusions? If that were true, they would be numerous enough to form a thick fog, as dense as iron.

–Pierre Pochet

X-rays are a hoax.

–Lord Kelvin

In every large community there will be found at least one physician willing to play up to his patients' psychological need for organicity. Thus do the caregivers themselves contribute to their patients' somatic fixations, plunging youthful and productive individuals into careers of disability.

–E. Shorter, 1995

The literature discussing the structure and function of the limbic system and its cortical projections (Figure 1, illustration section), an example of a neural network that uses a parallel distributed computational strategy, is complex and may be unfamiliar to many readers of this volume. These topics have been well discussed by M.-Marsel Mesulam (1985, 1990), and his works form a good foundation for the understanding of limbic physiology and its derangements.

An earlier version of this chapter appeared in Masi A (ed.) (1994) *Fibromyalgia and Myofascial Pain Syndromes*, London, Balliere-Tindall.

One can view the limbic neural network functioning as a computer, receiving intero- and exteroceptive stimuli (input), primarily via a bewildering array of chemically transduced messengers, integrating them with experiences and attitudes (processing), and selecting responses (output) that should ideally maximize the survival capabilities of the individual (Figure 2, illustration section).

The limbic system is a high-order functional regulator (integrative processing) in the brain, and has effects on fatigue, pain, sleep, weight, appetite, libido, respiration, temperature, blood pressure, memory, attention, concept formation, mood, vigilance, the immune and endocrine systems, and the modulation of the peripheral nervous system (to name a few). If there is limbic dysregulation, any or all of these functions could be deranged. Since there is a neurobiological mechanism for limbic functional disorders, I shall use the term "neurosomatic" to describe them.

Such a complex regulatory system could have many specific areas of vulnerability. Dysfunction could have a primary central etiology, or could occur in response to peripheral stressors of various sorts. Since the limbic system is involved in selecting adaptive responses to stress, and stress could be defined as any event that could alter actual or perceived homeostasis, the range of stimuli that could cause limbic dysregulation is large.

Not only could processing of sensory input be aberrant in CFS/FMS, resulting in dysfunctional responses, but the "weight" given to various sensations might be increased, perhaps accounting for phonophobia, photophobia, and odorant sensitivity, about which many patients complain (Figure 3, illustration section). The weight given to sensory input is called "sensory gating," and has been studied by examining the startle reflex, which is inhibited when the startling stimulus is preceded by a weak prepulse, a weaker version of the same stimulus. This phenomenon is termed prepulse inhibition (PPI), and has been studied in animals and schizophrenics. The technique has also been used to see whether men differ from women in the degree of inhibition of prepulses (Bickford, Luntz-Leybman, and Freedman 1993; Swerdlow, Wan et al., 1993; Swerdlow, Auerbach et al., 1993). Animal studies implicate the hippocampus and reticular formation in PPI, and women inhibit less well than men. The research on schizophrenics does not yield any consistent results. We are studying CFS patients using this technique, and found in a pilot study that all patients have decreased amplitude of the N-100 wave (Goldstein et al., 1994). If these results are validated they may represent a diagnostic test for CFS/FMS (see page 53). We have not been able to perform double-blind, placebo-controlled experiments because of lack of funding, but it is possible that some of the observed pharmacological effects of the medications used reproduce alterations in neurochemical and neurophysiological parameters caused by placebo administration (Peck and Coleman, 1991).

It is likely that FMS and the commonly comorbid anxiety, fatigue, migraine headaches, and irritable bowel syndrome (IBS) (Goldenberg, 1993) have a common neurobiological mechanism, which is almost certainly supraspinal. Pain, a major symptom of FMS as well as of IBS, CFS, and migraine headaches, has numerous descending inhibitory pathways from the brainstem (e.g., raphe nuclei, locus ceruleus, periaqueductal grey, reticular formation) as well as from higher centers such as the hypothalamus, thalamus, basal ganglia, limbic system, and cortical structures. The regulation of pain by higher centers is poorly understood (Tasker and Dostrovsky, 1989; Coderre et al., 1993), but will be discussed in the next chapter. The muscle fatigue of CFS appears to be central (Kent-Braun et al., 1993). Just as pain and fatigue are dysregulated, so are many other neural network functions. There is an increasing tendency to view FMS and CFS as variable presentations of the same pathophysiological process (Waylonis and Heck, 1992; Goldstein, 1993), which appears to be neurobiological. About one-third of CFS patients do not meet the tender point criteria for FMS.

Numerous neurochemical abnormalities have been described in CFS/FMS. A basic finding is a low level of central corticotropin-releasing hormone (CRH) (Demitrack et al., 1991). This polypeptide has other central nervous system (CNS) functions besides regulating proopiomelanocortin and adrenocorticotropic hormone (ACTH) secretion, and is involved in the regulation of the sympathetic nervous system as well as the prefrontal cortex (Fisher, 1989; Takamatsu et al., 1991). In contrast to patients with major depression, those with CFS have hypocortisolemia and increased serotonergic function (Cleare et al., 1995). Interleukin-1 beta (IL-1 beta), a pluripotential cytokine, regulates CRH secretion through interleukin-6

(IL-6) and prostaglandins E_2 and F_2 alpha (Rothwell, 1991). Cerebrospinal fluid (CSF) IL-1 beta levels were normal in a study of CFS patients (Lloyd et al., 1991), as well as in an FMS cohort (Russell, personal communication, 1995), suggesting antagonism of IL-1 beta effect. IL-1 beta is constitutively expressed in brain blood vessels (Wong et al., 1995). CRH is also stimulated by other agents (see following text). Postulating decreased IL-1 effect leaves the increased CSF substance P levels (Vaeroy et al., 1988) poorly explained, since IL-1 is known to stimulate substance P secretion (Martin et al., 1993). Substance P, however, inhibits the release of CRH (Larsen et al., 1993). It also unmasks connections in the dorsal horn and may be involved in the formation of new receptive fields (Hoheisel et al., 1993). The role of elevated substance P is further discussed in the next chapter. IL-1 beta appears to play various roles in the brain, constitutive or inducible. Chronic administration of IL-1 beta to rats increased NE concentrations in the paraventricular nucleus, median eminence, and hippocampus (Hokanson et al., 1995). It facilitates afferent sensory transmission in the primary somatosensory cortex (Won et al., 1995). Il-1 beta requires NE to induce Fos in the paraventricular nucleus, but can increase plasma corticosterone despite NE depletion (Dunn, Swiergel, and Stone, 1995).

Using the model of decreased central IL-1 beta effect resulting in decreased secretion of CRH, the peripheral immune activation found in CFS can be accounted for (Saperstein et al., 1992), since CRH is immunosuppressive by virtue of its stimulation of cortisol secretion as well as sympathetic activity in the spleen and regional lymphatic organs. IL-1 beta may, however, stimulate secretion of biogenic amines directly without prostaglandin involvement or elevation of CRH levels (Shintani et al., 1993). Recent evidence indicates that peripheral IL-1 beta induces corticosterone elevation and hypothalamic norepinephrine depletion by simulating peripheral vagal afferents rather than by affecting circumventricular organs or by gaining direct access to the brain (Fleshner et al., 1995). Modulating the activity of the central nervous system by stimulating peripheral nerves in various ways will be one of the central themes of this book.

We (Goldstein and Daly, 1993) have used exercise ergometry as a stressor in patients with CFS/FMS to compare IL-1 regulated functions pre- and post-exercise, as has been done by others (Griep, Boersma, and de Kloet, 1993). We failed to find the expected increases in cortisol, IL-1, IL-6, catecholamines, growth hormone, beta-endorphin, somatostatin, and core body temperature after exercise (Goldstein, 1993). These results were markedly different from those found in normal and anxious groups of exercising adolescents (Gerra et al., 1993). Hyperventilation was more common among the CFS patients who had greater than 11 out of 18 fibromyalgia tender points, as was a marked irregularity in tidal volume at maximal exercise, a finding not previously reported (see Figure 5, illustration section). The regulation of automatic respiration is a function of the limbic system (Munschauer et al., 1991), and this type of abnormality is more evidence of limbic dysfunction in CFS/FMS. An irregularity in tidal volume has also been recorded during REM sleep of patients with panic disorder (Stein et al., 1995).

We (Goldstein et al., 1995) and others (Ichise et al., 1992; Mountz et al., 1993) have found brain single photon emission computerized tomography (SPECT) with technetium hexamethyl propyleneamine oxime (HMPAO), a measure of regional cerebral blood flow (rCBF), to be abnormal in CFS. Patients with CFS/FMS in our study had the same regional hypoperfusion (anterior temporal, dorsolateral prefrontal, and right hemisphere worse than left) as CFS patients without FMS, and the FMS patients had more severe hypoperfusion. CFS/FMS patients had significantly different patterns of perfusion than a matched comparison group with depression. We consistently find rCBF measured using Xenon-133 (^{133}Xe) to decrease after exercise in this population (Mena, 1993), the opposite of what occurs in normals (Madsen et al., 1993).

Research increasingly points to a genetic propensity to develop CFS/FMS. We have found HLA-DR4 to be significantly increased in patients compared with normals ($P = 0.02$) (Goldstein, 1993), and others have (Klimas, 1993) or have not (Middleton, Savage, and Smith, 1991) confirmed these findings. HLA is the logo for the human major histocompatibility gene complex. DR4 refers to the genes of the DR4 chromosomal region. All clinicians seeing a large number of such patients note an increased familial incidence, with panic disorder (Hudson et al., 1992) being the familial comorbid disorder with the highest occurrence. Panic disorder is generally believed to have a predominantly limbic mechanism (Coplan et al., 1992). Biogenic amine levels in the cerebrospinal fluid of rhesus monkeys are under genetic control (Clarke et al., 1995). However, a hereditary predisposition to develop a certain illness may range from strong to weak. Those with a strong tendency to be afflicted with CFS/FMS may have had the disorder since childhood. Others may require one or more triggering stimuli such as child abuse, viral infections, surgery, pronounced physical or mental overexertion, childbirth, or emotional stress.

It is fairly well accepted that victims of child abuse are more likely to develop somatic symptoms as adults (Fry, 1993). Since the limbic system is the primary mediator of the stress response, it is reasonable to assume that functional changes, which may be long lasting, could occur in the neurons in this network (Teicher et al., 1993). The hypercortisolemia of prolonged stress may damage neurons in the cornu ammonis, area 1 (CA1) region of the hippocampus and alter the regulation of hippocampal corticosteroid receptors, an effect that may be ameliorated by the CNS calcium channel blocker nimodipine (Levy et al., 1993). Changes may occur not only in transmitters and receptors, but also in the second messenger cascade, transcription factors, peptides, proteins, and growth factors (Post, 1992). Waxing and waning of symptoms, common in neurosomatic disorders, may be related to variable production of compensatory factors such as thyrotropin-releasing hormone, CRH itself, and gamma-aminobutyric acid (GABA) or one of the subunits of the GABA receptor (Post, 1995). Hippocampal volumes, which are decreased in various conditions including post-traumatic stress disorder (Bremner et al., 1995), have been normal in the numerous CFS patients in whom I obtained hippocampal MRI views.

Viral infections affect patients differently, perhaps depending on how viral sequences are processed and presented. Some individuals may present an epitope that others do not. Viruses may produce a latent infection that does not cause an immune response (Joly, Mucke, and Oldstone, 1991), may alter secretion of only one neurotransmitter (Oldstone, 1989), or may cause "hit and run" infections in which long-lasting alterations of cellular function can occur after the virus has disappeared (Demitrack and Greden, 1991). A decrease in potassium-evoked 5-HT (serotonin) release from virus-infected cortical synaptosomes has been demonstrated (Bouzamondo, Ladogana, and Tsiang, 1993). Infection of mice with Newcastle disease virus, however, increases hypothalamic levels of serotonin and norepinephrine (Dunn and Vickers, 1994). A virally induced neurotransmitter deficit may be corrected with appropriate medication (Mehta, Parsons, and Webb, 1993). Latent herpes virus infections are well known to exist in nerve ganglia and to appear at times of stress (Bonneau et al., 1993). The trigeminal nerve, which can modulate limbic activity through projections to the pontine reticular formation and hypothalamus (Burstein, Borsook, and Strassman, 1993), is commonly involved in the production of herpes labialis, for example. Herpes simplex is the most common virus to infect the limbic system, usually in the anterior temporal cortex. Viruses may enter the limbic system via retrograde neuronal transport (Lavi, Fisman, and Highkin, 1988). Thus a viral infection could alter neuronal function in a genetically vulnerable person, who may already have some premorbid limbic-related disorders such as bruxism, IBS, and allergic rhinitis, in such a way that the function of the neural network could be further dysregulated, so that sensory gating (input) and processing abnormalities would produce more symptoms. The aspects of viral infection relevant to CFS/FMS are given in Table 2. Thus far, there is no single viral candidate for precipitating CFS, and multiple agents could be implicated.

Human immunodeficiency virus (HIV) glycoprotein 120 (gp120) blocks the CD4 receptor, which is also the vasoactive intestinal peptide (VIP) receptor. CD, or cluster of differentiation, refers to human lymphocyte surface molecules. CD4 binds to gp120. VIP stimulates the production of nerve growth factors (Buzy et al., 1992), as well as nitric oxide (Yamamoto et al., 1993) and IL-1 alpha and beta (Brenneman et al., 1992).

Gp120 can also block neuronal L-type calcium channels, a process that can be antagonized by nimodipine, a centrally acting dihydropyridine calcium-channel blocker (Stefano et al., 1993). Voltage-sensitive calcium channels have been divided into three subtypes, termed "L," "N," and "T" based on their conductancy and sensitivities to voltage. Only L-type calcium channel blockers are in clinical use today. VIP and IL-1 are important for neuronal survival (Brenneman et al., 1992). It has been suggested that antag-

TABLE 2. Aspects of viral infection relevant to CFS/FMS.

---

1. Infection is not lytic and does not cause structural alteration.

2. More than one virus may be involved. Two viruses may interact with each other and enhance virulence, a process known as transactivation, well known with human herpesvirus-6 and human immunodeficiency virus. Viral gene products and host gene products may interact as well.

3. Viral gene products and/or cellular products may affect bystander cells. These products may be cytokines, glycoproteins such as gp120 in HIV infection, or other transmitter substances. They may also cause systemic effects or immune activation if acting at a distance. A viral infection may also cause decreased secretion of a cellular product.

4. Superantigens may be produced. These are viral gene products that bind to the variable segment of the T-cell receptor and the major histocompatibility complex molecule, and cause fairly nonspecific immune activation. Bacterial exotoxins may also act as superantigens. Toxic shock syndrome and postinfectious arthritic disorders have been suggested as being caused by superantigens (Sissons, 1993).

5. A persistent CNS viral infection that does not provoke an immune response, a limbic encephalopathy, is also possible.

---

onism of VIP and IL-1 by gp 120 is responsible for the HIV cognitive/motor complex, which is often the first manifestation of the acquired immunodeficiency syndrome (AIDS). Since gp120 is currently being tested as an HIV vaccine, such may not be the case. Peptide T, a synthetic VIP analog, may be useful in blocking the central effects of gp120. The use of nimodipine in HIV encephalopathy is being investigated. Cognitive dysfunction could similarly occur in patients with CFS/FMS if a persistent or hit-and-run viral infection were implicated in the pathogenesis, or could even occur de novo.

Cytomegalovirus (CMV) has been detected in the frontal lobes on postmortem examination of schizophrenic patients (Hampel et al., 1994). A CMV-related recombinant virus has been isolated in many CFS patients and has been recovered on brain biopsy from patients with idiopathic neurologic diseases (Martin et al., 1994). Some patients with chronic fatigue syndrome have had an African green monkey cytomegalovirus sequenced from their blood. This finding raises the disturbing possibility that the attenuated poliovirus grown in green monkey cell culture in the early 1960s could have been contaminated and subsequently infected much of the population (Martin et al., 1995). This virus, when inoculated into cats, produces a diffuse encephalopathy, which is noninflammatory (Martin and Glass, 1995). Since this virus is not susceptible to existing antiviral agents (Martin, personal communication, 1995), neuroregulatory pharmacologic approaches are reasonable.

There is a genetic difference in HLA haplotypes that may determine which antigenic determinant of the Epstein-Barr virus (as well as other infectious agents) causes immune activation (de Campos-Lima et al., 1993). With variable epitopes, there would be variable immune responses, perhaps accounting for such conundrums as why only 5 percent of the population develops acute infectious mononucleosis. Similar considerations could apply to the development of CFS/FMS, Reiter's syndrome, and other postinfectious disorders.

What can the presumed pathophysiology of CFS/FMS as a limbic neural network disorder suggest about using pharmacological probes to explore therapeutic approaches?

LIMBIC REGULATION BY TRIGEMINAL NERVE MODULATION

The trigeminal nerve may be viewed as a major integrator of somatic and visceral input. Spinal, cervical, and some cranial nerves synapse with the spinal and mesencephalic trigeminal nerve tracts. The trigeminal nerve may produce expansion of the receptive field zones of wide dynamic range neurons and nociceptive-specific neurons under certain conditions, perhaps involving increased secretion of substance P, so that a greater number of neurons will be activated by stimulation of a receptive zone, causing innocuous stimuli to be perceived as painful (Dubner, 1992; Fromm et al., 1993). Most of this work has been done in the spinal cord dorsal horn, but could also apply to the rostral and caudal trigeminal nerve nuclei, especially the trigeminal subnucleus caudalis, which is considered to be the homologue of the spinal dorsal horn. This research has focused mainly on peripheral noxious stimuli, but has been applied to central processes such as deafferentation pain and phantom limb syndrome (Melzack, 1992).

There are numerous ways to modulate trigeminal nerve activity. The agent I use most frequently is an adrenergic ophthalmic solution such as naphazoline hydrochloride 0.1 percent (Vasocon, Naphcon, etc.). One drop is placed in each eye and the patient is assessed two to three seconds later. In about one-fifth of the patients there will be significant relief of pain and tender point sensitivity, as well as decreased fatigue and more mental clarity. CFS/FMS patients with prominent anxiety symptoms respond the best to this treatment, but anxiety is not essential for a good result.

I have tried to understand the mechanism of the above action by performing pre- and post-treatment ^{133}Xe brain SPECT. There is a significant diminution of rCBF after a drop in the first eye, which becomes profound after the second eye is instilled. The response is not ipsilateral, as would occur from stimulation of the trigeminal neurovascular system, which causes vasodilation in only one hemisphere. I have proposed that there is a multisynaptic pathway from the mesencephalic trigeminal tract to the pontine reticular formation, and/or to the hypothalamus and thalamic reticular nuclei, and subsequently to the cortex and the limbic system, perhaps the hippocampus (Goldstein, 1993). Sensory inputs produced by touch and pain are transmitted to the thalamus by separate pathways, but travel to the cortex in a single projection. When pain occurs, touch neurotransmission from the thalamus is inhibited by GABAergic interneurons in the thalamic reticular nuclei. Impairment of thalamic gamma-aminobutyric acid (GABA) secretion could result in touch sensation being perceived by the cortex as noxious, and could be one mechanism of central pain (Barinaga, 1992). There is also a direct projection from the trigeminal brainstem neurons of the rat to the hypothalamus (Malick and Burnstein, 1995). Benzodiazepines such as alprazolam enhance the effect of GABA and could act in the thalamus to reduce the central pain of FMS. GABA-mimetic medications should be even more effective (see sections on baclofen, gabapentin, and lamotrigine). Naphazoline may also stimulate trigeminal nerve glutamate secretion to inhibit release of substance P from trigeminal nucleus caudalis primary afferents (Cuesta et al., 1995).

The naphazoline-induced cerebral vasoconstriction may be due to the release of a neuroactive substance that also affects arterial tone. A transmitter secreted by the endothelium as well as by other cell types would be a likely candidate. The list of endogenous cerebral vasoconstrictors is shorter than that of vasodilators. It includes norepinephrine, neuropeptide Y, endothelin, thromboxane, IL-1 receptor antagonist protein, angiotensin II, vasopressin, and serotonin (depending on which serotonin receptor is involved [Matsui et al., 1991; Peticlerc et al., 1992; Uddman et al., 1993]). Nonadrenergic ophthalmic agents usually have no effect, except for proparacaine, which sometimes transiently reduces pain in FMS and has been touted as a treatment for trigeminal neuralgia (Zavonik and Fichte, 1991) and cluster headache. Proparacaine may work by decreasing excessive firing of low-threshold mechanoceptive neurons in the spinal trigeminal nucleus oralis (Fromm, 1991). Pilocarpine 0.5 percent is effective in some patients, although its onset of action is several minutes.

It is somewhat unusual in published reports of brain functional imaging to see a worsening of hypoperfusion correlated with symptomatic improvement, since cerebral metabolism and blood flow should be directly related. Regional rates of perfusion are tightly matched to the corresponding level of substrate demand for metabolic activity. However, imipramine produces cerebral hypoperfusion (Lottenberg, 1993), and endothelin increases cerebral metabolism with an uncoupling of blood flow, since it is a powerful cerebral vasoconstrictor (Gross et al., 1992). The hypermetabolic activation is mediated by L-type calcium channels and is inhibited by nimodipine, an effective treatment for CFS/FMS, suggesting that endothelin excess might contribute to neurosomatic symptomatology.

Case Report

A 46-year-old obese married Caucasian female accountant with type II diabetes mellitus had a history of migraine headaches since childhood. At age 42 she developed asthma and multiple chemical sensitivity with cacosmia, developing malaise after low-level chemical odorant exposure. Then at age 44 she developed typical CFS symptoms including fatigue, sleep disorders, cognitive dysfunction, and fibromyalgia. She had to stop working.

Ten seconds after using naphazoline 0.1 percent ophthalmic solution, one drop in each eye, all her symptoms were gone. She remarked that all the colors in the room seemed brighter. Many patients experience an attenuation of color perception caused by prefrontal dysregulation of the neural network in the early visual cortices (Damasio, 1994) with a nexus in V4 (Sadun, personal communication, 1995), to be specific. Area V4 of the visual cortex is a large region which has neurons that show complicated responses to wavelength but are fairly indifferent to movement. Dim vision occurs in dysautonomias such as the Shy-Drager syndrome. She was followed for six months and maintained her improvement, as long as she used the naphazoline once or twice a day. Her multiple chemical sensitivity resolved as well.

Any ocular alpha-adrenergic agent is effective, including alpha-2 agonists. I prefer to use naphazoline because it is so inexpensive, and has a long record of safety. Some tolerance usually develops to its effects.

Patients often look at me strangely when I suggest using eyedrops to treat a neurosomatic disorder, but are usually delighted when they are effective.

Sometimes patients become overstimulated by 0.1 percent naphazoline and complain of nervousness and insomnia ("I feel like I took six Vivarin!"). This problem can be simply resolved by diluting the product with normal saline until there are no adverse reactions. Over-the-counter (OTC) ocular vasoconstrictors (e.g., Clear Eyes) contain one-eighth the concentration of naphazoline found in prescription drops and may be suitable for the very sensitive individual. Most neurosomatic patients have no generalized benefit from the OTC agents.

POSSIBLE LIMBIC REGULATION BY ENDOTHELIN

Endothelin, a 21-amino-acid peptide, was discovered in 1988. There are three endothelins (ET-1, ET-2, and ET-3) and two endothelin receptor types (ET_A and ET_B). Endothelin receptors are found in neuronal, neuroendocrine, and endocrine cells as well as in endothelial cells. Endothelins promote the release of vasopressin, substance P, luteinizing hormone, follicle-stimulating hormone, prolactin, and growth hormone. Rapid development of sensitization to prolonged or repetitive stimulation with endothelin is usual, possibly by endocytosis of the endothelin-receptor complex (Stojilkovic and Catt, 1992). Tolerance to naphazoline ophthalmic solution is common, as it is to other agents that may stimulate endothelin secretion (see below). Perhaps pertinent to CFS/FMS, endothelin may or may not stimulate CRH neurons (Hirai et al., 1991; Yasin et al., 1994). Complicating the issue somewhat, ET-1, acting at the ET_B receptor, is vasodilatory, generating prostacyclin, nitric oxide, and an endothelium dependent hyperpolarizing factor distinct from nitric oxide (Haynes, Davenport, and Webb, 1993). Naphazoline, an alpha-adrenergic agonist, may of course act primarily by noradrenergic mechanisms.

ET-1, acting at the ET_A receptor, stimulates neuronal release of dopamine (Kurosawa et al., 1991), a neurotransmitter important in regulating mood and activity. The effect of dopamine on rCBF is somewhat similar to its action in the peripheral circulation. Low doses cause vasodilation and high doses produce vasoconstriction (Koyana et al., 1990; Grasby et al., 1993). The dopamine-releasing properties of ET-1 have thus far been studied only in relation to its production of ischemia, and can be attenuated by calcium channel blockers (Ooboshi et al., 1993) and hydralazine (Fuxe et al., 1992), both of which are sometimes effective treatments for CFS/FMS. Endothelin, acting at the ET_B receptor, is involved in both stimulatory and neurotoxic actions on striatal dopamine receptors, which are the result of release of glutamate acting at NMDA (N – methyl – D – aspartate) receptors on striatal dopaminergic nerve terminals (Kataoka et al., 1995). ET-1 given by intracerebroventricular injection to mice produces long-lasting, dose-dependent antinociception, which is not antagonized by naloxone (Nikolov et al., 1992). Because of the high density of endothelin receptors in the hypothalamus and limbic system, CSF endothelin levels were measured in patients with depression and in normal controls (Hoffman et al., 1989). Endothelin levels in the depressed group were about half of that of the control population. Endothelins are thought to be "paracrine factors normally involved in long-term cellular regulation, but which may be important in several pathologies, many of them stress-related" (Huggins, Pelton, and Miler, 1993). Numerous endothelin agonists have been synthesized (Huggins, Pelton, and Miler, 1993) and an agent with appropriate receptor specificity may be a useful treatment for neurosomatic disorders, unless elevated central endothelin levels are responsible for the baseline hypoperfusion seen in brain SPECTs of these patients, in which case centrally acting endothelin antagonists might be helpful. Peripheral endothelin antagonists would lower blood pressure, and could be hazardous in the neurosomatic patient. CSF endothelin levels are elevated in patients with fibromyalgia syndrome (FMS) (Goldstein, Russell, and Gilbert, 1995). Endothelin-1 has been found to stimulate the release of oxytocin and vasopressin, but not CRH (Yasin et al., 1994).

Migraine headaches are fairly common in neurosomatic patients, and plasma ET levels are elevated in migraineurs, even between crises (Farkkila et al., 1992). It has been suggested that ET-3 acts in neurogenic inflammation via prejunctional ET_B receptors, which promote the release of tachykinins such as substance P (Brandli et al., 1996).

LIMBIC REGULATION BY NITRIC OXIDE

Nitric oxide (NO) is the primary vasodilator in the brain. It "might serve as a diffusible signal within neuronal tissue that is necessary for the release of catecholamines and possibly other neurotransmitters evoked from axonal terminals. This proposed function for NO would be in addition to the three roles for the substance in vertebrate nervous systems—that is, regulation of local blood flow, regulation of synaptic efficacy, and segregation of axonal arbors on the basis of neuronal activity" (Hanbauer et al., 1992). NO synthase, a fairly ubiquitous enzyme, is heavily concentrated in the hippocampus (Valtschanoff et al., 1993) as well as in the rostral ventrolateral medulla, another site for sensory gating (Iadecola et al., 1993).

In the hippocampus, NO and another gaseous neurotransmitter, carbon monoxide, serve as retrograde messengers that produce activity-dependent presynaptic enhancement during long-term potentiation (Zhuo et al., 1993). Other putative retrograde messengers, more difficult to supply exogenously, include arachidonic acid and platelet-activating factor (Zorumski and Izumi, 1993). Long-term potentiation, which can last hours or days, refers to prolonged changes in a target neuron resulting from intense but brief trains of stimuli delivered to a presynaptic neuron. When I saw the profound regional cerebral hypoperfusion in CFS/FMS brain SPECTs, one of my first inclinations was to reverse it with NO. The best available marketed source of NO is nitroglycerin, which exerts its vasodilatory actions by conversion into NO. Giving CFS/FMS patients very low (0.04 mg) doses of sublingual nitroglycerin sometimes results in an amelioration of symptoms, especially pain, in about two minutes. It is also effective in central pain such as deafferentation syndrome and reflex sympathetic dystrophy. Patients with failed back syndrome sometimes respond to it. Tolerance to this effect of nitroglycerin often develops, but peripheral vasodilation still occurs.

One would expect considerable cerebral vasodilation on brain SPECT after nitroglycerin in neurosomatic patients, but such is not always the case. When the medication relieves neurosomatic symptoms there is actually vasoconstriction. NO is sometimes released by endothelin to decrease vasoconstriction, but NO does not stimulate endothelin release (Webb, 1991). This result again suggests that symptomatic improvement in CFS/FMS is not dependent on reversing hypoperfusion, and that post-treatment blood flow changes are epiphenomena. Perhaps contributing to this effect, human endothelial cells can synthesize and release inhibitors of NO production (Fickling et al., 1993).

Some of the agents I use are vasodilators, and it appears that their effect on rCBF in CFS/FMS patients is a summation of their intrinsic vasodilator capability and whatever vasoconstrictors are concomitantly released. Vasodilators may cause baroreceptors to reflexly stimulate NE (norepinephrine) secretion from sympathetic ganglia. This mode of action would not explain the ineffectiveness of compounds such as angiotensin-converting enzyme inhibitors or alpha blockers in treating neurosomatic disorders. Naphazoline, however, an adrenergic agonist in the eye, always results in cerebral vasoconstriction in patients who have a beneficial outcome, although this result is the end product of a multisynaptic pathway. Patients who do not respond to naphazoline have little or no reduction in their rCBF.

NO influences transmitter secretion from so many types of neurons that it is difficult to pin down a role for it in CFS/FMS.

Possible Roles for Nitric Oxide in CFS/FMS

Effects on NAPDH-Diaphorase Activity and Fos Expression in Brain Nuclei Following Nitroglycerin Administration

Nitroglycerin (NTG) exerts effects on the CNS which are mediated in part by the noradrenergic system. When NTG is administered to rats, there is Fos expression in brain nuclei which are known to contain NADPH-diaphorase, the enzyme which synthesizes nitric oxide. These structures include the locus ceruleus, parabrachial nucleus, nucleus tractus solitarus, spinal trigeminal nucleus caudalis, paraventricular and supraoptic nuclei. The regions of the latter two structures which expressed Fos were those which secreted *oxytocin* (OXT) and not vasopressin (Tassorelli and Joseph, 1995). There may be an OXT deficit in neurosomatic disorders, and OXT is often an effective treatment (see page 156). Recent neuroanatomic evidence has suggested a role for NO in processing sensory or nociceptive information in the medulla and spinal cord (Dun, Dun, and Forstermann, 1994; Lee et al., 1993). I shall demonstrate in subsequent chapters that a CNS NO and NE deficit in neurosomatic disorders impairs the proper interpretation of sensory input, resulting in sensations that are inappropriate to the stimulus situation, a lowered signal-to-noise ratio, and a reduction in neural plasticity. These deficits are at the core of neurosomatic disorders.

Effects on Glutamate Secretion

NO enters firing presynaptic neurons by retrograde diffusion, where it stimulates guanylyl cyclase, which produces cyclic guanosine monophosphate (GMP) (Kandel and Hawkins, 1992). The latter compound then induces glutamate secretion. NO diffuses only into neurons that are already secreting neurotransmitter, potentiating the signals in that particular microneural network, a process called long-term potentiation (LTP). LTP has been most studied in the hippocampus in relation to the making of new memories, the function most impaired in the neuropsychological testing of CFS/FMS patients (Sandman et al., 1993). Increasing "synaptic strength" in other types of neural assemblies may be an important aspect of CFS/FMS treatment. CFS/FMS may also be viewed as a synaptic convergence deficiency syndrome, convergence being defined as a process by which each neuron has stronger connections with fewer target cells (Greenough and Bailey, 1988). The role of NO in LTP could be an example of convergence. An impairment of its secretion could result in decreased neural plasticity (see page 39).

Serotonergic agents are often useful in CFS/FMS, and applications of serotonin in LTP paradigms mimics the behavioral and electrophysiological effects of LTP and produces a long-term enhancement of synaptic efficacy (Patterson, 1992).

Effects on Short-Term Memory

Short-term memory (encoding) is so poor in CFS and distractibility is so pronounced that we consider this deficit to be diagnostic (Sandman et al., 1993). LTP also occurs in the frontal cortex (Bear and Kirkwood, 1993), and impaired secretion of NO could detract from the precision of interneuronal communication in the region. Twelve FMS patients with few other symptoms besides pain were tested to see whether an encoding problem was present. All patients had evidence of this deficit, although none were aware of it (Goldstein and Sandman, 1990, unpublished). Encoding deficits often respond rapidly and dramatically to the treatments discussed in this book.

Anxiolytic Effects

NO is anxiolytic. Chlordiazepoxide has no effect when administered to mice pretreated with an NO synthase inhibitor, but chlordiazepoxide action returns when the mice are given L-arginine, a NO precursor (Quock and Nguyen, 1992). NO enhances NMDA-evoked release of [^{3}HGABA] via administration of its precursor, L-arginine (Jones et al., 1994).

Effects on Biogenic Amines

NO releases dopamine (Hanbauer et al., 1992), which could relieve fatigue and produce behavioral stimulation, as well as enhance cognition and attention. NO inhibits dopamine uptake. The ability of NO to diffuse across striatal membranes would enhance dopaminergic neurotransmission (Pogun, Baumann, and Kuhar, 1994) and may also inhibit [^{3}H] glutamate uptake. NO also increases the release of serotonin (Lorrain and Hull, 1993), and NMDA-induced release of [^{3}H] norepinephrine (Jones et al., 1994). This mode of action is unclear, however, since it is not affected by NO synthase inhibitors (Stout and Woodward, 1994). NO also selectively inhibits voltage-dependent calcium influx in neuronal cells through a cyclic GMP-dependent mechanism (Desole et al., 1994), i.e., NO is a calcium-channel blocker.

Effects on VIP

NO stimulates the secretion of VIP, and NO secretion is also stimulated by VIP (Grider and Jin, 1993). NO may be co-localized with VIP, and is found in the trigeminal ganglion.

Effects on Neuropeptide Y

Neuropeptide Y, a cerebral vasoconstrictor, is the neuropeptide with the highest concentration in the brain, and is released primarily in the limbic and cortical regions (Heilig and Widerlov, 1990). It is anxiolytic, co-localized in noradrenergic neurons, and is known to stimulate appetite and cause weight gain (independently of its effect on appetite) (Heinrichs et al., 1993). It has an inverse relationship with CRH, however, although it is co-localized with NE in presynaptic terminals. In certain circumstances neuropeptide Y releases NO (Kobari et al., 1993b) or is co-localized with it (Nozaki et al., 1993).

Effects on the Action of Opiates

Partly by its indirect dopaminergic effect, NO decreases morphine withdrawal symptoms in adult male rats (Adams et al., 1993). Morphine treatment stimulates NO synthesis (Ferreira, Duarte, and Lorenzetti, 1991). NO also accelerates tolerance to morphine (Babey et al., 1994). NO increases morphine-related behavioral changes in mice (Calignano et al., 1993), perhaps related to the finding that opioids increase dopamine release in the corpus striatum. Antinociception induced by intracerebroventricular NO may potentiate only beta-endorphin, but not mu, gamma, or kappa agonists. It is thus thought to be involved in descending pain inhibition (Xu and Tseng, 1993). Some of my fibromyalgia patients have reported that nitroglycerin significantly potentiates the effect and duration of their opioid analgesics.

Relationship with IL-1 Beta

Neuronal NO synthase is activated by a calcium-dependent mechanism, but can also be stimulated by IL-1 beta. It is not known for certain whether this latter mechanism is constitutive in the brain, but decreased regional levels of NO could be related to decreased IL-1 beta production or inhibition of its action by other cytokines or neuropeptides (Goldstein, 1993). Such a mechanism could also produce lower levels of CNS serotonin, dopamine, certain prostaglandins, IL-6, and CRH (Sandi and Guaza, 1995). IL-1 beta messenger ribonucleic acid (mRNA) and IL-1 receptor antagonist protein mRNA are densely localized in the dorsal raphe nuclei that synthesize serotonin (De Souza, personal communication, 1993). Perhaps related to the somnogenic action of IL-1 beta, inhibition of nitric oxide synthesis decreases both the amount and the duration of NREM (non-rapid eye movement) sleep in rats. It is thus thought that NO is involved in the maintenance of spontaneous sleep (Kapas, Fang, and Kruger, 1994). A modulatory effect of NO on ascending cholinergic reticular neurons was suggested to act on vigilance. Since NO is also stimulated by other somnogenic substances, such as GHRH (growth hormone releasing hormone), muramyl peptides, VIP and PGD_2 (prostaglandin D_2), NO might be a possible common mediator for the sleep-inducing effects of several sleep factors (Kapas, Fang, and Kruger, 1994). Decreased levels of citrulline, the end product of the manufacture of NO from arginine by NO synthase, are found in the spinal fluid of FMS patients (Russell, personal communication, 1995). Since spinal fluid IL-1 beta is normal in this group, and IL-1 beta induces NO synthase, a central NO deficiency may exist in CFS/FMS on the basis of NO synthase inhibition (Goldstein, 1993). Supporting this hypothesis is my clinical experience that high-dose L-arginine (the NO precursor) supplementation in neurosomatic patients has no effect on their symptoms.

The antinociceptive effect of NO in the brain is the opposite of what has been found in the spinal cord, where N-methyl-D-aspartate (NMDA) receptor activation is implicated in nociceptive processing (Meller and Gebhart, 1993). Many effects of NMDA receptor activation appear to be mediated by NO, since glutamate is a primary ligand for the NMDA receptor. Thermal hyperalgesia in animals is potentiated by NO, causing an increase in cyclic GMP and thus an increase in glutamate, and NMDA receptor antagonists and NO synthase inhibitors are being developed as novel analgesics (Woolf and Thompson, 1991). It thus appears that peripheral thermal pain processing is modulated by NO in a manner opposite to central pain, and certainly nitroglycerin has had no effect on peripheral noxious stimulation in my patients. A corollary to this hypothesis is that NO-modulated sensory gating in CFS/FMS occurs rostral to the dorsal horn. NMDA receptor antagonists given by the intracerebroventricular route have been shown to attenuate the antinociceptive effect of NMDA receptor antagonists, given intrathecally, which would primarily have a spinal site of action (Nasstrom, Karlsson, and Berge, 1993).

This explanation is similar to that proposed by M. B. Yunus, i.e., that the pain of fibromyalgia is a result of central sensory dysregulation (Yunus, 1992). Yunus conceives of a "heterogeneous neurohormonal dysfunction" as the primary problem and describes peripheral and supraspinal structures interacting at the level of the dorsal horn to cause sensory gating abnormalities. My view is that the dorsal horn is one of many sensory "gates" that might be dysfunctional, and that most of them are rostral to the spinal cord. This expansion of Yunus's basic concept would better explain the wide variety of symptoms and specific findings on functional imaging of the brain and neuropsychological testing.

Patients with myalgic encephalomyelitis, the British term for CFS, have been found to have red blood cells with an altered shape, so that they are nondiscocytic or "cup forms" (Simpson, 1989). Such red cells are less deformable than normal and are hypothesized to cause hypothalamic dysfunction by obstructing narrow vessels. At the proper concentration, however, NO can preserve or enhance red cell deformability (Korbut and Gryglewski, 1992).

Although NO is found mainly in parasympathetic neurons and can be potently stimulated by acetylcholine, it is also found in sympathetic postganglionic neurons and cell bodies, and is responsible for vasodilation when alpha-1 antagonists are used (Lewis et al., 1993). NO is also colocalized with substance P and calcitonin gene-related peptide, vasodilator substances produced in the trigeminal vascular system (Edvinsson, MacKenzie, and McCulloch, 1993).

I have noted for several years that CFS/FMS patients are more likely to have or to develop endometriosis than the normal population (Goldstein, 1990). CFS monocytes do not behave like monocytes from controls (Prieto, Camps-Bansell, and Castilla, 1992). This defect can be reversed in vitro with naloxone. One cause for endometriosis is the failure of monocytes/macrophages to ingest endometrium that is normally refluxed through the fallopian tubes during menstruation. The endometrial cells then disperse throughout the pelvis and abdominal cavity, cyclically bleed, but cannot be shed during normal menstrual flow. CFS patients may be more likely to have this defect, especially since the cytotoxicity of macrophages in the peritoneum is related to macrophage ability to produce NO (Sotomayor et al., 1993).

Female patients with CFS/FMS usually have premenstrual exacerbations of their symptoms. Most of the symptoms of late luteal phase dysphoric disorder are similar to those of CFS, and it is likely that this disorder has a limbic etiology similar to CFS/FMS.

Case Report

A 39-nine-year-old married white female data processor had been previously diagnosed as having schizoaffective disorder, but at the time of her first visit her mood was euthymic. She had been prescribed lithium carbonate and venlafaxine. She had a history of auditory hallucinations, agoraphobia, and drug abuse, and was an incest victim as a child. The typical CFS/FMS symptoms were present despite her psychotropic medications. She gave a history of 13 previous psychiatric hospitalizations.

Although most responding patients require very low doses of nitroglycerin, she did not. As she took incremental 0.04 mg sublingual doses her symptoms gradually improved. She had less pain, more energy, more "flexibility," less photophobia, and more cognitive clarity. At a total dose of 0.4 mg she was completely free of all symptoms and continued to feel normal with a nitroglycerin patch supplying 0.6 mg/hour. At a three-month follow-up, the nitroglyc-erin was not working quite as well, but was still very effective.

NEURAL PLASTICITY

"Neural systems adapt to the changing demands of their environ-ment by modulating both the intrinsic membrane properties of neu-rons and the strength of the synaptic connections between them" (Kennedy and Marder, 1992). In recent years it has been found that the adult brain has much more plasticity in its neuronal circuits than previously thought. Ongoing morphological changes occur in dendrites to modify the synaptic communication between neurons and glia. Neu-ral plasticity appears to be reduced in CFS/FMS, probably accounting for symptom exacerbation in situations which could potentially perturb homeostatic or allostatic mechanisms (see Chapter 3). In many re-spects, neurosomatic disorders could be viewed as disorders of neural plasticity. Synapse density of adult mammalian hippoccampal neurons has been found to fluctuate depending on the circulating levels of estradiol. In the adult primate estradiol valerate treatment resulted in a 39 percent decrease in the number of axosomatic synapses in the infundibular hypothalamic nucleus (Naftolin et al., 1993), a possible example of synaptic convergence. Such variations in synapse density could account for the cognitive dysfunction associated with late luteal phase dysphoric disorder and a decrease in the efficiency of synaptic gating and sensory input processing. The mechanism of this effect of estradiol is uncertain at present.

Stress can alter expression of various neurotrophins and their receptors in the brain, thus disturbing dendritic remodeling and retrograde neurotransmission. Wistar rats subject to immobilization stress had reduced levels of NGF, brain-derived neurotrophic factor and neurotrophin-3, as well as trkA and trkB mRNAs in the hippo-campus and medial septum. Such changes could impair learning and even possibly cause neuronal damage (Ueyema et al., 1995). NE production could be reduced by decreased NGF, although CSF levels of NGF in patients with FMS are elevated (Russell, personal communication, 1996).

EFFECTS OF NIMODIPINE IN CFS/FMS:
POSSIBLE MECHANISMS

Calcium channel blockers act at various sites at the L-type calcium channel to inhibit calcium influx during neuronal depolarization. Under certain circumstances, they may also inhibit calcium efflux. This property has been demonstrated for the calcium channel blocker nimodipine (Azmitia, Kramer, and Kim-Pak, 1993). L-type calcium channels are widely distributed in the brain and the central action of calcium channel blockers is well known in the prophylaxis of migraine.

One class of L-type calcium channel blockers is the dihydropyridines. These include isradipine, nifedipine, nicardipine, felodipine, nitrendipine, nisoldipine, amlodipine, and nimodipine. Each of these drugs is slightly different from the others. Amlodipine may be the second choice among dihdropyridines for neurosomatic disorders. It does not affect blood pressure or heart rate in the normotensive patient, is inexpensive, is dosed once a day, and improves memory in mice when given chronically (Reilly et al., 1995). Nimodipine is used primarily for its effects in counteracting cerebral vasospasm from subarachnoid hemorrhage, since it has fewer systemic hypotensive effects than other dihydropyridines and is more lipophilic, enabling it to cross the blood-brain barrier more easily. Nicardipine is a better cerebral vasodilator (Alborch et al., 1992), but it lowers blood pressure too much to be prescribed in the acutely ill patient with a ruptured aneurysm. It may be, however, that the neuroprotective effects of nimodipine in subarachnoid hemorrhage are not related to vasodilation, but to some other mechanism (Tettenborn and Fierus, 1993).

I have found nimodipine to be uniquely effective among the drugs of its class in managing CFS/FMS. It is also the most useful in treatment-resistant panic disorder (Gibbs, 1992), a related limbic dysfunction. Neuronal plasticity is related to calcium-dependent pre- and postsynaptic processes such as occur with LTP in the hippocampus (Gispen, 1993). Nimodipine strongly enhances the firing rate of single aged hippocampal neurons recorded in vivo, while two other calcium channel blockers, nifedipine and flunarizine, do not (Disterhoft et al., 1993). A 30 mg nimodipine capsule usually works in about 45 minutes. About 40 percent of patients experience relaxation, increased energy, a decrease in tender point sensitivity, improved exercise tolerance, and enhanced mental clarity. Calcium channel blockers of other types have previously been reported to be useful in panic disorder (Goldstein, 1985; Klein and Uhde, 1988) and in potentiation of opioid analgesics (Pereira, Prado, and Dos Reis, 1993). Nimodipine is also being investigated in treating HIV-1-associated cognitive motor complex. Calcium channel blockers potentiate the action of lidocaine (Taniguchi, Ichimata, and Matsumoto, 1993) and are analgesic as monotherapy when given epidurally (Dey et al., 1993) or topically in the eye (Chen et al., 1993). Some of my patients with developmental learning disorders have had remarkable improvement with nimodipine. The drug also has antidepressant effects, both in patients and in animal models (de Jonge, Griedl, and De Vry, 1993).

Besides binding to the CD4/VIP receptor, gp120 irreversibly binds to L-type neuronal calcium channels and inhibits cellular chemotaxis. This binding can be antagonized by nimodipine (Stefano et al., 1993). Gp120 also has a sequence homology to CRH that is related to induction of ACTH from lymphocytes by HIV (Stefano et al., 1993). It is possible that there could be endogenous analogs to gp120 sequences, or that such peptides could be neurotoxic gene products produced by other viruses that could trigger CFS/FMS. Obviously, a CRH agonist is not one of these products. The complex pathophysiology of the HIV-1-associated cognitive motor complex has been recently reviewed (Lipton and Gendelman, 1995). In many ways, such as overproduction of glutamate and interleukin-1 beta in the brain, it is the opposite of CFS. The drugs memantine (related to amantadine), nimodipine, and nitroglycerin have been suggested as therapeutic agents, since the final common pathway to neuronal injury is excess release of excitatory amino acids and calcium. Nitric oxide, a product of nitroglycerin, may in certain circumstances function as an NMDA antagonist (Lipton, 1993).

In almost all responders, nimodipine causes further vasoconstriction on post-treatment CFS/FMS ^{133}Xe brain SPECT, sometimes to a profound degree. This paradoxical effect is another demonstration that therapeutic benefit in CFS/FMS derives from release of a substance that has intrinsic vasoconstrictive properties. Nimodipine has been shown to release dopamine, serotonin, and acetylcholine (Azmitia, Kramer, and Kim-Pak, 1993; Fanelli et al., 1993; Rezvani et al., 1993). Of these transmitters, only serotonin can be vasoconstrictive in the human brain at physiological concentrations. Tolerance does not develop to the vasodilatory properties of nimodipine, but sometimes does to its amelioration of symptoms in CFS/FMS. Nimodipine does not cause release of any compound known to increase secretion of endothelin. Such agents include angiotensin II, thrombin, bradykinin, adenosine triphosphate (ATP), ACTH, platelet-activating factor, cytokines, vasopressin, and various growth factors including transforming growth factor beta (TGF-beta) (Stojilkovic and Catt, 1992) and insulin-like growth factor (IGF) (Matsumoto et al., 1990). None of these are known to be deficient in CFS/FMS except IGF. I have prescribed vasopressin in the form of desamino-D-arginine vasopressin (DDAVP) for numerous patients over the years with minimal results and have also combined it with fenfluramine as a secretagogue in an attempt to increase CRH secretion, with no effect. Vasopressin levels may be normal in CFS (Crofford et al., 1994), or decreased (Bakheit et al., 1993). TGF-beta, if anything, is elevated in CFS (Goldstein, 1990; Chao et al., 1991), and could possibly cause elevated CSF endothelin levels. Angiotensin-converting enzyme (ACE) inhibitors, such as captopril, are effective antidepressants (Zubenko and Nixon, 1984; Gard et al., 1994), which have some limited utility in ameliorating CFS/FMS symptoms, probably because captopril is an endopeptidase inhibitor that can increase concentrations of certain peptides, including the enkephalins. ACE inhibitors also increase bradykinin secretion, which increases endothelin levels as well as stimulating release of NO from endothelial cells. Captopril, the only ACE inhibitor to have a sulfhydryl group, is also the only marketed agent of its class with antidepressant properties, with the possible exception of enalapril. I have found losartan, a competitive antagonist of the angiotensin-1 subtype AII receptor (AII subtype receptor AT_1), to have anxiolytic properties. It sometimes helps neurosomatic symptoms in general. The AII subtype receptor AT_1 blockers may be useful as cognitive enhancing agents (Domeney, 1994; Wayner et al., 1993). Angiotensin-II also increases the secretion of endothelin (Stoljikovic and Catt, 1992).

Case Report

A 53-year-old Caucasian executive was well until he was involved in a stressful lawsuit six years prior to consulting me. During the trial he developed diarrhea and "tendinitis." Subsequently he became more and more fatigued, to the point of being unable to work. He consulted a psychiatrist and a psychologist who told him he had a physical problem, and several internists who assured him he was in good health. At the time he saw me he estimated that he had 25 to 30 percent of his premorbid energy levels. He had typical CFS symptoms as well as a history of a developmental reading disorder.

Thirty minutes after taking nimodipine 30 mg he felt "90 percent better." He also noticed that his ability to read was greatly improved. Whenever he tried to discontinue the nimodipine or forgot to take it, he relapsed. When seen one year after beginning nimodipine he stated, "I feel great. I'm like I was seven years ago!"

HYDRALAZINE

Reasoning that hydralazine, thought to dilate arteries by stimulating cyclic GMP (Nathanson, 1992), acts via a NO-type mechanism, I began to prescribe it for therapeutic trials in CFS/FMS. Responders reported amelioration of one or more target symptoms within an hour after a dose of 10 to 25 mg. Hydralazine has also been reported to potentiate the effects of nitrovasodilators in vascular smooth muscle prior to cyclate activation. It was hypothesized that hydralazine inhibited pyridoxal-dependent reactions inactivating sulfhydryl groups that are thought to be involved in the action of nitroglycerin (Unger, Berkenboom, and Fontaine, 1993). Indeed, methionine and cysteine, sulfur-containing amino acids, have been advocated for reversing nitrate tolerance, but have not been helpful in my CFS/FMS population. Hydralazine, of course, may work simply by lowering blood pressure and activating baroreceptors. My patients benefiting from hydralazine have also had worsening arterial vasoconstriction when studied by post-treatment brain SPECT.

Case Report

A 44-year-old Caucasian male flight attendant was well until two years prior to seeing me when he developed an acute diarrheal illness two weeks after being in Central America. Workup at a large multispecialty clinic was within normal limits. Since then he had complaints of hot flashes, dizziness, otalgia, disorder of initiating and maintaining sleep, tinnitus, fatigue, and weakness. He had an adverse reaction to metronidazole and had a lumbar puncture that showed elevated protein of unknown etiology. A CT (computerized tomography) scan of his brain was within normal limits. There was a past medical history of reflux esophagitis, and of being hospitalized 20 years previously for an adverse reaction to a flu shot. Prior to his illness he had been very active athletically but had to stop exercising after he became sick.

His main symptoms at the time he saw me were cognitive dysfunction, nonrestorative sleep, fatigue, dysequilibrium, blurred vision, benign fasciculations in his legs, myalgias, arthralgias, and night sweats. He was not working as a flight attendant at the time that I saw him, and was on disability.

Physical examination was unremarkable. The patient received trials of naphazoline eyedrops, nitroglycerin, nimodipine, pyridostigmine, mexiletine, and hydralazine. He felt markedly better 30 minutes after taking hydralazine, an improvement that persisted for the next 18 months. He described decreased muscle fatigue, increased cognition, less exercise intolerance, and restorative sleep. Since he still had some symptoms, especially diarrhea and bloating, he received trials of felbamate, risperidone, gabapentin, baclofen, and oxytocin. None of these had any effect. Tacrine 10 mg helped him to feel more relaxed.

At his last visit he was still working, even though he complained of diarrhea, some decrease in energy, and mild exertional intolerance. He stated that almost always, within 45 minutes of taking hydralazine, he has a "sense of energy," less muscle fatigue, and a lessening of all his symptoms except for diarrhea. The patient continues on hydralazine 25 mg three times a day.

PYRIDOSTIGMINE

Muscle weakness in CFS may sometimes be treated with pyridostigmine bromide in a manner similar to its use in myasthenia gravis. Surprisingly, pyridostigmine, a cholinesterase inhibitor that does not cross the blood-brain barrier, may alleviate mental "fogginess," increase energy, and reduce pain. This drug has been reported to increase secretion of growth hormone (Arvat et al., 1993) by potentiating growth-hormone-releasing hormone via a central cholinergic mechanism. Somatomedin C/IGF-1, a growth-hormone-related peptide, has been found to be low in patients with FMS (Bennett et al., 1992). As noted previously, IGF may increase the central secretion of endothelin. Pyridostigmine may also induce the adrenal glands to secrete more corticosteroids and catecholamines. It could further act by increasing peripheral sympathetic input to the CNS, and thus decrease global CBF (cerebral blood flow) on post-treatment brain SPECT.

MEXILETINE/LIDOCAINE

Mexiletine was introduced as a type IIb antiarrhythmic, with a major site of action in the brain. It is related to lidocaine and tocainide, and has few serious adverse reactions in low doses. More recently, mexiletine has been used successfully for neuropathic pain, particularly dysesthesias. Its mode of action is unknown, but it may act by increasing central CRH secretion (Calogero et al., 1990). Lidocaine and procaine act as local anesthetics at sodium channels, but their action in the hypothalamus to stimulate CRH is independent of their effect on sodium conductance. Lidocaine blocks the reuptake of norepinephrine, GABA, and choline. Mexiletine also inhibits the release of substance P from mouse spinal nociceptive terminals (Kamei et al., 1992). Dorsal roots are more sensitive to lidocaine than peripheral nerves, and mexiletine may exert its effect on neuropathic pain at this site (Schwartzman, 1993). It also decreases CBF in CFS/FMS patients as assessed by brain SPECT. Intravenous lidocaine, useful in neuropathic pain, is also an effective treatment for FMS (Posner, 1994). When it acts only as an analgesic, CBF is increased. When symptoms globally improve, CBF is decreased as with all other rapidly acting agents.

Intravenous (IV) lidocaine treatment of fibromyalgia syndrome significantly improved the visual analog scale for pain in a group of fibromyalgia patients as compared to a control patient group who received placebo (Posner, 1994). I find IV lidocaine 200 to 300 mg in 500 ml of normal saline to be a rapidly effective analgesic in

FMS patients. The effects sometimes last for days or weeks, perhaps by inducing long-term potentiation (see p. 65), and often global symptoms are improved. About half of my patients respond to this treatment after being refractory to all oral agents. IV lidocaine is the most effective single treatment I currently prescribe. It has the unusual property of greater symptom relief and duration of action with each successive use, plateauing after four infusions, and lasting three to seven days. Intranasal 4 percent lidocaine has been recommended for rapidly aborting migraine headache (Kudrow, Kudrow, and Sandweiss, 1995). I use it in a spray bottle and find it helpful in about half of my patients.

Case Report

A 54-year-old married Caucasian female consulted me for a three-year history of CFS/FMS that had begun abruptly. She complained of diffuse pain, exhaustion, heartburn, panic attacks, weakness, sleep disorders, cognitive dysfunction, and headaches. Prior to seeing me she had been extensively evaluated and had unsuccessful trials of every class of psychotropic medication. She was often bedridden and sometimes could not walk because of pain, fatigue, and weakness.

During the succeeding three years an enormous number of treatment trials were completely unsuccessful. She remained on high doses of alprazolam to ameliorate her panic disorder.

One day her husband carried her into the office. She had been unable to walk around her yard or perform self-care. She was given lidocaine 200 mg in 500 ml of normal saline by infusion over two hours. She stated at its completion: "I feel 100 percent better." She then went to the reception room and did a tap dance for the patients. The benefits from the infusion persisted for 7 to 14 days. It relieved many of her symptoms, not just her pain.

CONCLUDING REMARKS

A possible mechanism of action for the medications discussed in this chapter would be stimulation of NE release with subsequent enhancement of CRH secretion and decrease of substance P levels. CRH might also be stimulated directly. Since CRH enhances peripheral sympathetic neurotransmission when given centrally, it may cause cerebral arterial vasoconstriction directly or do so by causing release of norepinephrine. The stimulation by IL-1 of CRH was blocked by NO in one experimental model (Rivier, 1993), and such a result could not support a facilitatory role of NO in CRH secretion, at least by an IL-1-dependent process. NO, however, may also enhance CRH secretion (Sandi and Guaza, 1995). Local anesthetics have also been shown to inhibit uptake of choline, norepinephrine, and GABA in several human- or rat-derived clonal cell lines (Lukas and Bencherif, 1993). If endothelin is not involved, stimulating the secretion of the co-localized vasoconstrictors NE and NPY (neuropeptide Y) by CFS/FMS treatment may be a final common pathway for the beneficial outcome. Excess endothelin could have deleterious effects, and stimulate the secretion of substance P.

Many other medications are useful in treating neurosomatic disorders. Some have been discussed in *Chronic Fatigue Syndromes: The Limbic Hypothesis* (Goldstein, 1993). Others will be mentioned subsequently in this book. Double-blind, placebo-controlled testing of these drugs has not been performed because of lack of funding, but the clinician may wish to try them, as I do, sequentially in individual patients.

The basic point that I wish to convey, however, is that most, if not all, disorders of regulatory physiology have important limbic components. Thus far they seem to involve sensory gating and processing of sensory input, and are probably multifactorial in etiology. The regions of the limbic neural network most affected, and the way in which the function of the neuronal machinery is deranged, markedly influence patient symptomatology. The rapid response to the medications described here and the concomitant profound post-treatment alteration in brain SPECT suggests, at least on a neurophysiological basis, that many neurosomatic disorders may be improved by ameliorating state-dependent deranged neural network function.

Chronic Fatigue Syndrome Pathophysiology

I think that we are beginning to see the biology of the twenty-first century, and it is a biology of complexity.

–Edward S. Golub
The Limits of Medicine (1994)

All diseases of Christians are to be ascribed to demons.

–St. Augustine

In the past two years I have been better able to understand chronic fatigue syndrome (CFS) and related neurosomatic disorders as being caused by abnormalities in the way the brain processes sensory information. All sensory information except smell travels through the brainstem to the thalamus, the most sophisticated gating structure of the central nervous system, before being relayed to isotypic sensory cortices. Smell is transmitted directly to the piriform cortex of the limbic system and by an indirect relay through the mediodorsal thalamic nucleus to the orbitofrontal and insular cortices. The isotypic sensory cortex has no direct connection with the limbic system, because there is no survival value for alterations of primary sensory perceptions such as shape, place, and tone by the affective state of the organism. Subsequently, sensory information is interpreted by unimodal and heteromodal association cortices, as well as limbic areas such as the hippocampus and amygdala. The dorsolateral prefrontal cortex (DLPFC) appears to be the most important of the heteromodal association areas for new learning, and for neurosomatic disorders that are probably unique to human beings. The DLPFC has been termed a "supramodal" association area that "monitors and judges the activities of the cognitive networks and selects preferred responses that are influenced, to a considerable extent, by limbic (internal) input" (Benson, 1993). As a result of dysfunctional sensory processing, responses might not be appropriate to a given stimulus situation, e.g., a patient might feel burning pain or severe weakness for no apparent reason, perspire profusely when he is not warm, or gain 30 pounds in six weeks without changing eating habits. I originally thought that this process occurred primarily in the limbic system, but recent evidence implicates the prefrontal cortex (PFC) as the main player, and its dysfunction may then cause abnormalities of limbic regulation.

Primates, and especially humans, have a tremendous expansion of cortical volume compared to other animals. Three areas in particular have grown remarkably: (1) the prefrontal cortex, (2) the inferior parietal cortex, and (3) the middle temporal gyrus. In humans, the DLPFC, and the volume of white matter underlying it, located in the superior frontal lobes, is vastly larger than that of the apes, and much larger than that of chimpanzees (Fuster, 1989; Altman, 1995). Along with erect posture, the opposable thumb, and the ability to speak, the DLPFC sets us apart from "lower" life-forms. What is the function of this region of the brain?

Until recently, the role of the DLPFC was understood by lesion studies, beginning with the interesting case of Mr. Phineas Gage. Gage was a railroad worker who in 1848 was involved in an accident in which a metal rod went through his forehead, supposedly into his DLPFC. He had no sensorimotor abnormalities, but had a marked personality change. He was "no longer Gage" (Harlow, 1868). Formerly a reliable, conscientious individual, he became dissolute and irritable. Further studies of patients with DLPFC lesions revealed that the DLPFC controls so-called "executive functions." These include organization, planning activities that involve sequential tasks, motivation and drive, self-analysis, and neural regulation. The DLPFC is also involved in memory encoding, or the making of new memories. Gage's lesion actually involved the left and right prefrontal cortices in the ventromedial (orbitofrontal) regions, rather than the dorsolateral. These findings suggest that the regions of the frontal lobes "are interconnected and act cooperatively to support reasoning and decision making" (Damasio et al., 1994). Gage's behavior may be more appropriately attributed to the "orbitofrontal disinhibition syndrome"

(Duffy and Campbell, 1994; Damasio, 1994). The increased volume of white matter in the PFC is probably an indication of an increase in intrinsic and extrinsic connectivity.

The orbitofrontal cortex (OFC) gates interoceptive information, consistent with its primarily receiving limbic-hypothalamic projections, while the DLPFC receives projections mainly from heteromodal association areas. The DLPFC and OFC have rich intracortical connections (Weinberger, 1993). A circuit from the anterior cingulate, which connects to the medial striatal/nucleus accumbens region, sends major afferents to the rhinal areas and hippocampus and minor afferents to the OFC and amygdala, among other structures (Mega and Cummings, 1994). "Processing in the anterior cingulate circuit enables the intentional selection of environmental stimuli based on the internal relevance those stimuli have for the organism. Input about that internal relevance is provided by the activity of the orbitofrontal cortex" (Mega and Cummings, 1994). Thus, one would expect to find anterior cingulate, OFC, and insular dysfunction in patients with irritable bowel syndrome (IBS), and generalized somatosensory dysfunction, especially tactile (Schneider, Friedman, and Mishkin, 1993). OFC hypoperfusion has been found in every IBS patient we have studied with brain SPECT (Goldstein and Mena, 1995). IBS patients experiencing pain from colonic balloon distension at a pressure that was not algesic in normal controls all exhibited PET activation of the left DLPFC and anterior cingulate, suggesting an altered perception of the saliency of this sensory input. Cholinergic fibers, possibly projecting from the solitary tract, lateralize to the left PFC (Silverman et al., 1996-submitted for publication).

Localization studies, the staple of neurologists, are not particularly helpful in understanding neurosomatic illnesses such as CFS. These illnesses are neural network disorders in which brain circuits do not function properly, but there is no destruction, or even structural alteration, of brain tissue when examined with standard microscopic and structural imaging techniques. CFS is a disorder of brain function, and can be best studied with brain functional imaging.

Techniques such as brain single photon emission computed tomography (SPECT), positron emission tomography (PET), quantitative EEG (electroencephalogram), and evoked response mapping in CFS consistently show or suggest hypofunction of the DLPFC and often the hippocampus. Fibromyalgia syndrome appears virtually identical to CFS in patients who have brain SPECT imaging (Goldstein, Mena, and Yunus, 1993). Although the location of regional cerebral blood flow (rCBF) decrease is the same in both groups, CFS/FMS patients have worse regional hypoperfusion than those with CFS who lack the requisite number of tender points (Goldstein, Mena, and Yunus, 1993). Depression imaged by PET and SPECT is somewhat similar, but usually involves the left DLPFC, as does schizophrenia, although different subregions or neuronal populations (Guze and Gitlin, 1994) may be involved in schizophrenia. The anatomy of these connections is complex, and involves the striatum, globus pallidus/substantia nigra, and thalamus, which then project back to the frontal cortex (Mega and Cummings, 1994). Some groups believe that left DLPFC hypoperfusion is indicative of psychomotor poverty (schizophrenia) and psychomotor retardation (depression). Much of the resultant symptomatic differences may result from varying types of striatothalamocortical dysfunction (e.g., Dolan et al., 1993).

Hypoperfusion of the right DLPFC occurs more frequently in CFS/FMS than in depression. The right caudate and both thalami may also be selectively hypoperfused in CFS/FMS, as seen on SPECT done with MRI (magnetic resonance imaging) coregistration for precise anatomic localization of deficits (Alexander et. al., 1994). The dorsal caudate projects to the DLPFC, the ventral caudate to the OFC. Emphasis is shifting from the linguistic processing specialization of the left hemisphere versus the right hemisphere processing of nonlinguistic information. "The right hemisphere is critical for processing novel situations and the left hemisphere is key to the processes mediated by well-routinized representations and strategies. The left frontal systems appear to be critical for the cognitive selection driven by the content of working memory and for context-dependent behavior, the right frontal systems for cognitive selection driven by the external environment and for context-independent behavior. The crucial role of the right hemisphere in processing cognitively novel situations underscores the importance of the right frontal systems in task orientation and in the assembly of novel cognitive strategies" (Goldberg, Podell, and Lovell, 1994). Hemispheric differences in efficacy of types of information processed may be partially explained by the tendency of the left hemisphere to process outputs from neurons with relatively small receptive fields. The right hemisphere, in contrast, tends to process outputs from neurons with relatively large overlapping receptive fields. These differences are most noticeable when input must be classified in some way, and may depend on the type of attention paid to different tasks (Brown and Kosslyn, 1993). Possible biochemical correlates to this specialization include the lateralization of norepinephrine (NE) pathways to the right hemisphere and dopamine (DA) to the left hemisphere (Glick, Ross, and Hugh, 1982). NE is critical to cognitive novelty and dopamine to cognitive routinization (Tucker and Williamson, 1984). The relevance of the right DLPFC to neurosomatic symptom generation will be discussed below. A misperception of cognitive novelty may be present. "Activation" brain SPECT scans, performed on CFS patients while they are doing calculations, inappropriately decrease rCBF the right hemisphere, especially the right dorsolateral prefrontal cortex in many patients, a region involved in dealing with a novel stimulus. This finding corroborates the hypothesis of cognitive novelty misperception in CFS (Goldstein and Mena, 1995). The left hemisphere is usually activated when performing a well-learned task, and the left parietal lobe normally has increased rCBF when the subject is doing calculations. This increase is rarely seen in CFS patients.

Poverty of speech has been associated with lesions of the left angular gyrus. This cortical area is multimodal, and its functions in humans include visuospatial orientation and attention (Dolan et al., 1993). PET studies have found activation of the DLPFC to be associated with decreased rCBF in the left angular gyrus. This region is thought to be a part of a distributed neural network involved with tasks that require "willed action" (Frith et al., 1991). There are also reports of hypofunction of the inferior parietal cortex (also called the angular gyrus) and the medial temporal gyrus in many psychiatric disorders. These two uniquely human regions appear to be part of a distributed neural network, which may malfunction in various multicausal ways to produce inappropriate sensations, behavior, emotions, and physiologic regulation. Auditory evoked responses, a method to record the path of a sound stimulus as it is transmitted through the central nervous system, suggest an abnormality in sensory processing in a DLPFC-hippocampal-superior temporal auditory cortex circuit in patients with CFS (see

Figure 16, illustration section). Direct connections from specific areas of the primate prefrontal cortex to the superior temporal auditory region have been demonstrated (Romanski, Bates, and Goldman-Rakic, 1995). There is decreased amplitude of the N-100 wave, which appears to be a trait marker, since it does not change with treatment in CFS (Goldstein et al., 1994; Donati et al., 1994). N-100 amplitude is decreased in dementia, and is either decreased or increased in depression. "Attention becomes effortful with increased working memory load, needs for interference control, or difficulty of target detection" (Breiter et al., 1995). Effortful attention depends on a large-scale distributed neural network implicated for selective attention, most components of which are independent of the sensory modality employed. When subjects attend to an auditory stimulus, there is an enhancement of activation in the auditory cortex (Grady et al., 1995). Such enhancements are probably diminished or paradoxically decreased in neurosomatic disorders. A course of ECT (electroconvulsive therapy) restores decreased N-100 amplitude to normal in depression, but antidepressant treatment does not (reviewed in Rimpel et al., 1995). Decreased amplitude of the N-100 wave could be a marker for LC (locus ceruleus) hypofunction, and involves early sensory/attentional processes, perhaps an impairment in improving the signal-to-noise ratio. It is not a distinctive marker for impaired extinction of perception of novelty, as is seen in prepulse inhibition. The regulatory role of the OFC in modulating dopamine secretion in the ventral striatum has been studied in regard to prepulse inhibition of the acoustic startle response in rats. Since it is thought that OFC dopamine (DA) exerts an inhibitory control over striatal dopamine systems, large doses of 6-hydroxydopamine were injected into the OFC of rats. The reduction in prepulse inhibition correlated with the extent of DA depletion (Bubser and Koch, 1994).

It thus appears important to know the function of the PFC in a neural network. This region of the brain is unique in that it regulates its own neurotransmitter input from brainstem nuclei. It sends excitatory neurons, which secrete glutamate, to regulate the output of brainstem nuclei, which produce biogenic amines, especially dopamine and norepinephrine (NE). Readers may recall that for some time I have postulated a glutamatergic deficit in CFS (Goldstein, 1993), although glutamatergic projections may affect behavior differentially depending on the structures involved, and the degree of receptor stimulation (Svensson, Carlsson, and Carlsson, 1994). There may also be deficits in norepinephrine, dopamine (Russell et al., 1992), neuropeptide Y (NPY) (Crofford et al., 1994), oxytocin, and nitric oxide. Elevations in CSF substance P (SP) found in FMS (Russell et al., 1994), may be due to sympathetic denervation hypersensitivity. SP also inhibits CRH release from hypothalamic slices in vitro (Faria et al., 1991), and may be involved in the CFS CRH deficiency (Demitrack et al., 1991).

Sectioning of the superior cervical ganglion (SCG) in rats resulted in a 55 percent increase in SP-immunoreactivity. SP was also increased by a nicotinic cholinergic ganglionic antagonist. Treatment with the alpha blocker phenoxybenzamine, which increases sympathetic activity, reduced ganglion SP. It was suggested that impulse activity of preganglionic nerves decreases ganglion SP in principal ganglion neurons through a transsynaptic process (Kessler and Black, 1982). Furthermore, adrenalectomy in rats raised levels of SP and somatostatin (SOM) in rat lumbar dorsal root ganglia. Administration of a high dose of corticosterone failed to prevent the increase of these peptides, suggesting that severed fibers from the adrenal medulla might be responsible (Covenas et al., 1994).

Finally, an inbred Wistar rat strain, "GH," has reduced numbers of sympathetic motor neurons. In these rats, SP concentrations in the SCG, spinal cord, iris, and trachea are twice those of normal rats, but other areas such as ear skin, atrium, and sympathetic neurons compete for nerve growth factor (NGF), and the reduced number of sympathetic neurons in certain locations made more NGF available for SP neuron proliferation (Bakhle and Bell, 1994). Transgenic mice that overexpress NGF have sympathetic hyperinnervation of immune organs with resultant reduction in immune responsiveness, as measured by the mitogen response to concanavalin A (Carlson et al., 1995). The highest levels of the SP receptor (NK-1), detected using the potent antagonist ligand [^{3}H]-LY303870 were seen in noradrenergic areas such as the LC and the BNST (Gehlert et al., 1995).

In many circumstances, SP and NE act synergistically, rather than as functional antagonists. These actions involve rates of neural transmission rather than information processing. SP continuously infused into the nucleus of the solitary tract enhanced the baroreceptor reflex response, the same result as was obtained by elevating the concentration of norepinephrine at this medullary nucleus. It has been suggested that "the enhancement of the baroreceptor reflex response by substance P may invoke an increase in the concentration of noradrenaline at the nucleus tractus solitarii via presynaptic mechanism" (Chan et al., 1995).

SP has been shown to produce antinociception indirectly through activation of the pontospinal noradrenergic pathway (Yeomans and Broudfit, 1990). SP also suppresses the activity of alpha-2 receptors at the medullary nucleus reticularis gigantocellularis (Len et al., 1994) and mediates the slow depolarization of sympathetic ganglion cells following the stimulation of visceral afferent fibers by distension of hollow organs (DeGroat, 1989). SP is a vasodilator (via release of NO), while NE is a vasoconstrictor. SP is involved in the facilitation of the excitatory efficacy of afferent input (Yaksh and Malmberg, 1994).

I have been astounded to see vasodilators such as nitroglycerin and nimodipine routinely cause global hypoperfusion on post-treatment brain SPECT in CFS patients, perhaps via vasoconstrictor neurons from the sympathetic superior cervical ganglion (SCG), and possibly the locus ceruleus (LC). We have found a mean decrease of 7 percent in global CBF in 18 CFS treatment responders given nimodipine acutely (Goldstein and Mena, 1994). *All medications tested that acutely improve CFS symptoms cause global cerebral hypoperfusion.* PET studies of healthy women experiencing transient happiness demonstrated widespread reductions in rCBF, especially in the bilateral temporoparietal and right frontal cortices, suggesting that reduction in rCBF is not deleterious (George et al., 1995). Transient sadness, however, caused an increase in rCBF, predominantly in limbic and paralimbic areas.

Paradoxical responses in blood pressure have been reported in certain autonomic neuropathies, such as peripheral autonomic degeneration (Bradbury-Eggleston syndrome). In patients with this disorder, clonidine, pindolol, and hydralazine have raised blood pressure and produced general functional improvement; the latter two agents are effective in neurosomatic disorders. Syncope of unknown etiology frequently responds to theophylline, an antagonist of the vasodilatory adenosine receptor (Robertson, 1993). Stress responses in patients with diseases of the sympathetic nervous system have been recently reviewed (Ziegler, Ruiz-Ramon, and Shapiro, 1993).

Electroconvulsive therapy (ECT) reduces global CBF as assessed by [133]Xenon SPECT. Particularly in patients who responded to the treatment, reductions occurred after the first convulsion, and two months after completion of the course of treatment (Sackheim et al., 1994). Thus the global and regional CBF deficits observed in depression are trait markers, and ECT results in additional perfusion reductions. It may be, however, that rCBF in the left DLPFC increases with ECT, although a post-ECT reduction in PFC CBF was the topographic change most consistently related to superior clinical outcome in one large study (Nobler et al., 1994).

In another study (Scott et al., 1994), SPECT, using a higher-resolution tracer, ^{99m}Tc-exametazime, performed 45 minutes after a single treatment with ECT in depressed humans, showed decreases in transmitter uptake in the inferior anterior cingulate cortex. The magnitude of the change was directly correlated with the severity of the depression as measured by the Hamilton depression rating scale. The physiologic meaning of this change in rCBF was "uncertain" according to the authors.

An experiment by the same group compared SPECT in major depression before and after successful treatment with antidepressants. They found *increases* in tracer uptake confined to the basal ganglia and inferior anterior cingulate cortex, as well as increases in the right thalamus and right posterior cingulate cortex. No changes were seen in the neocortex, surprisingly. Increased activity in dopaminergic circuits was cited as a plausible mechanism (Goodwin et al., 1993). This result contrasts to the findings of Sackheim's group that response to antidepressant treatment deepens hypofrontality, although more posterior areas demonstrated increased perfusion (Nobler et al., 1995). In normal subjects studied by PET, fluoxetine, after a single dose, caused decreased metabolism in amygdaloid complex, hippocampal formation, and ventral striatum. It also caused increased metabolism in the right superior parietal lobe (Cook et al., 1994). Fluoxetine is also well known to decrease caudate and orbitofrontal glucose metabolism in obsessive-compulsive disorder (Baxter et al., 1992). It may be a property of all antidepressant drugs that they increase extracellular dopamine in the prefrontal cortex (Tanada et al., 1994). Furthermore, ECT increases the synthesis of NPY in rats (Bolwig, 1994; Stenfors, Mathe, and Theodorsson, 1994). NPY is a powerful vasoconstrictor and is associated with numerous regulatory functions, including anxiolysis. Anxiolysis, which can be dissociated from the well-known effects of NPY on increasing ingestive behavior, may be related to stimulation of Y_1 receptors in the central nucleus of the amygdala (Heilig et al., 1993). Decreased NPY levels have been found in the frontal lobes of persons who committed suicide, suggesting a role for this substance in depression, as well (Grundemar and Hakanson, 1994). Prepro-NPY-mRNA levels increased tenfold in one experiment after ECT (Bolwig, 1994). NPY was persistently elevated in the left brain only one week after ECT (Stenfors, Mathe, and Theodorsson, 1994). Neuropeptide Y is colocalized with NE in noradrenergic neurons, and has little vasoconstrictor effect singly in vitro. In vessels primed by alpha-agonists, however, it is a potent and long-acting vasoconstrictor (Grundemar and Hakanson, 1994). NE and NPY stimulation may be the mechanism for producing global hypoperfusion and symptomatic improvement in patients by rapidly acting agents in the neurosomatic treatment protocol.

Activation of LC neurons, which project widely throughout the brain, could serve the same function as the SCG neurons and induce a state in which forebrain circuits could be tuned to provide the greatest possible discrimination between optimal and nonoptimal inputs, perhaps activating the right PFC more than the left. There are target-specific columns for sympathetic preganglionic neurons in the thoracic spinal cord of the rat that are spatially arranged in three distinct groups, the most medial of which projects to the SCG. The PFC has a monosynaptic glutamatergic projection directly to this column (Pyner and Coote, 1994; Bacon and Smith, 1993). Furthermore, after bilateral superior cervical ganglionectomy in rats, changes were noted in levels of serum growth hormone (GH), prolactin (PRL), thyrotropin-releasing hormone (TRH), and somatostatin (SOM), thus providing an argument for the physiologic relevance of projections from the SCG to the medial basal hypothalamus (Cardinal et al., 1994). Pyridostigmine, which does not cross the blood-brain barrier, still increases the secretion of growth hormone, as well as growth hormone-releasing hormone (Arvat et al., 1993), perhaps by stimulating the SCG. Signal-to-noise increase in target areas should correspond to increasing synaptic strength and modulate the system in global, state-dependent cognitive processes that would include determining information salience as well as encoding new memories (Berridge, Arnsten, and Foote, 1993). One function of the LC/noradrenergic system is modulation of behavioral state. It can enhance the processing of relevant stimuli and increase the signal-to-noise ratio. In primates, the PFC is the major region that inhibits the processing of irrelevant stimuli (Knight et al., 1981), and dysfunction of the region may cause diminished amplitude of the N-100 wave in CFS patients. LC dysfunction can also cause decreased levels of PFC dopamine (Svensson, 1994).

Noradrenergic fibers from the LC suppress weak inputs and enhance strong inputs, thus increasing the efficiency of feature extraction from sensory input and deciding what is relevant from one set of information to another. NE induces neuronal membrane hyperpolarization, thus making it harder for weak excitatory input to reach spike threshold, but strong input that does reach threshold will cause more spikes in the presence of NE. This enhancement occurs through the blockade of a calcium-mediated potassium current (Nishimura et al., 1995). LC hypofunction could therefore produce attention deficit disorder because an individual's ability to decide what is salient when exposed to sensory input would be impaired. It would also explain the common complaint of CFS patients that it is difficult to drive on the freeway or go to shopping malls, because they are impaired in their ability to filter out irrelevant stimuli. The sympathetic control of the cerebral circulation has been well reviewed (Edvinsson, MacKenzie, and McCulloch, 1993; Ohta et al., 1991). Vessels in the carotid territory are innervated primarily by fibers from the SCG. The stellate ganglion innervates the vertebrobasilar artery, and the LC has a vasoconstrictive effect on intraparenchymal, but not pial, vessels (in the cat). Some find that severe anxiety causes decreased rCBF, while mild anxiety causes vasodilatation (Mathew, 1995).

The neurochemical network involved in the production of neurosomatic symptoms thus appears as shown in Diagram 1.

DIAGRAM 1

Norepinephrine (NE) is cosecreted with neuropeptide Y (NPY). NE increases the signal-to-noise ratio of sensory input. Substance P (SP) in many respects has an opposite effect. NE and NPY are decreased in FMS, while SP is increased. Both NE and SP neurons compete for nerve growth factor (NGF). If noradrenergic nuclei are not stimulated sufficiently by glutamatergic afferents from the prefrontal cortex, SP neurons will "win" the competition for NGF, contributing to a misinterpretation of sensory input by the FMS patient.

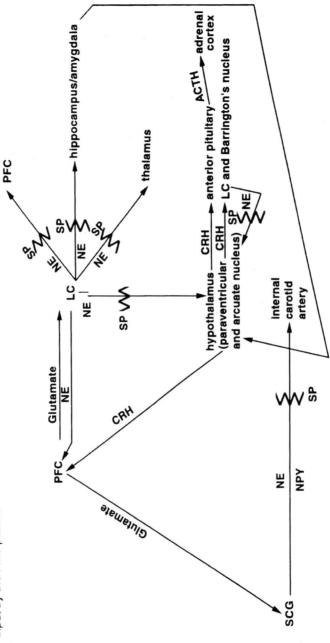

Case Report

A 44-year-old white male had felt fatigued as long as he could remember, and had self-described "brain fog" that impaired his ability to work. He had gotten through school with difficulty, and was threatened with job loss because of poor performance. As often occurs, he felt nearly normal 30 minutes after taking a medication on the CFS/FMS therapeutic protocol, in his case pyridostigmine. What makes his case informative, however, is that he, an individual with a latent Horner's syndrome, developed unilateral mydriasis, a phenomenon caused by stimulation of postganglionic fibers from the superior cervical ganglion (SCG) in the nondilated eye. Stimulation of preganglionic cholinergic neurons, synapsing on upregulated receptors, might produce the release of norepinephrine (NE), neuropeptide Y (NPY), and causing the global hypoperfusion on brain SPECT that commonly occurs when there is a rapid response to treatment (see Figure 20, illustration section). It is also typical in CFS patients to see pupillary dilatation lasting up to a week after instillation of a mydriatic, again suggesting denervation hypersensitivity. Sympathetic pupillodilator fibers arise in the posterolateral hypothalamus and descend uncrossed to the eighth cervical and first and second thoracic segments, where they synapse with the lateral horn cells. Preganglionic fibers from these cells ascend through the second ventral thoracic root and synapse in the SCG. Some of these preganglionic fibers are cholinergic. They join the first division of the trigeminal nerve and reach the eye as the long ciliary nerve to the pupillary dilator muscle.

Vasoactive substances may also alter behavior. The role of the SCG and other autonomic ganglia in causing behavioral change has been previously considered by other researchers. Peripheral beta-adrenergic stimulation of sympathetic ganglia increases encoding in rats; peripheral beta blockade impairs it (McGaugh et al., 1993). Endothelin, NPY, and NO may be released subsequently (Stojilkovic and Catt, 1992), when sympathetic ganglia are stimulated.

In considering the role of the amygdala in memory storage (McGaugh et al., 1993) it was found that opioid antagonists and

GABA antagonists enhance memory in rats. Unfortunately, in neurosomatic patients with amnestic disorder, naltrexone, an opioid antagonist, facilitates memory and improves symptoms only occasionally, while flumazenil, a benzodiazepine antagonist, has not benefitted any of the ten neurosomatic patients without panic disorder to whom I have administered it. In fact, the GABA$_B$ agonist baclofen, recommended by the FDA for use as a muscle relaxant, is often quite helpful in relieving neurosomatic symptoms and has not impaired the memory of any of my patients. Furthermore, cholinergic agents attenuate the memory impairment caused by GABA and opioid agonists (Castellano and McGaugh, 1991). An effective oral central cholinergic agonist is not available. Tacrine, a cholinesterase inhibitor marketed for patients with Alzheimer's disease, probably acts by noncholinergic mechanisms (Vorobjev and Sharonova, 1994), while pyridostigmine, another cholinesterase inhibitor used in myasthenia gravis, does not cross the blood-brain barrier. Some believe that at therapeutic doses tacrine acts only as a cholinesterase inhibitor, and does not have other actions unless high concentrations are achieved (Davis and Powchik, 1995).

The release of NO makes the function of neuronal assemblies more efficient, decreasing the symptoms of the neurosomatic disorders. NO, secreted by brainstem thalamic axons, produces arousal patterns in thalamocortical cells (Steriade, 1993). The chemical neuroanatomy of the sympathetic ganglia, which contain numerous neuropeptides, has been recently reviewed by Elfvin, Lindh, and Hokfelt, (1993).

NE depletion could account for the fragility in encoding that we see in CFS patients, since this state enhances the disruption of irrelevant stimuli in new learning paradigms in rodents. This phenomenon is independent of GABAergic inhibition (Edeline and Manunta, 1995), although NE, via the alpha-1 receptor, can stimulate GABAergic neurons (Alreja and Liu, 1995). In the prefrontal cortex and hippocampus, GABA can facilitate noradrenergic release through a presynaptic GABA mechanism (Suzdak and Gianutsos, 1985). The DLPFC, if lesioned bilaterally in monkeys, impairs performance in a delayed response task, a test of working memory (Goldman-Rakic, 1987). Such monkeys are especially vulnerable to interference from irrelevant stimuli (Bartus and Levere, 1977).

Several of my male patients have complained that they feel exhausted for several days after ejaculating. Although little is known about the central neurochemistry of orgasm, it appears that NE facilitates it, and that NE is depleted after ejaculation (Rodriguez-Manzo and Fernandez-Guasti, 1995). If a male neurosomatic patient were deficient in NE prior to sexual activity, ejaculation could thereby worsen his symptoms.

Case Report

A 43-year-old Caucasian female developed CFS/FMS symptoms after the onset of a left Horner's syndrome attributed to fibromuscular dysplasia, since she had a previous history of this disorder in her renal arteries. She had also been hospitalized for Prinzmetal's angina. After an excellent therapeutic response to oxytocin, gabapentin, baclofen, and felbamate, she relapsed several months later after the felbamate was discontinued due to reports that felbamate caused aplastic anemia. During further therapeutic trials she received an injection of Kutapressin, which caused mydriasis in her right eye. She also experienced a worsening of her symptomatology coincident with the mydriasis, illustrating the marked variability of response to autonomic interventions among patients with CFS/FMS. This patient, although she was hypertensive, subsequently had a good response to doxazosin and clonidine. Treating dysautonomia as a primary disorder is not usually a successful strategy, although dysautonomia, which includes fluctuating low blood pressure, is a common finding in neurosomatic disorders (Goldstein, 1993; Rowe et al., 1995).

Two alpha-1 agonists are in phase III trials. Midodrine is used for neurogenic orthostatic hypotension and does not cross the blood-brain barrier (Jankovic et al., 1993). It is well tolerated and effective when compared to placebo. Modafinil is a central alpha-1 postsynaptic agonist with vigilance-promoting properties. It has been prescribed for disorders of excessive sleepiness, for which it is somewhat less effective than dextroamphetamine and methlyphenidate (Billard et al., 1994). Since there appears to be an alpha-1 noradrenergic deficit in many neurosomatic disorders, midodrine and modafinil may be effective therapeutic agents.

The alpha-2 antagonist, yohimbine, is sometimes effective in the patient who responds to stimulants. It increases norepinephrine secretion by blocking the presynaptic alpha-2 autoreceptor. Patients who have anxiety disorders often feel dysphoric from yohimbine.

We are currently studying the CFS population with pupillometry. CFS patients and controls were blindly instilled with 0.05 percent tropicamide into the conjunctival sac. All patients demonstrated pupillary dilation (mean = 3.5 mm) and few controls did so. We are now testing tropicamide in various dilutions to establish optimal sensitivity and specificity to test for noradrenergic upregulation. Pupillometry may provide a rapid, inexpensive test for neurosomatic disorders on the principle of noradrenergic denervation hypersensitivity. We are matching the CFS patients by their Schirmer tests to a dry eye control group to rule out the possibility that ocular sensitivity may have been caused by inadequate tear secretion (Sadun, personal communication, 1995). A differential response to enhancing noradrenergic transmission in rats has been attributed to the manner in which the amygdala and hippocampus gate information in and out of the nucleus accumbens (Roozendaal and Cools, 1994). In another pupillometry experiment, my CFS patients differed only modestly from controls in the degree of dilatation they demonstrated after instillation of diluted phenylephrine, a pure alpha agonist. Since tropicamide is anticholinergic, perhaps there is also an element of cholinergic denervation hypersensitivity in neurosomatic disorders, which would account for the therapeutic effect of 0.5 percent (or less) pilocarpine in certain patients.

Alpha-2 agonists such as clonidine are reported to improve performance in encoding paradigms, but have not been particularly effective in my patient population, perhaps because doses needed to stimulate the post-synaptic alpha-2 receptor are fairly high and would cause hypotension (Arnsten, Cai, and Goldman-Rakic, 1988). Clonidine has, however, improved word fluency in patients with Korsakoff's syndrome while increasing rCBF in the PFC (Moffoot et al., 1993). Alpha-1 agonists have a neuronal excitatory function. This excitation results from a ligand-modulated voltage- and calcium-dependent potassium current causing depolarization in the pontine reticular formation, thalamus, and spinal cord. Theoretically, an ideal drug to treat neurosomatic disorders would be a selective alpha-1 agonist. Although none are currently marketed in the United States (they are in clinical trials), two of these agents are available in Europe. Midodrine is a safe, effective treatment for neurogenic orthostatic hypotension (Jankovic et al., 1993). It has a peripheral mode of action. Symptoms that are significantly improved include dizziness, weakness, fatigue, syncope, low energy level, impaired ability to stand, and depression.

Modafinil is described as a "central putative alpha-1 postsynaptic agonist with vigilance-promoting properties" (Billiard et al., 1994). It has been investigated for the treatment of narcolepsy and hypersomnia and is effective in alleviating these disorders. It has no effect on cataplexy. Modafinil induced significant increases in anesthetized rats in aspartate, glutamate-glutamine, inositol, and creatine-phosphocreatine, as determined by magnetic resonance spectroscopy (Pierard et al., 1995). Except for creatine-phosphocreatine, these are all substances that should benefit the neurosomatic patient. Hopefully, selective alpha-1 agonists should stimulate NE by raising signal-to-noise ration of sensory input.

Beta agonists cause depolarization in the hippocampus, thalamus, and cortex (Stevens, McCarley, and Greene, 1994). Using this model, tacrine and intravenous immunoglobulin, which also block potassium channels, should also have neuronal excitatory properties.

A recent experiment in CFS patients found that meclobemide, a selective MAO-A (monoamine oxidase A) inhibitor, was more effective than the serotonin reuptake inhibitor, fluoxetine (Hickie and Wilson, 1994). The authors attributed this improvement to preferentially augmenting catecholaminergic neurotransmission, since they believe meclobemide has little effect on serotonergic neurotransmission, a conclusion that does not seem warranted (Freeman, 1993).

The most powerful vasoconstrictor in the body is the neuropeptide endothelin, which has the singular property of dissociating cerebral blood flow from metabolism, i.e., endothelin increases metabolism while it decreases blood flow (Gross et al., 1992). Endothelin increases the secretion of glutamate (activating the N-methyl-D-aspartate [NMDA] receptor), dopamine, and nitric oxide (Stojilkovic and Catt, 1992). Glutamate may be deficient in the DLPFC in CFS; we are now attempting to measure it with magnetic resonance spectroscopy (MRS). Nitric oxide (NO) is a retrograde neurotransmitter that is involved in the making of new memories (long-term potentiation, or LTP) by increasing synaptic strength and synaptic convergence. LTP is a robust form of synaptic plasticity that has been demonstrated to occur in the hippocampus, where it is involved in making new memories (encoding), and also takes place in the neocortex (Bear and Kirkwood, 1993). A brief, high-frequency stimulation can result in enhanced synaptic transmission for days or weeks. LTP in the CA1 region of the hippocampus is induced by synchronous presynaptic activity, probably from several neurons that depolarize a post-synaptic site, allowing calcium ions to pass through NMDA receptor channels. The NMDA receptor is one of three major receptor groups at which glutamate acts (Kandel, 1994).

One way to strengthen a synaptic connection is for the post-synaptic neuron to secrete a transmitter (carbon monoxide [CO] and NO are two such transmitters) that diffuses in a retrograde manner into firing presynaptic neurons to increase their secretion of glutamate (Snyder, 1994). Presynaptic neurons that are not firing are not affected by these retrograde neurotransmitters. NO may not be as important in stimulating corticotropin-releasing hormone (CRH) secretion (low in CFS) as is CO. Both NO and CO are involved in LTP (Shinomura, Nakao, and Mori, 1994), but CO is more important in stimulating the secretion of CRH (Parkes, Kasckow, and Vale, 1994), and thus one could postulate a CO deficiency in CFS. There are other putative retrograde transmitters, such as arachidonic acid, NGF, and platelet-activating factor. Recently, a more general model of nonsynaptic diffusion neurotransmission (NDN) has been proposed (Bach-y-Rita, 1993a) as a complementary mechanism to classical synaptic transmission. Neurotransmitters such as the biogenic amines participate in NDN, especially in neuron assemblies where sustained rather than immediate action is required.

Neurotrophins (NT) such as nerve growth factor (NGF) are involved in synaptic plasticity as retrograde messengers (Thoenen, 1995). They are secreted by a NT-synthesizing postsynaptic neuron. If the presynaptic neuron has NT receptors (called tyrosinekinase positive or Trk+), presynaptic secretion of transmitters such as glutamate or acetylcholine will be enhanced. If there are no Trk + receptors on the presynaptic neuron, such an event will not occur. Thus NTs, functioning as retrograde messengers, can enhance synaptic efficacy in selected neuronal systems. Since NTs are also growth factors, they can increase dendritic sprouting in active Trk +

neurons thus enhancing neuronal connectivity in firing ("activity-dependent") neurons. Activation of neurons in this system occurs by glutamate via the NMDA receptor, and can be modulated by cholinergic, serotoninergic, and adrenergic mechanisms. Thus, NTs are "selective retrograde messengers that regulate synaptic efficacy" (p. 593).

Endothelin levels in the cerebrospinal fluid of patients with major depression are half those of normal (Hoffman et al., 1989), as are those of NPY (Heilig et al., 1993) in one experiment. In another experiment endothelin and NPY levels were normal in depression (Mathe et al., 1994). We have measured CSF endothelin levels in patients with FMS and find a trend to elevated concentrations compared to normals (Goldstein, Russell, and Gilbert, 1995). One way in which endothelin may increase metabolism is by increasing the expression of immediate early genes (IEGs) such as c fos, a process that is greatly enhanced by addition of a dihydropyridine calcium channel blocker, manidipine, related to nimodipine (Huang, Simonson, and Dunn, 1993). Immediate early genes encode regulatory proteins that control the transcription response of cells to environmental stimuli. Their expression is stimulated within 30 minutes after many different kinds of cellular activation. Elevated endothelin levels may account for the regional hypoperfusion seen in baseline CFS/FMS brain SPECT, and also after exercise and cognitive activation stress. In these situations, endothelin might be elevated disproportionately to NE and could be responsible for neurosomatic dysfunction, especially since it induces the secretion of substance P, which widens receptive fields and increases the "gain" of neuronal assemblies. It has been suggested that elevated levels of endothelin found in the postmortem brains of patients with Alzheimer's disease are etiologic in the decreased regional cerebral blood flow found in the disorder (Minami et al., 1995).

A paper that has influenced my thinking about the neural network function of the PFC is titled "A Connectionist Approach to the Prefrontal Cortex," by Daniel R. Weinberger of the National Institute of Mental Health (1993). The DLPFC, the area rostral and medial to the motor and premotor areas, sends projections to all areas of the central nervous system (CNS) except for the isotypic sensory and motor cortices and subcortical sensorimotor relay nuclei. There is even a monosynaptic pathway from a specific prefrontal area in the rat, which descends via the corticospinal tract to a central sympathetic area in the thoracic spinal cord (Bacon and Smith, 1993). This finding suggests that the PFC can directly modulate its own autonomic input from regions caudal to the brainstem, such as the SCG. In a method determined by genetic and experiential (learning) factors, the PFC determines the "saliency," or importance, of preprocessed interoceptive and exteroceptive sensory input, and "gates," or controls, the amount of information that subsequently goes into and samples what comes out of processing centers such as the hippocampus and amygdala but does not affect the processing itself (Weinberger, 1993). The DLPFC is critical for gating distracting sensory input, and dysfunction of this region produces attentional problems of various sorts (Chao and Knight, 1995).

The input and output pathways of the amygdala and their relation to stress situations have been recently reviewed (LeDoux, 1994). This system has been best studied in the context of auditory fear conditioning. Auditory stimuli are transmitted to the acoustic thalamus and thence to the lateral amygdala (LA) either directly or via the auditory cortex. Hippocampal projections to the LA determine "contextual conditioning," i.e., how handling of the input will be altered by environmental and experiential factors. Because of the possible predominance of right DLPFC dysfunction in neurosomatic disorders, many situations may be erroneously interpreted as being those for which none of the pre-existing strategies in the subject's cognitive repertoire readily applies, producing anxiety and other inappropriate responses. The LA then projects to the central nucleus of the amygdala (CE), where processing of the information occurs. The CE projects to the brainstem areas involved in autonomic and somatomotor hippocampal response control. The PFC further modulates amygdalar input and output, which appears dysregulated in neurosomatic disorders.

The CE also projects to the paraventricular nucleus (PVN) of the hypothalamus directly and via the bed nucleus of the stria terminalis (BNST). Lesions of the CE or BNST prevent release of CRH from the PVN in certain stress situations. Unlike other areas of the brain, the CE responds to elevated cortisol levels by increasing CRH mRNA. Microinjection of the CRH antagonist, alpha-helical CRH_{9-41}, reverses stress-induced behavioral suppression (Koob et al., 1994). An increased glucocorticoid receptor signal at the level of the hippocampus is associated with decreased levels of hypophyseal CRH because of increased sensitivity to circulating cortisol (Meaney et al., 1994).

HLA typing has demonstrated characteristic haplotypes in CFS (Goldstein and Terasaki, 1990; Keller et al., 1994) and indicates a genetic predisposition to develop neurosomatic disorders. Neonatal stressors can alter central information processing in children for years afterward, causing an increase in somatic symptoms (Grunau et al., 1994), abnormalities in rodent hippocampal CRH receptors (Nemeroff, Owens, and Weiss, 1994), and changes in adrenal responsiveness to stress for the entire life of the organism. Minimal stressors such as 15-minute periods of maternal deprivation for a total of 4.5 hours in the first three postnatal weeks of rats can cause lifelong HPA (hypothalamic-pituitary-adrenal) dysfunction (Mikuni et al., 1994). Stress research has understandably, but unfortunately, been overly focused on the HPA axis.

Victims of childhood sexual abuse have a higher incidence of behavioral, learning, and somatization disorders as adults. Sexually abused girls have higher levels of morning and lower levels of afternoon plasma cortisol than a control group (Putnam et al., 1991). A group of sexually abused girls recruited from a prospective longitudinal investigation had an attenuated plasma ACTH response to ovine CRH when compared with control girls recruited from the same study (DeBellis et al., 1994). This result contrasts with adult rats that were exposed to neonatal separation for 180 minutes/day as neonates. They exhibited a marked increase in hypothalamic CRH mRNA and had reduced efficiency of glucocorticoid negative feedback (Plotsky and Meaney, 1993).

Prenatal stressors in the materno-feto-placental unit may also produce effects that last into adulthood. Prenatal administration of dexamethasone caused an increased serotonin concentration in the cerebral cortex and hypothalamus of 14-week-old rats. It also enhanced corticosterone secretion induced by open field stress in seven-week-old rats (Mikuni et al., 1994). Such events as using dexamethasone to enhance fetal lung maturity, and prenatal maternal stress or infection could have the same effects (Trautman et al., 1995). Induction of an immune response in a pregnant rat affects fetal brain development. Adult offspring of such rats have an increased HPA axis responsiveness to psychological stress and a decreased number of corticosteroid receptors in the limbic system (Reul, 1994).

Such events early or possibly later in development could alter the function of the PFC through

$$\text{hippocampal} \rightarrow \text{PVN} \rightarrow \text{CRH} \overset{\nearrow \text{PFC}}{\underset{\searrow \text{SCG}}{\rightarrow \text{LC}}}$$

circuits, which could strongly influence the judgments of saliency by which gating of processing areas is regulated. The genetic predisposition to develop such a dysfunction may range from weak to strong and would interact with the type and severity of the environmental stressors.

Organisms that are stress-resistant have higher levels of LC activity than those that are stress-susceptible and also, perhaps as a corollary, have higher levels of striatal and mesolimbic dopamine concentrations (Weiss and Scott, 1994). Stress-susceptible individuals may have decreased LC cell numbers (Freeman, Karson, and Garcia, 1993), which can be regenerated to an extent by the antidepressant desipramine (Kitayama et al., 1994). They also reveal genetically determined decreases in CSF 5-hydroxyindoleacetic acid. Decreased CRH and decreased PFC glutamate input to the LC and dopaminergic A10 nucleus could account for the stress susceptibility. A severe susceptibility to stress may account for a lifelong neurosomatic disorder. In other individuals illness would have to be triggered or kindled later in life after the brain had undergone further development.

It is quite a novel idea that increasing the noradrenergic function of the LC has an anxiolytic effect and could ameliorate the symptoms of neurosomatic disorders. This finding emerged independently from my own work, primarily in the experiments of Jay M. Weiss and his group (Weiss et al., 1994), in rats. In several experimental situations, they found that augmenting synthesis of NE by stimulating tyrosine hydroxylase was effective in preventing stress-induced behavioral depression. Tyrosine hydroxylase activity was not increased in areas of the brain where dopamine was synthesized and central DA levels were not elevated.

When rats were placed in conditions that elicited anxious or mildly fearful behavior, activation of the LC-NE system in various ways decreased behavioral measures of anxiety, while decreasing the activity of the system had the opposite effect, and elicited anxiety-related responses. Anxiogenic effects of CRH infusion into the LC area are attributed to peri-LC neurons such as Barrington's nucleus, which has a much higher concentration of CRH and its receptors than does the LC. A circuit involving the LC, PFC and central-lateral thalamic nuclei has been found to modulate the emotional integration of nociceptive responses. The LC, known to contribute to spinal analgesia, has thus been shown to regulate supraspinal analgesia as well (Sanchez-Moreno, Condes-Lara, and Alvarez-Leefmans, 1995).

The idea that CRH is anxiogenic in and of itself has been suggested by numerous studies (e.g., Smagin, Swiergel, and Dunn, 1995; Shibasaki et al., 1993; Skutella et al., 1994). It thus remains difficult to explain why patients with low central CRH are still subject to panic attacks, and why CFS patients routinely improve during pregnancy, when placental secretion of CRH into the maternal circulation is very high (Goland et al., 1992), unless increasing CRH results in increased NE secretion, as has been shown experimentally. The LC is also activated by excitatory amino acids (EAAs) (Weinberger, 1993; Page and Valentino, 1994), and LC function may vary depending upon the nature of the stimulus, which may be neurochemically mediated by complex EAA projections from the nucleus paragigantocellularis (Ehnis and Aston-Jones, 1988).

Noradrenergic tone has been demonstrated to have several modulatory effects on immunologic organs. Epilepsy prone Balb/c mice were found to have elevated splenic NE levels and suppressed IgG production relative to an epilepsy resistant strain. The effect of NE on IgG production was found to be mediated by the beta-2 adrenergic receptor (Green-Johnson et al., 1995).

Lewis rats are susceptible to autoimmune disorders, but have denser noradrenergic innervation of the spleen and thymus than Fischer 344 or Sprague-Dawley rats. Lewis rats are much more likely to develop autoimmune disorders after sympathectomy (Dimitrova and Felten, 1995). This finding suggests that if sympathetic regulation were impaired in a genetically predisposed individual, an autoimmune disease might develop.

Some researchers believe the site of action of antidepressant drugs to be in the LC. They find that long-term antidepressant treatment in major depression, in which CRH is elevated, decreases the activity of the HPA axis and blocks activation of the hypothalamic CRH system induced by chronic stress (Curtis and Valentino, 1994). Drugs that decrease LC tyrosine hydroxylase (TH) are beneficial in melancholic depression while those that increase LC TH are helpful in atypical depression (Brady, 1994) and possibly neurosomatic disorders.

It thus seems that we have come full circle to the biogenic amine hypothesis of William Bunney and John Davis, proposed in 1965, i.e., that antidepressants should enhance noradrenergic function. The fact that not all of them do, that there is a lack of temporal correlation between NE increase and antidepressant effect, and that cocaine and amphetamine, which raise NE levels, are not effective antidepressants (nor are they very good for neurosomatic disorders) still remains to be explained (Curtis and Valentino, 1994). If cholinergic function is increased in neurosomatic disorders, we may even resurrect the theory that there is reciprocally dysfunctional central ACh (acetylcholine) and NE neurotransmission (Janowsky et al., 1972; O'Keane and Dinan, 1994).

Since I have previously postulated an interleukin-1 deficiency in CFS, it is interesting to note that locus ceruleus and hippocampal levels of tumor necrosis factor alpha (TNF-alpha) increase after desipramine administration. TNF-alpha acutely decreased [^{3}H] norepinephrine release. By day 14 of desipramine, potentiation of [^{3}H] norepinephrine release was observed by administration of TNF-alpha. This process could be reversed by the alpha-2 adrenergic receptor antagonist idazoxan, suggesting that TNF-alpha induced regulation of norepinephrine release is associated with the alteration of alpha-2 adrenergic autoreceptor responsiveness (Ignatowski and Spengler, 1994). Increased levels of TNF-alpha should *increase* CRH secretion, but this substance was not measured.

Studying the hypothesis that early childhood abuse may alter the course of limbic system maturation, children and adolescents who had been physically, psychologically, and sexually abused were admitted to an inpatient psychiatric unit and studied neuropsychologically (Teicher et al., 1993). Abnormalities (as compared to nonabused controls) were found in the left frontotemporal regions in the physically/sexually abused children as determined by conventional EEG and BEAM (quantitative spectral EEG plus auditory, visual, and somatosensory evoked responses). Psychologically abused or neglected children showed abnormalities in the left temporal region only (Ito et al., 1993). We studied 100 CFS patients with the BEAM technique and found left temporal abnormalities in spectral average, as well as in long latency visual and auditory evoked responses, especially the n-120 wave, a marker for selective attention. Frontal abnormalities were uncommon. We did not screen patients at that time for a history of child abuse (Goldstein, 1993), but have done so for the last three years finding a rate of about 40 percent.

Childhood stress increases cortisol levels, which can affect hippocampal function and structure (Sapolsky et al., 1990; McEwen, 1994). Adverse early rearing also affects the response of adults to the noradrenergic probe yohimbine, with deleterious sequelae to stress responsivity (Caplan et al., 1994) as a result of dysregulated catecholamine secretion (McCarty, 1994).

The above findings about the effects of early experience "reflect a naturally occurring plasticity whereby the early environment is able to 'program' rudimentary, biological responses to threatening stimuli" (Meaney et al., 1994). These responses, in a naturalistic setting, should have adaptive value later in life, especially in regard to social subordination (vide infra, Sapolsky). Differences in coping styles are thus partly genetic, and partly due to variations in parental care and early life stress. Exaggerated or insufficient HPA axis responses to defend a homeostatic state in a stressful situation could result in behavioral and neuroimmunoendocrine disorders in adulthood, particularly if stimuli that should be nonstressful were evaluated for saliency inappropriately by the PFC in humans or by basal forebrain structures in lower animals. These considerations lead directly to the important studies of Robert Sapolsky. They also refer to the relatively new concept of "allostasis," the physiologic regulation of states that are not in equilibrium.

The work of Robert Sapolsky is rather unique, and is helpful for an understanding of neurosomatic disorders. Sapolsky recently summarized his research for the layman in an excellent book titled *Why Zebras Don't Get Ulcers: A Guide to Stress, Stress-Related Diseases, and Coping* (1994). It is his study of coping with psychosocial stress and its neurobiological correlates that makes his work so valuable. He has also reviewed the subject for the professional (1994a).

Sapolsky considers why some events are stressful for certain individuals and not for others, a matter I have discussed in relationship to contextual responses of the hippocampus and salient responses of the PFC. He proposes that "foremost among psychological stressors is a lack of control, which can cause a stress response in and of itself." Locus of control issues have been studied in neurosomatic disorders and have been found to be important in how CFS patients deal with their symptoms (Heider et al., 1994; Lewis, Cooper, and Bennett, 1994).

Attributional styles in a cognitive-behavioral paradigm were compared between a depressed CFS group and depressed controls. The CFS patients tended to attribute their symptoms to external causes (e.g., viruses) while the depressed controls experienced inward attribution (Powell, Dolan, and Wessely, 1990). Such an attributional style has been related to alexithymia and somatization "whereby somatic symptoms become metaphors for emotional distress" (Wise and Mann, 1994), but those who believe they have postviral fatigue do not have a somatic attributional style in general (Cope, David, and Mann, 1994) and feel powerless only in relation to the nature and intensity of their CFS symptoms.

A related psychological stressor involves lack of predictability. Lack of control and predictability are exemplified by the decreased use of medication with patient-controlled analgesia, which enables an individual in pain to control when he or she receives intravenous analgesic. Other important modulators of stress in humans and nonhuman primates, which Sapolsky has studied in a naturalistic setting, include ability to displace aggression, degree of social affiliation (being in a variety of protective relationships), and the ability to interpret events as improving rather than deteriorating. All of these stressor classes are associated with HPA axis activation and its potentially deleterious effects if maintained chronically.

Sapolsky examines dominance hierarchies in nonhuman primates, and finds that the subordinate individuals have the most stressful lives, both physically and psychosocially. All stressors involve "marked absence of control, predictability, or outlets for frustration." These evoke hypersecretion of CRH, however, which may not be the usual case in neurosomatic disorders (Demitrack et al., 1991). Abnormal dexamethasone suppression tests are common in this population, who have also been found to have elevated sympathetic tone (McCarty, 1994) and reproductive dysfunction.

Most relevant to pathophysiology, however, are Sapolsky's observations about the physiologic correlates of personality styles:

1. Individuals who are unable to differentiate between neutral and threatening stimuli have the highest basal cortisol concentrations.
2. Those who are most apt to initiate aggression have the lowest cortisol levels.
3. Highly affiliative baboons have low cortisol levels.
4. Those who by subsequent behavior can distinguish between an interaction that they have "won," as opposed to "lost," also have lower cortisol levels. An impaired ability to make such a distinction is analogous to attitudinal and interpretational impairments found in depressed patients in the cognitive behavioral paradigm.

Sapolsky notes that these behaviors are stable over time and thus reflect aspects of individual personality. He believes that some behavioral and psychological plasticity exists in humans if appropriate stress management techniques are utilized. Sapolsky's work dovetails nicely into the concept of "allostasis," the regulation of the internal milieu through dynamic change in a number of hormonal and physical variables that are not in a steady-state condition (Sterling and Eyer, 1981). Homeostatic mechanisms, in contrast, are driven by deviation in one variable and a subsequent response to stabilize it. "Allostatic load" is the price the body pays for containing the effects of arousing stimuli and the expectation of negative consequences. This subject has been recently reviewed (Schulkin, McEwen, and Gold, 1994) and I shall attempt to summarize it in relationship to neurosomatic disorders.

A recurring theme in allostasis research, as in Sapolsky's, is that chronic negative expectations and subsequent arousal increases allostatic load. Persons who always anticipate adversity should be depressed (Beck, 1979) and/or anxious and have HPA activation. Stress hormones are further elevated by perceived lack of predictability of events and lack of personal control over them, so that the world becomes a threatening place. The role of the amygdala in this process has been emphasized (LeDoux, 1994; Schulkin, McEwen, and Gold, 1994).

The activation of the amygdala is known to lead to the anticipation of fearful events (LeDoux et al., 1987). A recent finding has been that elevated glucocorticoids *increase* CRH expression in the amygdalar CE, which could potentiate fear and anxiety. CRH expression is increased by glucocorticoids in other extrahypothalamic sites that may comprise a neural network: the parabrachial and solitary nucleus of the lower brainstem, the central gray, the BNST, Barrington's nucleus, and the prefrontal cortex (Imaki et al., 1991). "Our hypothesis is that activation of CE CRH may set the context for expecting adverse events, and perhaps the induction of chronic arousal pathology over long periods of time and allostatic load" (Schulkin, McEwen, and Gold, 1994). This network receives dense projections from brainstem and hypothalamic sites and sends regulatory efferents back to these structures.

The amygdala receives information from all neocortical sites and integrates external events with internal signals (Kapp et al., 1992; LeDoux, 1994). CSF CRH is elevated in depression, schizophrenia, and obsessive-compulsive disorder (OCD). Glucocorticoid-CRH interactions may mediate both homeostatic and allostatic regulation. They can regulate homeostasis (vegetative functions, feeding, sex) at the level of the paraventricular nucleus by glucocorticoids, and allostatic functions by the action of CRH in extrahypothalamic sites. Furthermore, hippocampal changes can ensue from prolonged elevation of glucocorticoids (McEwen, 1994) producing further elevation of PVN CRH because of loss of hippocampal CRH inhibition.

How, then, to explain neurosomatic disorders in which CRH is decreased? One possibility is that hippocampal inhibition is *increased* because glucocorticoid receptors are upregulated and/or CEA (central nucleus of the amygdala) activation is decreased. I tend to favor an increase in hippocampal inhibition. The fact that another level of contextual neuroendocrine regulation by the PFC in humans has been added must be of some importance. PFC glutamatergic hyposecretion to the LA may decrease CE CRH levels. An increased sensitivity of lipocortin secretion (which inhibits CRH secretion) to exogenous glucocorticoids could also be a factor (Taylor et al., 1993). The most parsimonious explanation is that central alpha-1-adrenoceptor activation of CRH neurosecretory cells is impaired (Coplan et al., 1995), a rationale that is confounded if CSF vasopressin levels are normal (Whitnall, Kiss, and Aquilera, 1993). CFS patients may even have elevated vasopressin levels. I have treated a CFS patient with inappropriate ADH (antidiuretic hormone) secretion. Her findings and response to treatment were similar to those of others with normal vasopressin levels.

We consistently see abnormalities in CFS patients that could be related to dysregulation of the DLPFC-hippocampal circuit. These abnormalities in cognitive testing and auditory evoked response measurement have been mentioned previously, and could contribute to hippocampal dysfunction. The finding of noradrenergic denervation hypersensitivity in these patients may relate to LC hyposecretion, which could be functional, caused by decreased glutamatergic input from the PFC, or anatomic, as seen in decreased LC neuronal number in stressed animals (Freeman, Karson, and Garcia, 1993). It could, of course, also be due to a chronic viral infection, which could decrease levels of transmitter substances. Resolving this conundrum will greatly advance the understanding and management of the neurosomatic disorders.

Dopamine projections to the PFC, studied in animals, are specifically activated by mild stress (Kalivas and Duffy, 1989). Repeated activation of this region in the developing brain, which is the last to mature, not being completely myelinated until puberty (Fuster, 1993), could conceivably result in prolonged dysfunction. Furthermore, the PFC in humans, which gates sensory input according to its saliency every millisecond, must learn what is salient over time and integrate those experiences and attitudes with a genetic developmental predisposition. In this biopsychosocial model there would be numerous events or persistent environmental situations that could alter assessment of saliency. Looking at DLPFC function from the model of cognitive-behavioral therapy, DLPFC dysfunction would be responsible for negative expectations. When this hypothesis has been tested electrophysiologically, however, the P-300, which is thought to index the updating of neurocognitive models that are concerned with the prediction of future events, has been normal in one study (Sara, Vankov, and Herve, 1994) but decreased in amplitude in another (Saletu et al., 1993).

All information processed in the limbic system is referred to one neocortical site, the PFC. Some types of short-term memories are made in the hippocampus and then are strengthened by recurrent hippocampal neuronal firing during slow-wave sleep (Wilson and McNaughton, 1994). REM sleep is also vital for consolidation of new memories (Karni et al., 1994). After a time, the information is transferred to distributed networks in the neocortex, perhaps as a result of strengthening a microneural assembly in the hippocampus and also by activating the medial thalamus, which then activates portions of the cortex (Barinaga, 1994). All these areas, as well as the basal forebrain, can activate each other in feedforward or feedback circuits. This observation would explain the common CFS synaptic impairment in making new memories through LTP. Because of insufficient presynaptic glutamate secretion, the magnesium block might not be removed from the NMDA receptor (input) (Mayer, 1994) and thus synaptic strength of the relevant microneural assembly, enhanced by NO, would also be reduced (output).

Magnesium (Mg) ions in the extracellular fluid enter the pore formed by NMDA receptors to produce an ion channel block, thus strongly attenuating excitatory neurotransmission. The binding site for Mg is within the membrane electric field, and thus the blocking action of Mg is highly voltage dependent, and is regulated by the membrane potential. The ion channel of NMDA receptors is permeable to Na (sodium), K (potassium), and Ca (calcium) ions. If enough glutamate molecules attach to adjacent non-NMDA receptors, ionic flux (primarily Ca influx) is sufficiently increased so that Mg leaves its binding site. These events are regulated to an extent by extracellular Mg ion concentration (Mayer, 1994).

NO, a gas, rapidly diffuses into local presynaptic neurons, which are firing in order to increase their secretion of glutamate by stimulating guanylyl cyclase and ADP (adenosine diphosphate)-ribosyl transferase. How a memory is encoded subsequently is poorly understood. This process could be most simply gated by regulating presynaptic glutamate secretion (input) and retrograde neurotransmitter (e.g., CO or NO) production (output) in hippocampal areas where encoding might occur.

Encoding can be distinguished from "stimulus recognition," the ability for subjects to choose between items that had been presented earlier and new ones of the same class. The storage and retrieval of these items responsible for "delayed recognition" has shifted away from the hippocampus and amygdala to the rhinal sulcus (Mishkin and Murray, 1994). Ablation of this area alone in monkeys produces a visual recognition loss comparable to complete medial temporal ablation (Meunier et al., 1993). There is a circuit connecting the higher-order sensory processing areas reciprocally with the rhinal areas, the medial dorsal nucleus of the thalamus, and the orbitofrontal cortex (Mishkin and Phillips, 1990). There may also be a loop to the nucleus basalis, since acetylcholine is involved in recognition memory. It now appears that the participation of the amygdala and hippocampus is needed only for delay intervals greater than ten minutes. Bilateral temporal infarction, including left rhinal infarction, produces severe retrograde and anterograde amnesia in humans; the rhinal lesion appears to be involved with the retrograde amnesia (Schnider, Regard, and Landis, 1994).

Case Report

A 66-year-old Caucasian male had been well until four years previously when he began to suffer episodes of profound fatigue associated with anterograde and retrograde memory loss, including procedural memory. Formerly a highly successful specialized auto mechanic, he also forgot how to repair cars and had to leave his occupation. He was amnesic for large periods of his life extending into childhood. Multiple consultations yielded the diagnosis of a variant global amnesia and the episodes were finally halted by diphenylhydantoin, but his memories were not restored. Brain MRI was normal and brain SPECT showed frontotemporal hypoperfusion bilaterally. Functional brain imaging has been little used in global amnesia and the limited findings are not consistent (Evans et al., 1993). An EEG was normal, although sleep EEGs, which have shown bitemporal abnormalities in another patient with retrograde amnesia (Kopelman, Panayiotopoulous, and Lewis, 1994) were not done. He consulted me, saying that he felt exhausted all the time, that his life was ruined, and that he was going to kill himself if he could not be helped. Twenty minutes after receiving ten units of oxytocin IM (intramuscularly) he had regained much of his energy. The next morning he remembered how to repair automobiles, as well as many past events, perhaps indicating a need for protein synthesis for synaptic remodeling of neural circuitry and the need for sleep to self-reactivate the neuronal circuits of long-term memory (Kavanau, 1994; Nguyen, Abel, and Kandel, 1994). As he continues oxytocin, he regains more of his memory. Pindolol, a beta-adrenergic antagonist and 5-HT_{1A} (serotonin 1A) agonist, has enhanced memory reacquisition, but has also produced hypomania in this patient. His DLPFC lesions may cause glutamatergic hypofunction and may be attenuated by glycine (Myhrer and Johannesen, 1994), as are negative symptoms in schizophrenia (Javitt et al., 1994). Post-treatment brain SPECT revealed a global worsening of hypoperfusion, a phenomenon seen after all rapidly acting successful treatments.

Case Report

Pseudoseizures respond to oxytocin also. A 38-year-old divorced Caucasian female medical transcriber was well until three years prior to seeing me, when she became depressed, suicidal, and anxious as a result of marital dysfunction, requiring a three-day psychiatric hospitalization. She was well thereafter until having a silicone gel breast explantation for capsular rupture. Subsequently she developed typical CFS/FMS symptoms, along with dystonic movements, stuttering, and lapses of consciousness. Extensive neurologic workup, including video-EEG monitoring, was normal except for bilateral frontotemporoparietal hypoperfusion and posterior cingulate hyperperfusion on SPECT. Trials of clonazepam, lorazepam, nortriptyline, phenytoin, and benztropine were not beneficial. She had no response to naphazoline or nitroglycerin. Nimodipine mildly relieved all her symptoms. One hour after ten units of oxytocin she was alert and had no fatigue, no pain, and no further posturing or grimacing. A minimal speech dysfluency remained, which responded well to gabapentin.

Many, if not all patients with pseudoseizures have a comorbid diagnosis of panic disorder (Snyder et al., 1994). This association ties in nicely with the hypothesis that anxiety disorders are at the core of many somatoform disorders (Sheehan and Sheehan, 1982), but does nothing to explain the neurologic basis of the disorder.

Hypochondriasis also overlaps with panic disorder, but the two conditions are clinically distinct (Barsky, Barnett, and Cleary, 1994). Pseudoseizures are common (Eisendrath and Valan, 1994), and are seen in patients who have models for seizure disorder (often epileptics themselves), who have had a childhood loss, or who have been diagnosed with personality or somatoform disorders. Secondary gain is not a prominent feature, and the diagnosis should be suspected in the presence of the above features plus absence of self-injury, incontinence, or an elevated postictal prolactin level. The relationship of pseudoseizures to child abuse and dissociation (Bowman, 1993) is uncertain. Patients with pseudoseizures respond well to a neurosomatic treatment protocol.

If the DLPFC alters glutamatergic secretion in the hippocampus it could gate input; changing NO production could gate output. On a larger scale, encoding and problem solving occur in the hippocampus and DLPFC, and could be perturbed in CFS. Attentional mechanisms, often dysregulated in CFS, involve the inferior parietal cortex, and stimulus recognition, the process by which a novel stimulus becomes familiar, involves the rhinal cortex of the medial temporal lobe. These structures may also be gated by the PFC, as well as by the thalamic reticular nucleus, which regulates pain transmission to the neocortex. The thalamic reticular nucleus connects various thalamic relay nuclei. In the case of neurogenic pain, a lesion of somatosensory networks from nerve to cortex, it has been proposed that there is an imbalance between ventrolateral and ventroposterior nuclei, resulting in an overinhibition of both by the thalamic reticular nucleus (Jeanmonod, Magnin, and Morel, 1993). The pain of CFS/FMS would be more central than neurogenic, and since there are no demonstrable thalamic lesions, the PFC may be more responsible for dysregulating information from parallel thalamic circuits.

Since the thalamic reticular nucleus undergoes developmental plasticity, however, postulating an intrinsic dysregulation of this structure in some patients with neurosomatic disorders seems reasonable. "[T]he reticular nucleus plays an important part in organizing the earliest connections between cortex and thalamus and . . . the developmental sequence may explain the complex connections found in the adult" (Mitrofanis and Guillery, 1993). This development has been reported in detail in the ferret (Mitrofanis, 1994).

Most peripheral neurons pass through one or more thalamic relay nuclei. But these relays receive their heaviest innervation not from the periphery, but from returning corticothalamic fibers. Each thalamic nucleus receives projections from the cortical area to which it sends its axons, as well as from other, functionally related cortical areas. All corticothalamic axons must pass through the reticular nucleus, which is innervated by collateral excitatory branches from these axons of passage. In general, the reticular cells provide an inhibitory GABAergic innervation back to the thalamic nucleus that provides their input. Reticular cells also receive afferents from various brainstem centers and from the cholinergic basal forebrain, relating reticular activity to level of arousal (Williamson et al., 1994). There is also an important disinhibitory projection to the reticular nucleus from the globus pallidus externa (Parent and Hazrati, 1995).

In general, administering benzodiazepines to augment thalamic GABAergic activity is ineffective. This lack of efficacy may occur because there is a large subset of thalamic GABA receptors that are insensitive to benzodiazepines, perhaps because they have a lower level of the gamma-2 subunit in the receptor. Cortical GABA receptors have a higher concentration of gamma-2 subunits, which confer benzodiazepine sensitivity to GABA receptors. The benzodiazepine receptor is located in the alpha subunit of the GABA receptor. There are three types of alpha GABA receptors, which vary in concentration between cortex and thalamus (Oh et al., 1995). These findings may explain why GABA-releasing agents are superior to benzodiazepines in many neurosomatic patients.

This book is not the place to extensively review thalamic neurophysiology, and will focus primarily on the reticular nucleus, which I believe contributes heavily to the neural network dysfunctions characteristic of the neurosomatic disorders. For a review of thalamic neurophysiology I refer you to *Thalamic Networks for Relay and Modulation* (1993), edited by D. Minciacchi et al., and published by Pergamon.

The reticular nucleus is important during the transition from waking to sleep. During this period it changes its firing mode from rhythmic bursts to single spikes (Steriade, Domich, and Oakson,

1986; Steriade, 1993). This transition is initiated primarily by inputs from the basal forebrain and various brainstem ascending systems. The discharge pattern is regulated by the inhibitory activity of thalamic GABAergic interneurons, which are controlled by the reticular nucleus. The reticular nucleus may be considered as a "pacemaker" for the thalamus, and is able to influence thalamic activity in a global manner. Reticular nucleus dysfunction could impair sleep onset and sleep maintenance by blocking spindle generation, which causes prolonged inhibitory post-synaptic potentials (IPSPs) in thalamocortical cells, thereby obliterating afferent signals despite no changes in their presynaptic components (Steriade, 1994). The cortex and reticular nucleus also play a major role in the genesis of delta oscillation, in which thalamocortical neurons are even more hyperpolarized than during spindle generation. If brainstem cholinergic inputs and PFC glutamatergic neurons are not sufficiently deactivated during sleep, such hyperpolarization and delta wave generation may not occur properly, accounting for frequent awakenings (Steriade and McCarley, 1990). Vivid dreams and nightmares reported frequently by CFS patients could be a result of overstimulation, or underinhibition of pontine cholinergic neuronal input that is involved in the generation of REM sleep, in which dreaming occurs. The OFC is the primary prefrontal input to the basal cholinergic nuclei (Mesulam and Mufson, 1984).

Crick (1984) suggests that the reticular nucleus is involved in selective attention by focusing a particularly active thalamic input to the cortex "like an internal attentional searchlight." The reticular nucleus is a thin sheet of cells wrapped around the dorsal thalamus. Reticular topographic maps are similar to thalamic maps (Crabtree and Killackey, 1989).

Pathways between thalamic nuclei and the cortex are guided and reorganized during development by the reticular and the associated perireticular nucleus. These nuclei are much larger during development than in adult life (Mitrofanis, 1992). The perireticular nucleus has been described as a "sorting mechanism" (Mitrofanis and Guillery, 1993), separating fibers that have different properties. The reticulothalamic pathway is among the earliest afferents the thalamus receives, and its neurons may function as guideposts, or "pioneer" neurons for later corticothalamic and thalamocortical connections.

It has been recently demonstrated that the reticular nucleus (RT) provides an "information highway" for crosstalk between the thalami on the two sides of the brain, usually to intralaminar and ventromedial nuclei, via the intrathalamic commissure. The "RT could influence the activity of wide territories of the cerebral cortex and basal ganglia of both hemispheres" (Raos and Bentivoglio, 1993). Thus the reticular nucleus may be said to have two important functions. It can focus selective attention and can regulate development of connections between the thalamus and cortex.

The potential role of the reticular nucleus in neurosomatic disorders should be obvious. Thalamocortical and corticothalamic connections could be made inappropriately by combined genetic factors and developmental stressors. The reticular nucleus itself could be dysregulated in its sensory gating functions by a dysfunctional PFC. This pathophysiology could account for many of the somatic symptoms experienced by neurosomatic patients (e.g., pain, dysesthesias, feeling hot and cold, sleep disorders) and could explain how these symptoms could "move around" from place to place in an apparently non-neuroanatomic manner.

The functional neuroanatomy of the other thalamic areas as related to neurosomatic disorders is too complex to cover in this book (see Figure 19, illustration section). Nuclei deserving mention include the centromedian, the parafascicular, and especially the intralaminar nuclei, which help to modulate levels of awareness. They can bring the entire basal ganglia-thalamocortical system to a higher level of activity or a state of readiness (Groenewegen and Berendse, 1994). The fatigue of neurosomatic disorders might be caused by dysregulation of the intralaminar nuclei. Input from the caudal reticular formation or from the rostral reticular nucleus can initiate such coordinated activity. It seems unnecessary to postulate a primary deficit in the reticular formation in neurosomatic disorders. The midline-intralaminar nuclei in humans are important for spontaneous and reactive behavior and are involved in affective aspects of sensory information (Guberman and Stuss, 1983). The midline-intralaminar nuclei project to additional afferent sources of the basal ganglia-thalamocortical circuits such as the hippocampus and amygdala, and can further regulate the activity of this neural network (Groenewegen et al., 1990).

The anterior thalamic nuclei functionally integrate brainstem and hypothalamic activity and transmit it via the mammillary bodies to the cingulate gyrus and Papez circuit. "The dorsomedial nuclear ensemble has complex relations with orbitofrontal and dorsolateral prefrontal cortices. The executive role of these cortical areas and their projections caudally through septum, hypothalamus, and mesencephalic reticular core are beginning to be recognized as central to personality structure" (Scheibel, 1994).

Thalamic abnormalities in schizophrenia have been detected by using magnetic resonance average imaging (Andreasen et al., 1994). Decreased thalamic size was noted, as well as abnormalities in the medial dorsal and lateral regions. Schizophrenic psychopathology "can be readily understood as the result of abnormalities in filtering stimuli, focusing attention, or sensory gating" (Andreasen et al., 1994). Interestingly, the abnormalities are primarily right-sided, and occur in areas that project to the frontal and parietal regions, which have linked circuitry when certain higher cognitive functions are performed (see section on cerebellum in the next chapter) (Mega and Cummings, 1994).

After information is learned, other cortical areas instead of the DLPFC are involved in retention of this material. I believe that a model of thalamic reticular-PFC dysregulation, developed from cognitive neuroscience, applies to the regulation of other kinds of sensory information, thus largely resulting in inappropriate perceptions and neural regulation.

An important paper published in 1995 by Karen D. Davis and colleagues (Davis et al., 1995) describes evocation of visceral pain by thalamic microstimulation in humans. Stimulation ventroposterior to the thalamic ventrocaudal nucleus evoked visceral pain like that which had previously been experienced by the patients, a phenomenon that relates to the propensity of neurosomatic patients to experience pain in the sites of old injuries when relapsing, or to the persistence of pain in peripherally traumatized sites long after healing should have occurred. Various patients experienced pain reminiscent of appendicitis, dyspareunia, childbirth, ulcer pain, and maxillary sinusitis. "These observations of sensations perceived to arise from internal organs are suggestive of a memory trace of a previously severe painful experience" (Davis et al., 1995).

Many rapidly acting CFS treatments may increase endothelin secretion by noradrenergic-NPY mechanisms, and endothelin increase then results in increased glutamatergic neurotransmission from the PFC, as well as stimulating the secretion of NO from endothelial cells. It is endothelial, and not neuronal, NO that is responsible for LTP (O'Dell et al., 1994). The reduction in rCBF seen in treated patients with neurosomatic disorders, however, may be an epiphenomenon of the changes in symptoms and behavior, since both acute hypoperfusion and clinical improvement seem to be related to enhanced release of vasoconstrictor substances. In this regard, it is interesting to recall that electroconvulsive therapy (ECT) in depressed patients results in a decrease of global cerebral blood flow (Sackheim et al., 1994), except perhaps in the left DLPFC, where it may increase (Vasile, 1994). ECT also elevates CSF NPY levels (Bolwig, 1994). Endothelin could subsequently modulate classical neurotransmitter secretion as well as increasing running activity and energy substrate mobilization by increasing PFC glutamate secretion to the ventromedial nucleus of the VMH. Acting at the kainate glutamatergic receptor of the VMH in concert with norepinephrine (NE), PFC neurons may thus regulate the integration of exercise and energy metabolism (Minokoshki, Okano, and Shimazu, 1994). Dysfunction of this network could then be responsible for metabolic abnormalities found in CFS exercise ergometry such as low anaerobic threshold, as well as in changes of mitochondrial function and possibly structure. Anaerobic threshold refers to the point at which muscles start making energy from glucose without using oxygen. Mitochondria, cellular organelles involved in energy production, participate in this process.

The central nervous system mobilizes energy stores just prior to exercise through noradrenergic mechanisms. The locus of control of central energy metabolism is in the limbic system, primarily in the VMH, which also regulates various stress hormones, particularly glucocorticoids. Injecting $GABA_A$ antagonists or glutamate agonists into the VMH elicits running activity (Narita et al., 1993). The $GABA_A$ system presynaptically inhibits glutamate release in the VMH. Thus the VMH can integrate both exercise and energy metabolism at the same time.

Furthermore, the VMH has been shown to be intimately concerned with the regulation of glucose uptake in skeletal muscle via the sympathetic nervous system even after muscle contraction has been blocked by pancuronium bromide. Adrenal demedullation had no effect on this process (Minokoshi, Okaro, and Shimazu, 1994). The VMH also increases glucose uptake in brown adipose tissue (BAT) and in the heart. The functional activity of glucose transporters in these organs was increased by VMH stimulation but not by insulin. The VMH is thought to be the major hypothalamic component of the sympathetic nervous system (Saito, Minokoshi, and Shimazu, 1989). Stimulation of other hypothalamic nuclei does not alter skeletal muscle glucose uptake.

The effect of VMH sympathetic efferents on mitochondrial function, or abnormally raised lactate levels following work rates at a lowered anaerobic threshold in patients with chronic fatigue syndrome, has not been studied, but it is reasonable to postulate a central mechanism for this phenomenon as well.

An important recent paper relates fatigue to activity of non-nociceptive myelinated and unmyelinated nerve fibers (termed ergoreceptors) during muscular contraction induced by stretch, pressure, or metabolites (Williams et al., 1995). Fatigue is also related to skeletal muscle contractions that are associated with "central command: inputs from higher centers to brainstem autonomic areas" (Mitchell, Kaufman, and Iwamoto, 1983). Neurokinin A- and substance P-like substances were increased in the lateral reticular nucleus, the solitary tract, the vestibular nucleus, the ventrolateral medulla (VLM), and the periaqueductal gray (PAG) after isometric skeletal muscle contractions. Tachykinins (neurokinin A and B, and substance P) were not released after passive hindlimb contraction and were thought to be released in response to ergoreceptor activation. Release of tachykinins continued in the VLM in the postcontraction period, a response that has also been observed in the dorsal horn (Duggan et al., 1991).

The levels of substance P (SP) have repeatedly been found elevated in CSF of FMS patients. The paper by Williams et al. (1995) provides a plausible mechanism for inappropriate post-exertional fatigue based on dysregulation of the functional neuroanatomy of this neuropeptide and the functionally related neurokinin A. SP is secreted in excess and the duration of the secretion persists after muscle contraction ceases.

Rats who have VMH lesions initially show acutely depressed NK (natural killer cell) function (Katafuchi et al., 1994), cited as one of the hallmarks of CFS in the early days of its investigation. Many manipulations of the brain have this effect, but all either involve the sympathetic nervous system (SNS) innervating the spleen, or involve both the SNS and the HPA axis. VMH lesions also decrease GH levels. GH enhances NK activity. An immediate effect of VMH ablation is to increase sympathetic activity in the splenic nerve much like an injection of IL-1 beta would, both of which decrease NK function. Six weeks after VMH ablation, when sympathetic function decreases (or beta endorphin plasma levels increase), NK function rises. It would be of heuristic value, based on the VMH mechanisms cited above, to conclude that NK function abnormalities in CFS were of neuroimmunoendocrine etiology and not due to a primary immune dysfunction.

It is likely that CRH plays a role in VMH function (Terao, Oikawa, and Saito, 1993). Interleukin-1 beta stimulates CRH secretion. Postulating a blockade of IL-1 beta stimulation of CRH in CFS, we tested numerous endogenous hormones and regulatory functions pre- and postmaximal exercise ergometry (Goldstein and Daly, 1993). These included cortisol, catecholamines, growth hormone, beta endorphin, and core body temperature. The expected postexercise elevation of these hormones was significantly blunted, and most surprising of all, core temperature did not change, and sometimes even went down! Catecholaminergic neurons supply the major afferent innervation of the hypothalamus. They arise from the ventral noradrenergic bundle originating from A1 to A2 brainstem nuclei, and to a lesser extent from the locus ceruleus. CRH neurons are under a strong catecholaminergic control, and activation of CRH gene expression following IL-1 beta injection peripherally is greatly inhibited by a 6-hydroxydopamine lesion of the ventral noradrenergic bundle (Parsadaniantz et al., 1995).Thus an inability to appropriately increase NE secretion will impair an increase in CRH production. CRH may not elevate basal temperature as much as it does stress- induced temperature, particularly that induced by exercise; this effect is eliminated by CRH antibody (Rowsey and

Kluger, 1994). In other words, exercise-induced temperature elevation is not a result of heat generated by increased activity, but is
neurohormonally mediated. The elevation is related to a change in
the thermoregulatory set-point, and is not mediated by prostaglandins, since it is not affected by sodium salicylate. Similar mechanisms may be involved in the temperature intolerance commonly
experienced by CFS/FMS patients. CRH directly affects PFC function and increases arousal without increasing ACTH or catecholamines (Shibasaki et al., 1993). CRH receptors are located in the
PFC as well as the LC (Swanson et al., 1983). CRH increases
prefrontal NE, either by acting directly on the LC or on presynaptic
prefrontal terminals. A CRH antagonist attenuates stress-induced
PFC NE release (Swiergel, Takahashi, and Kalin, 1993). A CRH
deficiency state could have a similar effect. A major brain stem
center involved in micturition is Barrington's nucleus, which is
modulated by rostral inputs. It is rich in CRH neurons (Valentino et
al., 1994), and a CRH deficiency could be responsible for some of
the symptoms of interstitial cystitis (IC), another neurosomatic disorder, which manifests elevated levels of urinary SP (Clauw et al.,
1994). Interstitial cystitis may be caused by CRH-noradrenergic
denervation hypersensitivity in the bladder mucosa and submucosa.
Other researchers, however, have found increased sympathetic innervation and related neuropeptide synthesis. IC patients had an
increased number of neurons positive for NPY and VIP. SP and
CGRP (calcitonin gene-related peptide) neuronal numbers were
normal, compared to a control group. It was thought that the increase in NPY and VIP neuronal numbers in IC was associated with
increased sympathetic innervation of the bladder (Hohenfellner et
al., 1992). This view would coincide with the increasingly popular
opinion that IC is a reflex sympathetic dystrophy (RSD) of the
bladder, the end product of SNS stimulating arterial contraction,
which causes pain, which further stimulates the SNS, etc. (Fleishmann, 1994).

Others find a decrease in NPY in IC bladders and suggest that
Hohenfellner's results are related to his using hydrodistended bladders, which have acutely decreased, but chronically increased, NPY
levels (Ruggieri et al., 1994). They suggest that reduced NPY disin-
hibits nociceptive afferents that express algesic peptides such as SP

and CGRP, and are associated with activation of silent C-fibers. Reduction in NPY fits better with a noradrenergic denervation hypersensitivity model.

Although there may be a central noradrenergic deficit in IC, there may be a peripheral sympathetic overactivity. If IC is really a variety of RSD, then there should be overexpression of nerve growth factor (NGF), which would induce alpha-1 sympathetic neurons to inappropriately innervate sensory nerves (Davis, Albers et al., 1994), or increase SP levels in the absence of sufficient noradrenergic fibers (Bakhle and Bell, 1994). NGF levels in IC have not been measured. Nevertheless, a central component still must exist because of the generally poor results of bladder denervation procedures in IC (Irwin and Galloway, 1994).

When examining the IC patient, I palpate the pelvic muscles vaginally to exclude pelvic myofascial pain syndromes (Travell and Simons, 1993). No IC researcher whose work I have read has applied the neurosomatic paradigm to the illness except Daniel T. Clauw, and most of them fruitlessly (thus far) diagnose and treat IC as an end-organ disorder without attempting to elicit the common history of symptoms such as fatigue, diffuse pain, and cognitive dysfunction. The psychological distress of IC is thought to occur in reaction to the illness and not to be a causative factor (Ratliff, Klutke, and McDougall, 1994).

Models of peripheral nerve injury reproduce many of the behavioral pain manifestations that are seen in RSD patients. Constriction of the sciatic nerve in rats produces enlarged receptive fields in the dorsal horn, and the threshold for neuronal firing in these regions decreases (Schwartzman, 1993). This model, however, results in a decrease in SP, the opposite of what is seen in FMS (Bennett et al., 1989). Nevertheless, enlargement of receptive fields of central pain processing neurons in laminas I and II of the dorsal horn in experimental RSD is associated with increased dynorphin levels. Since a pain-projecting neuron may receive afferents from several spinal segments, RSD pain could be perceived as nondermatomal, even at the dorsal horn level. Its perception at the thalamocortical level is probably dysregulated as well. At the spinal level, experimental RSD and its resultant central sensitization can be ameliorated by NMDA antagonists and SP blockers (Yamamoto and Yaksh, 1992).

RSD has also been relieved by ECT (King and Nuss, 1993). In general, I find ECT to relieve symptoms of depression in my neurosomatic patients, all of whom have required continuation antidepressant therapy to prevent relapse (Riddle and Scott, 1995). Other manifestations of neurosomatic disorders are ameliorated transiently, if at all.

Analgesia at the supraspinal level often has opposite mechanisms to that at the level of the dorsal horn. In this regard, it has been demonstrated that dynorphin A (dynA) augments nociceptive behavior induced by administration of NMDA intrathecally. Dynorphin-related peptides may thus stimulate the NMDA receptor indirectly by a non-opioid mechanism, perhaps involving NO, since dynA can suppress opioid withdrawal and tolerance in experimental animals (Shukla and Lemaire, 1994). Since the pathophysiology of neurosomatic disorders is almost exclusively supraspinal, such patients may have a dynA deficiency contributing to lack of NMDA receptor activation.

The highest density of dynorphin-immunoreactive cell bodies in the brain was found in the hypothalamus, followed by the central nucleus of the amygdala, the hippocampus, and the striatum. Striatal dynA is stimulated by dopamine acting at D_1 receptors modulated by striatal GABAergic interneurons. Prescribing dopamine agonists such as L-dopa, pergolide, or bromocriptine rarely benefits the neurosomatic patient, although selective D_1 agonists are not yet clinically available. The level of striatal prodynorphin mRNA and peptide levels is greatly increased by ECT (Angulo and McEwen, 1994). Dynorphin is also found in substantial quantities in the sympathetic ganglia although very little is located in the SCG of the guinea pig (Elfvin, Lindh, and Hokfelt 1993).

Summing up, PFC function could be rapidly changed by many triggering agents in the predisposed individual: viral infections that alter neuronal function, immunizations that deplete biogenic amines (Gardier et al., 1994), organophosphate or hydrocarbon exposure, head injury, childbirth, electromagnetic fields, sleep deprivation, general anesthesia, or stress: physical (e.g., marathon running), mental, or emotional.

PFC glutamatergic hyposecretion appears to be related to most neurosomatic and circadian rhythm disorders. Glutamate is the neurotransmitter of the retinohypothalamic tract, mediating the entraining effects of light in the suprachiasmatic nucleus (SCN) (Shirakawa and Moore, 1994). This action of glutamate is potentiated by serotonin and vasoactive intestinal peptide (Huang and Pan, 1993). There is also a pathway from the ventral lateral geniculate nucleus to the SCN. This pathway, in hamsters, does not entrain circadian rhythm by photic stimulation, but does so instead by activity, or locomotion. Its effects are mediated in part by NPY, which can cause three-hour phase advances when injected into the SCN without increasing locomotor activity (Biello, Janik, and Mrosovsky, 1994). If NPY secretion is dysregulated in neurosomatic disorders, circadian rhythm disturbances may be one of the symptoms.

The PFC could maintain chronic pain states; central pain may be caused by a microneural assembly that did not adequately remodel itself after the peripheral injury resolved. Many CFS/FMS patients complain of old injuries or wounds hurting again during relapse. The PFC could be involved in chronic low back pain (Bacon et al., 1994), as well as repetitive strain injury and other myofascial pain syndromes, all of which may be viewed as central pain syndromes. The DLPFC could integrate the "physical" and the "mental." Because the DLPFC is important in synthesizing new behaviors from previous information, attitudes, and expectations, its function could explain placebo reactions, the neurochemistry of which may be mimicked by many of the medications I use for CFS, as well as culturally derived symptom choice, called "culture-bound syndromes" in the *Diagnostic and Statistical Manual of Mental Disorders*, Fourth Edition (DSM-IV). Although the pharmacology of the placebo response has been little studied, placebo responders in depression can be distinguished from placebo nonresponders by their higher platelet serotonin uptake site density (Sheline et al., 1995). DLPFC pathophysiology could explain somatoform disorders, as well, including hysteria, which may sometimes be caused by left hemisphere internal capsule structural lesions (Drake, 1993), which could alter thalamocortical neurotransmission. Doubtless most neuroimmunoendocrine disorders (comprising at least a third of a textbook of internal medicine) are influenced by the PFC, and could, in a basic sense, be considered disorders of information processing.

Case Report

A 44-year-old married Caucasian disabled female was diagnosed as having systemic lupus erythematosus (SLE) 17 years previously. She had patchy alopecia, a malar rash, synovitis and marked photosensitivity which prevented her from being in the sun for very long. Her double-stranded DNA antibodies were positive, and she had recently had a lip biopsy consistent with Sjogren syndrome. She developed fairly typical symptoms of CFS/FMS five years before seeing me after a viral infection. Many lupus patients have fibromyalgia.

She had good responses to nitroglycerin, nimodipine, and gabapentin. She felt more energetic, her tender points were gone, and she had much more mental clarity. I asked her to take a walk to test her exercise intolerance and when she returned she stated that for the first time in seventeen years she could walk in the sun without symptoms of photosensitivity. Over the next three months all signs of lupus resolved and her anti-ds DNA test became negative.

Probably this patient improved because her medications enhanced central and peripheral noradrenergic neurotransmission, with resultant immunosuppression. The role of the autonomic nervous system has been little studied in lupus (Wallace, personal communication, 1995), but it is a basic principle of psychoneuroimmunology that postganglionic noradrenergic fibers regulate the function of the spleen and lymph nodes, and even individual fixed immunocytes. Pertinent to this case, splenic norepinephrine is decreased in a mouse genetic model of human SLE (Breneman et al., 1993), and lymph node substance P is increased in rheumatoid arthritis (Felten et al., 1992). It is reasonable to assume that a neurosomatic treatment protocol could ameliorate autoimmune disease, and I have applied for a grant to test this hypothesis in a controlled experiment in patients with SLE.

NE depresses the response of the postsynaptic neuron to weak inputs and increases the response to strong inputs, thereby improving the signal-to-noise ratio of the neuron to excitatory synaptic inputs. The mechanism of the depression of the response to weak inputs is mediated by a noradrenergic blockade of a calcium-mediated potassium current, causing a much larger "gain" in the input-to-output conversion. Thus weak excitatory input will not reach spike threshold, but "strong input that does reach threshold will cause even more spikes than it would in the absence of NE . . ." (Nishimora et al., 1995).

The possibility thus exists that a mechanism for allergic and auto-immune disorders may be decreased by signal-to-noise ratio in lymphocyte function, so that self-antigens and irrelevant antigens will produce an inappropriate immune response. We are currently measuring lymphocyte function and calcium-mediated potassium currents in vitro while varying the noradrenergic environment.

Conversely, infections and disorders of decreased immunity may be ameliorated by decreasing noradrenergic function. Such an approach was used with some success (sympathetic blockade) by the Russians in the early 1900s (Speransky, 1943).

The Possible Roles of the Cerebellum and Basal Ganglia in Neurosomatic Neural Network Dysfunction

False facts are highly injurious to the progress of science, for they often endure long; but false views, if supported by some evidence, do little harm, for everyone takes a salutory pleasure in proving their falseness; and when this is done, one path towards error is closed and the road to truth is often at the same time opened.

–Charles Darwin
The Descent of Man

A recent experiment involved the injection of herpes simplex virus 1 (HSV-1) into the DLPFC of monkeys and tracing its axonal spread (Middleton and Strick, 1994). Surprisingly, two of the areas labelled were the cerebellum and globus pallidus, suggesting that these two structures may be constituents of a cognitive neural network. What evidence can be adduced to support this assertion?

First, let us examine the controversy about the role of the cerebellum in cognition. A debate about this topic was published in 1993 (*Trends in Neuroscience* 16[11]: 444-454), and I shall review the opinions of the participants, as well as relate them to neurosomatic medicine.

The cerebellum has traditionally been viewed as a motor mechanism, but it becomes activated when functional brain imaging is used to study cognitive and language tasks in humans (Ryding et al., 1993). Like previously mentioned areas of the cerebral cortex, the lateral part of the cerebellum, primarily including the macrogyric part of the dentate nucleus, has enlarged tremendously in hominid evolution (Passingham, 1975). One party in the controversy believes that the lateral cerebellum can improve cognitive and language function (Leiner, Leiner, and Dow, 1993).

A newly evolved part of the cerebellum, the neodentate, has grown to enormous size in humans. Its target structures are the brainstem, the thalamus, and the cerebral cortex. A corticocerebellar neural network has been demonstrated with connections to the pons, red nucleus, inferior olive, and the thalamus. The primary target of neodentate projections is the frontal lobe, particularly the dorsolateral prefrontal area, and Broca's language area in the inferior prefrontal cortex. These areas, particularly Broca's, are involved in the process of word finding (Tonkonogy and Goodglass, 1981), a task with which neurosomatic patients often have difficulty.

Twenty million nerve fibers on each side of the brain are contained in projections from the frontal cortex to the pontine nuclei, which project directly to the cerebellar cortex (Tomasch, 1969). To quote Leiner, Leiner, and Dow (1993), "We contend that, in the brain of all vertebrates, the cerebellum can improve the performance of any other parts of the brain to which it is reciprocally connected." Limbic connections can modulate vegetative and emotional functions, and cortical connections can improve the cognitive process of human language. There are two-way communications between the cortex and the cerebellum, as there are between the cortex and the thalamus, to improve the coordination for performance of cognitive and language tasks.

Adults assigned the task of generating a cognitive association between a noun and a verb (e.g., "needle" and "sew") were found to activate the inferolateral cerebellum, which is also activated during mental counting and mental imagery (Ryding et al., 1993). PET in CFS patients at a baseline state has revealed hypometabolism of the anterior cerebellum (Lottenberg, 1993); this finding has not been demonstrated by SPECT. Motor tasks, including speech, activate the paramedian part of the cerebellum (Peterson and Fiez, 1993). The thesis of a cognitive cerebellum is rebutted by the assertion that massive cerebellar infarcts do not cause impairment in language function, and that the projection of the cerebellum to the prefrontal cortex primarily involves the frontal eye fields (Broadman area 8), which are an oculomotor area in humans (Glickstein, 1993). It has been traditionally asserted that the function of the massive enlargement of the cerebellum is motor learning, and not cognitive skills.

Another critic (Bloedel, 1993) responds that the cerebellum is primarily involved in motor learning *and the cognitive processes* related to motor planning, motor performance, and updating body schema. Only the last of these processes may be involved in bulimia, a condition sometimes comorbid with neurosomatic disorders. The activation of cerebellar structures during cognitive tasks may not have a functional implication, since cortical afferents during cortical seizures may activate the cerebellum without any reciprocal activity of cerebellar efferents (Davis and Bloedel, 1984). The cortex may stimulate the cerebellum, but a functional circuit may not be involved.

Leiner, Leiner, and Dow (1993) further propose that "the evolution of cerebellar capacities in the human brain could have been a prerequisite for the evolution of human language." The dentate nucleus in the monkey has a somatotopic representation of the animal's body parts, with the head being represented in the lateral aspect (Thach, Goodkin, and Keating, 1992). What movements, they ask, can the enormously enlarged neodentate control in humans? It may "target the cerebral prefrontal cortex, which contains symbolic representations of information, or ideas, or concepts." They view the neodentate acting as a computer to control the traffic of such symbols in a neural network, a creative, if reified, idea. Data is cited that implies that the neodentate computer could carry out such operations as "counting, timing, sequencing, predicting and anticipatory planning, error-detecting and correction, shifting of attention, pattern generation, adaptation, and learning." Many of these abilities are impaired in neurosomatic disorders. Leiner et al., contest the assertion that cerebellar changes do not produce language deficits, and give clinical examples of problems with word generation and learning (Bloedel, 1993). Recent reviews concluded that cerebellar contributions to nonmotor cognition are uncertain and require further study (Daum and Ackermann, 1995; Barinaga, 1996).

My view, based on our PET data (Goldstein and Lottenberg, in Goldstein, 1993), and influenced by the work of R.F. Thompson and his group, is that the corticopontine cerebellar system contributes to cognitive function and other aspects of neurosomatic disorders. Cerebellar dysfunction, however, has not been reported in functional brain imaging of most conditions discussed in this book, and we have never seen it in hundreds of brain SPECTs performed on our CFS/FMS patients. Thompson and his colleagues have convincingly shown that acquisition of a conditioned eyeblink response in rabbits and rats is dependent on an intact cerebellum (Nordholm et al., 1993). How this finding relates to neurosomatic disorders is unclear to me, but should involve long-term potentiation. One study has found left cerebellar abnormalities in depressed ill patients versus controls who were studied by PET during a spatial matching test. A failure of the affectively ill patients to activate the left DLPFC, while activating a wider region of the temporoparietal cortex, was observed. The depressed subjects also uniquely activated the left cerebellum, a finding noted in statistical tables, but not discussed by the authors (George et al., 1994). Conditioned responses are acquired in rats with the aid of locus ceruleus (LC) firing in the presence of stimulus novelty (Sara et al., 1994). One would expect activation of a LC-cerebellar pathway, perhaps through the parabrachial nucleus, during this process. The pathway might hypofunction in neurosomatic disorders due to decreased LC activity producing impaired selective attention to relevant sensory stimuli.

Magnetic resonance imaging was used to examine the role of the cerebellar dentate nucleus in cognitive processing in humans (Kim, Ugurbil, and Strick, 1994). Seven subjects demonstrated bilateral activation of the dentate during attempts to solve a pegboard puzzle. This activation did not occur when the pegs were simply moved by the subjects, suggesting that cortical projections of cerebello-thalamic fibers go elsewhere than the frontal eye fields.

Injecting HSV-1 into area 46 of a cebus monkey labels ipsilateral neurons in the internal segment of the globus pallidus as well as the contralateral dentate nucleus of the cerebellum (Middleton and Strick, 1994), and "define(s) an anatomical substrate for the involvement of basal ganglia and cerebellar output in higher cognitive function." These results substantiate the existence of cortico-striato-thalamo-cortical (CSTC) circuits, or "loops," which would have a cognitive rather than a motor function. CSTC functional neuroanatomy has been recently reviewed (Parent and Hazrati, 1995).

The way that I conceptualize the CSTC loop in CFS/FMS and possibly other neurosomatic disorders is that PFC hypofunction results in decreased glutamatergic excitatory afferents to the caudate and VTA (ventral tegmental area) dopaminergic nuclei. Caudate hypofunction reduces pallidal inhibition, since striato-pallidal GABAergic and dopaminergic projections are inhibitory. The globus pallidus sends inhibitory GABAergic projections to the mediodorsal thalamus, which in turn sends excitatory glutamatergic projections to the PFC (and receives excitatory glutamatergic reciprocal projections from the PFC) (Alexander and Crutcher, 1990) (see Figure 19, illustration section). Thus inhibitory transmission from the globus pallidus would be increased.

OCD is infrequently seen in neurosomatic patients and is characterized by OFC and caudate hypermetabolism. Caudate hypermetabolism should release more GABA to inhibit the pallidum, and pallidal outflow inhibits thalamocortical excitation. Thus OCD is characterized by increased thalamocortical excitation, adapting the schema of Drevets and Raichle (1992). Brain SPECTs in my CFS patients with and without OCD are identical.

The matter is unfortunately complicated by multiple dopaminergic projections to the cortex and striatum, and by a direct loop from the caudate to the globus pallidus interna and substantia nigra pars reticulata. There is also an indirect loop from the caudate to the globus pallidus externa and thence to the subthalamic nucleus via inhibitory GABAergic fibers and subsequently by excitatory glutamatergic fibers to the globus pallidus interna (GPi)/substantia nigra (SN) pars reticulata. The subthalamic nucleus relays pallidal output to the substantia nigra, and also projects back to the globus pallidus externa via EAAs acting at non-NMDA receptors (Soltis et al., 1994). The indirect loop combines enkephalin with GABA and expresses D_2 receptors. The direct loop utilizes substance P (SP) with its GABA projection to the pallidum and expresses dopamine D_1 receptors (Mega and Cummings, 1994), which stimulate dynorphin A secretion (Angulo and McEwen, 1994). The elevated levels of SP found in FMS should result in increased activity of the direct loop, if they are not just a local phenomenon. DA levels should be decreased in this model and thalamocortical excitation should be inhibited. This model resembles that of Parkinson's disease, in which, however, SP levels are decreased (Cramer et al., 1991). CSF SP levels have not been measured in OCD.

Caudate hypofunction has been associated with both depression and mania and may relate to the hemispheric laterality of the lesion, or involve which dysregulated afferents the caudate receives and to which structures it projects. The differential degree of dopaminergic innervation from the SN and VTA may also play a role.

The D_1 receptors of the direct loop stimulate adenyl cyclase and are therefore excitatory. They release more GABA and thus inhibit the GPi and SN, resulting in thalamocortical excitation, presumably desirable in neurosomatic disorders although Drevets and Raichle (1992) believe excessive thalamocortical excitation can cause "abnormal reverberatory activity that maintains the fixed cognitive and emotional set of depression." Could inadequate thalamocortical excitation cause neurosomatic disorders?

Lesions of the caudate in Huntington's disease (HD) and stroke have produced OCD, as has damage to the GP (globus pallidus) by various insults, including carbon monoxide poisoning. These lesions reduce pallidal inhibition of thalamocortical projections to produce OCD (Cummings, 1994), much better conceptualized as a reverberating circuit than the depression mechanism postulated by Drevets and Raichle (1992). GP insults would decrease inhibition of the subthalamic nucleus and increase dopaminergic output of the basal ganglia.

A loss of dopamine input from the striatum, as seen in Parkinson's disease, decreases thalamocortical activation by decreasing the inhibitory outflow of the direct loop and increasing activity of the excitatory indirect loop (Stoof, Drukovich, and Vermeulen, 1993). Reduced dopaminergic input from the VTA in Parkinson's disease is associated with increased depression and dementia (Torack and Morris, 1988). Since the SN is apparently functionally intact in neurosomatic disorders, differential VTA input to the direct and indirect loop may determine the degree, and possibly the type, of thalamocortical excitation.

The role of the basal ganglia in nociception and pain has been reviewed (Chudler and Dong, 1995). It has only been recently appreciated that the basal ganglia, besides being involved in motor functions, also process non-noxious and noxious somatosensory information. The functional significance of such processing is beginning to be understood.

It appears that basal ganglia neurons encode stimulus intensity but not location. The receptive fields of these neurons are very large, often including the entire body (Carelli and West, 1991;

Schultz and Romo, 1987). Such a diffuse representation would suggest that the basal ganglia could be involved with a diffuse central pain disorder such as fibromyalgia. Nociceptive neurons in the ventrolateral OFC also have large (whole body) bilateral receptive fields (Backonja and Miletic, 1991).

Striatal neurons may be involved in gating sensory information to higher motor areas such as the intralaminar thalamic nuclei and premotor cortex from several different modalities to coordinate behavioral responses. These modalities may also contribute to the perception of the saliency of the sensory input (Chudler and Dong, 1995), leading to motoric response.

The basal ganglia have been shown to be perhaps the most important structures for nociception. Microinjection of morphine and enkephalin into the SN results in dose-dependent, naloxone-reversible analgesia produced by the mu opioid receptor. Systemic morphine analgesia can be reversed by intranigral naloxone microinjection (Baumeister, 1991). Dopamine release by nigral stimulation, and intranigral microinjection of GABA, have effects similar to morphine (Baumeister, Anticich, et al., 1988; Baumeister, Hawkins, et al., 1988).

Case Report

A 45-year-old white male physician had severe Parkinsonian dyskinesia, right side worse than left, and worsening on-off phenomenon, refractory to medical therapy. He also had fibromyalgia. A brother had a similar history. A stereotactic left pallidotomy was performed, which markedly decreased his dyskinesia on the right side (Laitinen, Bergenheim, and Hariz, 1992).

His fibromyalgia was at first very much improved. He had no pain at all for a few days and had good balance and flexibility. His energy was greatly increased, and he was able to hop on one foot. As do most pallidotomy patients, after one week postoperatively he became fatigued about 5:00 p.m. This problem lasted for eight weeks and then resolved. He reports that his energy level is now slightly better than preoperatively as long as he takes L-dopa and pergolide. The fibromyalgia has decreased by 75 percent on the right side but is back to preoperative levels on the left.

A left ventroposterolateral pallidotomy would involve the globus pallidus externa and, by inhibiting GABAergic fibers, would increase caudate and thalamocortical activation, in the same manner as does OCD. The ventrolateral globus pallidus comprises the globus pallidus externa (GPe) in the region that receives projections from the body of the caudate. The GPe receives an inhibitory projection from the ventromedial caudate to the lateral subthalamic nucleus, which then sends excitatory neurons to the GPi and the substantia nigra pars reticulata. Thus a pallidotomy could increase the analgesic efficacy of the substantia nigra. Neuronal fibers are then sent to the medial section of the ventral anterior thalamus as well as an inferomedial sector of the magnocellular division of the mediodorsal thalamus. The circuit then closes with projections from this thalamic region to the lateral OFC (Mega and Cummings, 1994).

Pain is a frequent component of Parkinson's disease and is not directly related to motor phenomena. It can occur in areas contralateral to motor abnormalities and can precede the appearance of motor abnormalities by several years (Koller, 1984). There is no correlation between the degree of pain and motoric dysfunction, and antiparkinson medication does not reliably relieve pain when it relieves motor symptoms (Lees, 1987). Changes in nociception have not been reported in Parkinson's patients after pallidotomy, but increased pain thresholds have been noted after adrenal medullary transplant into the caudate nucleus (Penn et al., 1988).

Basal ganglia circuits of possible relevance to neurosomatic disorders include those involving the caudate. Although we (Goldstein et al., 1995) do not see caudate dysfunction on functional brain imaging using SPECT, others have reported SPECT hypoperfusion of the thalamus and caudate in FMS patients (Alexander et al., 1994; Mountz et al., 1995), which we also have found by PET (Goldstein and Lottenberg, 1993). Patients with unilateral neuropathic pain were found to have a contralateral decrease in thalamic activity as studied by PET (Iadarola et al., 1995). The degree of caudate hypoperfusion is directly related to patient report of pain, but occurs whether depression is present or not. This effect would be the opposite of obsessive-compulsive disorder (OCD), i.e., an *increase* of the inhibitory effect of the globus pallidus on the thalamus and thalamocortical excitation (Cummings, 1994).

The PFC supplies the striatum with glutamatergic fibers. When the DLPFC is stimulated, striatal dopamine and acetylcholine are released (Taber and Fibiger, 1993). This effect occurs phasically, not tonically. Efferents from the PFC synapse directly onto tyrosine hydroxylase-containing neurons of the ventral tegmental area (Seasack and Pickel, 1992) and the substantia nigra (Gerfen et al., 1982). Stimulation of the PFC could also evoke striatal dopamine (DA) release via the intralaminar nuclei of the thalamus projecting to the PFC and thereby activating striatal collaterals to evoke DA release (Cesaro et al., 1979). This process probably takes place when the PFC is evaluating the saliency of a novel stimulus (Weinberger, 1993). Secondary post-stroke unipolar depression has been associated with pallidothalamic lesions. The magnocellular mediodorsal (mcMD) thalamus, which projects to the orbitofrontal cortex, is inhibited by the globus pallidus. Disinhibition of the mcMD, reinforced by right cerebellar lesions, may result in post-stroke depression. Post-stroke bipolar disorder may involve the same regions except for the globus pallidus, which can have the normal oscillation of its functions dysregulated by lesions of the substantia nigra or cerebellum, structures involved in thalamic tremor (Lauterback et al., 1994).

The neuropsychiatric sequelae of caudate injury have been recently discussed (Salloway and Cummings, 1994). They include depression, mania, apathy, disinhibition, obsessive-compulsive disorder (OCD), and deficits in planning, sequencing, attention, and free recall. Lesions of the globus pallidus can cause OCD, Tourette's syndrome, apathy, irritability, mania, and amnesia.

Lesions in the medial caudate can cause apathy and depression; inferior lesions produce disinhibited behavior (and project to the OFC); dorsolateral lesions impair executive function (and project to the DLPFC); and bilateral dysfunction has been seen in most patients with mania. Hypoperfusion in the right caudate is most common in patients with neurosomatic disorders (Alexander et al., 1994).

Deficits in mood regulation are prominent symptoms in patients with neurosomatic disorders. Seeking a neuroanatomic locus for mood regulation, Helen S. Mayberg, MD, at the University of Texas Health Science Center, has published results of PET studies of mood-disordered patients with basal ganglia disease (Mayberg, 1994). I shall summarize the findings of this creative investigator.

Mayberg notes that lesion-deficit correlations with structural brain imaging "consistently support an association between lesions disrupting frontostriatal or basolimbic pathways and depressed mood." Functional brain imaging also demonstrates this relationship. Mayberg and her colleagues have used PET to examine depressed and nondepressed patient populations with basal ganglia disorders to find out what differs between the two groups and to relate these findings to patients examined with primary depression.

Three basal ganglia disorders were studied: Parkinson's disease (PD), Huntington's disease (HD), and unilateral ischemic lesions of the striatum. The goal was to match patients as closely as possible except for the presence or absence of mood symptoms.

The pathophysiology of depression in Parkinson's disease is thought to involve loss of dopamine (DA), serotonin (5-HT), and norepinephrine (NE) neurons and subsequent degeneration of their cortical and subcortical projections, although other mechanisms are possible. Mayberg and her colleagues found "bilateral caudate and orbito-inferior frontal hypometabolism in the depressed PD patients compared with both non-depressed patients and control subjects. These results are consistent with, although not identical to, findings in poststroke depression and primary affective disorders."

Mayberg cites the paper of Cantello et al., (1989), which reports that depressed PD patients, in contrast to nondepressed PD patients, do not have the expected euphoric response to intravenous methylphenidate, probably because of degeneration of ventral tegmental area (VTA) dopaminergic neurons in a circuit with the nucleus accumbens. Her observation is an important contribution to the treatment of neurosomatic disorders. She also notes that dopamine agonists have little effect on the depression or cognitive function of PD patients. It may be that levodopa replacement in humans, as in rats, selectively improves nigrostriatal dopaminergic function but does not usually affect the mesolimbic or mesocortical systems.

Only a minority of CFS/FMS patients respond to stimulants (pemoline, methylphenidate, dextroamphetamine). They virtually never are improved by the dopamine agonists (levodopa, pergolide, bromocriptine), although their CSF HVA (homovanillic acid) levels are low (Russell et al., 1992). *There is no evidence of a neuronal degenerative process in CFS, and the dopaminergic hypofunction may be due to decreased glutamatergic input from the PFC to the VTA* (Weinberger, 1993). I have found a "dopaminergic cocktail" of bupropion, ergoloid mesylates, amantadine, and deprenyl sometimes to be an effective therapy, even when these agents are not beneficial singly. The primary metabolic product of bupropion, however, has a noradrenergic action. The mechanism of action of amphetamine and cocaine is thought by some to be located in the striatum. The pharmacology involves a dopaminergic activation of a glutamatergic system that in turn activates a GABAergic system. "Because the GABAergic system represents the major efferents from the striatum, the evidence suggests that the motor-stimulatory effects of amphetamine and cocaine result from a disinhibition of inhibitory systems in the thalamus, resulting in facilitation of excitation in the cortex" (Karler et al., 1995).

CSF 5-HIAA (5–hydroxyindoleacetic acid) levels, reflecting central serotonin levels, were slightly depressed in CFS/FMS patients (Russell et al., 1992), but were normal in another study (Bearn and Wessely, 1994). PD patients who are depressed have decreased CSF 5-HIAA levels, but nondepressed PD patients have normal levels (Kostic et al., 1987; Mayeux et al., 1988). The same principle might apply to CFS/FMS patients. If the slightly low CSF 5-HIAA found in a pooled CFS/FMS sample was the result of specimens from depressed and nondepressed patients, serotonin may also have a primary mood-regulating effect in some patients with neurosomatic disorders as well. It is fairly common for a patient to report that an SRI (serotonin reuptake inhibitor) improved his/her depression, but had no effect on other symptoms. The relationship of serotonergic neurons to those that secrete other transmitters is complex. The serotonergic system modulates distributed neural networks functioning in parallel rather than actually mediating individual responses. A stimulus does not directly produce a serotonergic response, but secretion alters the "gain" of a widespread neural circuit. 5-HT (serotonin) has been implicated in controlling feeding behavior, thermoregulation, sexual behavior, sleep, and pain modulation (Leonard, 1992).

5-HT transmitter interactions will continue to be investigated since all three monoamines have multiple subtypes, pre-and post-synaptic receptors, and interactions with other neurotransmitters (such as glutamate, GABA, and NO, and many neuropeptides and hormones). Summarizing a vast literature, one could say that NE acting at the alpha-1 receptor stimulates mesolimbic DA release, while 5-HT does not, at least not by a first-order synaptic mechanism (Chen and Reith, 1994). ". . . NE terminals in the medial prefrontal cortex regulate extracellular DA in this region. This regulation may be achieved by mechanisms involving an action of NE on receptors that regulate DA release (heteroceptor regulation) and/or transport of DA into noradrenergic terminals (heterotransporter regulation) (Gresch et al., 1995). 5-HT exerts an inhibitory action on DA neurons in the VTA through the 5-HT_{1C} receptor subtype (Prisco, Pagonnone, and Esposito, 1994). Dopamine deficiency in the VTA may be anxiogenic. Antagonizing the 5-HT_2 receptor increases only mesocortical dopamine secretion (Svensson et al., 1995), perhaps explaining the action of risperidone in neurosomatic disorders. 5-HT, probably acting at the 5-HT_{1A} presynaptic autoreceptor, inhibits the glutamate-induced secretion of NE in the locus ceruleus (LC), suggesting that the NE denervation hypersensitivity could be treated by a 5-HT_{1A} antagonist (Aston-Jones et al., 1991) (see section on pindolol, p. 165). Dopamine, acting at the D_1 receptor, may have a tonically inhibitory action on 5-HT growth and sprouting (Whitaker-Azmitia, Quartermain, and Shermer, 1990). 5-HT neurons projecting to the nucleus accumbens and VTA have an excitatory effect on mesolimbic DA neurotransmission (Van Bockstaele, Cestari, and Pickel, 1994), but 5-HT inhibits DA secretion in other regions (Dubovsky, 1994). A selective 5-HT_{2A} receptor antagonist increases dopamine efflux in the prefrontal cortex of the rat (Schmidt and Fadayel, 1995).

It may be too simplistic to assign mood-elevating effects primarily to serotonin. Noradrenergic antidepressants lose their effectiveness when patients are given alpha-methyl-paratyrosine, and SRIs do not work when patients are acutely depleted of tryptophan, a serotonin precursor. These findings suggest that the antidepressants' mechanism of action is post-synaptic, since NE reuptake inhibitors do not differ from SRIs in their clinical efficacy. Furthermore, tryptophan depletion in drug-free depressed patients does not acutely worsen their depression (Delgado et al., 1994).

Mayberg refers to the work of Walle Nauta (1971) in her assertion that "the major cortical outflow to the dorsal raphe originates in the orbitofrontal cortex." What is the function of these neurons? Do they regulate serotonergic neurotransmission back to the orbitofrontal cortex (OFC) or to other regions of the brain? The PFC has relatively few serotoninergic fibers (Azmitia and Whitaker-Azmitia, 1991), although their projections are diffuse (Papadopolous and Parnavelas, 1991). The modulatory function of serotonin (5-HT) on neuronal rate of firing is still important in the PFC, however. The 5-HT agonist, fenfluramine, which sometimes relieves neurosomatic symptoms with or without a concomitant adrenergic agonist, produces increased PFC metabolism in normal human volunteers studied by PET (Broadman areas 47, 46, 45, and 10), and a relative decrease in the occipitotemporal regions. There was a trend for the right side to be more activated than the left (Kapur et al., 1994). The changes seen could have been due to a direct effect of 5-HT, or to secondary changes in the DA and/or NE function of the PFC. An increase in temporo-insular activity was seen on the left side only. Thus, even though 5-HT projections to the cerebral cortex are diffuse, the functional effects of a 5-HT challenge are regionally specific. Mayberg hypothesizes that PD mesocorticolimbic dopaminergic denervation affects the OFC, causing a second-order degeneration of serotonergic cell bodies of the dorsal raphe. Do these nuclei require tonic OFC input to maintain their viability? There is a direct synaptic contact between serotonergic nerve fibers and the vast majority of sympathetic preganglionic neurons that send axons either to the superior cervical ganglion or to the adrenal medulla. Thus serotonin input may be sympathoexcitatory (Jensen et al., 1995).

Huntington's disease (HD) is characterized by loss of spiny neurons in the caudate and putamen as well as neurochemical changes in the globus pallidus and substantia nigra. Forty percent of HD patients have depression, which often precedes the characteristic involuntary movements and dementia. CSTC abnormalities have been proposed to account for the cognitive dysfunction and mood disorder. Matching depressed and nondepressed HD patients, Mayberg and her colleagues found OFC and thalamic hypometabolism as seen on PET to differentiate the two groups. This pattern is similar to that of the Parkinson's disease (PD) patients. Degeneration of the dorsomedial caudate, found in most HD patients, suggests Mayberg, could cause anterograde or retrograde degeneration of CSTC pathways, resulting in loss of thalamic, OFC, or DLPFC neurons. This postulate is reasonable to me although it is the ventral caudate that projects to the OFC. According to the work of Walle Nauta (1971), the amygdala, which receives massive projections from the OFC, should also be hypometabolic, but the hippocampus should not be. Hippocampal circuitry is more involved with the DLPFC, although hippocampal-amygdalar interactions are increasingly being discovered.

Turning to stroke studies, starting with the work of R.G. Robinson and his colleagues (including Mayberg) in the mid-1980s, poststroke depression has been associated primarily with left frontal and left basal ganglia lesions. Early after left brain injury, there are decreases in central monoamines, more so than if the stroke occurred on the right. Looking for clues that an injury remote to brainstem or VTA monoaminergic nuclei might still cause these nuclei to degenerate or hypofunction, Mayberg and colleagues (1990) cleverly divided the patients into those with strokes in motor nuclei of the basal ganglia (mainly putamen) or nonmotor nuclei (anterior caudate). Those with putamen lesions had widespread areas of ipsilateral hypometabolism in the cortex and thalamus as seen on PET. Those with caudate lesions had ipsilateral hypometabolism of the frontal, temporal, or cingulate cortex, i.e., focal rather than hemispheric metabolic changes. Interestingly, those with manic symptomatology all had right-sided caudate lesions. DLPFC hypometabolism was not noted in this group, whereas functional studies of primary depression characteristically demonstrate left DLPFC hypoperfusion (SPECT) or hypometabolism (PET) (Dolan et al., 1993; Goldstein et al., 1995). Left DLPFC hypofunction is thought by some to relate to the symptoms of psychomotor retardation or poverty of affect (Guze and Gitlin, 1994), but right DLPFC or caudate hypoperfusion seen on SPECT in CFS/FMS is present whether the patient is depressed or not.

Mayberg's group (1994) compared PET scans of patients with primary and secondary depression and found the commonality of anterior temporal-OFC hypoperfusion, with greater reduction in rCBF in the patients with basal ganglia disease. Mayberg (1994) proposes a unifying view of secondary depression based on her unique experimental paradigms. She implicates two circuits, (1) OFC-basal ganglia-thalamic and (2) basotemporal-limbic, linking OFC to anterior temporal cortex via the uncinate fasciculus. Dysfunction of these circuits, she suggests, could occur by:

1. Degeneration of the VTA with disruption of mesolimbic dopaminergic projections causing relative functional deafferentiation.
2. Primary degeneration of the amygdala.
3. Cell dropout in the frontal cortex.
4. Anterograde or retrograde degeneration of CSTC circuits as a result of caudate degeneration. The earliest degenerative changes in the brain in HD occur in the central portion of the head of the caudate nucleus (Von Sattel et al., 1985), which is the termination of projections from area 46 of the dorsolateral prefrontal cortex (Weinberger, 1993).
5. *Secondary changes in brainstem monoamines from dysfunction of the OFC, "the major outflow to the mesencephalon"* (Mayberg, 1994).

I take issue only with above suggestion 5. Why is the left DLPFC implicated in most functional brain-imaging studies of primary depression? The dorsal caudate nucleus receives projections from this region. What is the role of the right DLPFC hypoperfusion that we (Goldstein et al., 1995) find in CFS/FMS patients over the age of 45 in this schema? Why is the right caudate hypoperfused in CFS/FMS (Alexander et al., 1994)? Why do depressed CFS/FMS patients not differ at all on brain SPECT from those CFS/FMS patients who are not depressed by DSM-III-R criteria? Does the OFC *really* provide the major cortical outflow to the mesencephalon, or is that from the DLPFC almost equal? "Both subdivisions project to brain aminergic nuclei, although orbital mesial projections are probably more abundant" (Weinberger, 1993). The issue remains moot at this time since virtually nothing is known about PFC regulation of serotonergic neurotransmission in the primate brain (Jacobs, 1995).

I hope that in future work Mayberg and her colleagues further investigate right and left hemispheric involvement in their patients, as well as the role of the DLPFC in depression and related neurosomatic disorders. The powerful research paradigm they have developed could illuminate the functional neuroanatomy of many other conditions.

Another group (Drevets and Raichle, 1992) has been investigating neuroanatomical circuits in depression. Using PET measurements of rCBF, they reported the atypical finding of *increased* blood flow in the left PFC, left amygdala, and left medial thalamus, and decreased flow in the left medial caudate in patients with familial pure depressive disorder (FPDD), a subtype of unipolar major depression. The area of the PFC they analyzed was primarily orbitofrontal. They did not find the characteristic left DLPFC hypoperfusion.

Their work implicates two interconnected circuits:

1. limbic-thalamo-cortical, involving the amygdala, mediodorsal nucleus of the thalamus, and ventrolateral and medial prefrontal cortices;
2. limbic-striato-pallidal-thalamic, which involves the striatum as well as the components of circuit 1.

Drevets and Raichle believe their data to be compatible with the neural model of depression proposed by Swerdlow and Koob (1987). They hypothesize that underactivation of forebrain DA systems resulted in "enhancement of limbic-thalamo-cortical positive feedback [which] leads to the perseveration of a fixed set of cortical activity manifested by the emotional, cognitive, and motor processes of depression." They attribute decreased caudate blood flow to decreased activity at striatal DA receptors. This abnormality could result from decreased PFC glutamatergic stimulation of these receptors.

Since the striato-pallidal-thalamic projection is inhibitory, decreased activity of this circuit may disinhibit the excitatory loop composed of the mediodorsal thalamus, PFC, and amygdala, increasing their synaptic activity, which could be represented by increased rCBF in these structures. All these findings could be related to the mesocortical DA deficiency. This mechanism is very neat, but the findings of increased blood flow in the ventral PFC, medial thalamus, and amygdala have not been confirmed by others.

Drevets and Raichle suggest that antidepressants modulate limbic-thalamo-cortical activity. They enhance DA activity both by increasing secretion and receptor sensitivity, which would directly suppress the postulated increased neuronal activity in the PFC and amygdala, as well as enhancing pallido-thalamic transmission to indirectly decrease activity in the limbic-thalamo-cortical circuit.

They consider SRIs and MAOIs (monoamine oxidase inhibitors) to also have an antidepressant effect by increasing serotoninergic function. SRIs and MAOIs may do so by reducing the sensitivity of presynaptic 5-HT autoreceptors on raphe neurons and increasing the sensitivity of postsynaptic 5-HT neurons. Both of these mechanisms have been implicated in the pathophysiology of depression (Delgado et al., 1994), but a complex postsynaptic dysfunction in 5-HT utilization is increasingly favored.

Sleep and Arousal
Generating Systems

Science must begin with myths, and the criticism of myths.

–Sir Karl Popper

Sleep shall neither night nor day
Hang upon his pent-house lid;
He shall live a man forbid:
Weary se'nnights nine times nine
Shall he dwindle, peak and pine.

–William Shakespeare
Macbeth, I, iii, 19

Since feeling tired, fatigued, or sleepy is a primary complaint of neurosomatic patients, a review of the functional neuroanatomy of sleep and arousal and its possible perturbations will help to understand neurosomatic pathophysiology and treatment.

A persuasive hypothesis about the function of sleep has recently been advanced (Benington and Heller, 1995). The topic has also been reviewed elsewhere (Gioiditta, 1995). Slow-wave sleep (SWS) is said to promote the restorative nature of sleep and induce the replenishment of astrocytic glycogen stores that are progressively depleted during waking. Transient, local decreases in cerebral glucose produce reductions in cellular energy that cause increased synthesis of adenosine from AMP (adenosine monophosphate), stimulating adenosine receptors and so producing thalamocortical EEG manifestations of increased sleep need. Thus adenosine release is increased by accumulated sleep need and the magnitude of adenosine release in NREM sleep determines the intensity of EEG SWS.

Adenosine is an inhibitory neurotransmitter that acts primarily nonsynaptically by diffusion and facilitated transport. Its levels are inversely related to ATP, which is a K^+ channel blocker. Reduction in ATP and increase in adenosine hyperpolarizes cells by increasing potassium conductance, which could promote sleep onset and potentiation of NREM sleep. Wakefulness depletes brain glycogen and increases adenosine release as a result.

> Adenosine release during sleep may be an adaptation to facilitate sleep maintenance. High levels of adenosine release during sleep would cause neurons to be tonically hyperpolarized even when release of acetylcholine and other excitatory neuromodulators is transiently increased, thereby increasing the arousal threshold and facilitating an immediate return of sleep after transient disturbances. Disorders of sleep maintenance could, in fact, be caused by defects in adenosine metabolism. (Benington and Heller, 1995)

The locus of this defect in neurosomatic disorders may be the biosynthesis of S-adenosylmethionine, the precursor to S-adenosylhomocysteine (SAH), which forms adenosine via SAH-hydrolase. S-adenosylmethionine has been shown to be an effective treatment for FMS in three double-blind studies (Grassetto and Varotto, 1994). Alternatively, the nocturnal release of excitatory neuromodulators could be fairly sustained (night sweats, bruxism, nocturnal panic attacks, nightmares), overcoming the adenosine effect. Substance P, known to be elevated in CFS/FMS CSF, is a candidate neuromodulator to produce this arousal. The subthalamic nucleus, pivotal in the control of basal ganglia output, helps to regulate mitochondrial oxidative metabolism. Its dysfunction may decrease production of ATP (Blandini and Greenamyre, 1995). ATP production elsewhere in the brain, and even in other organs, could be affected by a similar type of neural dysregulation.

There are two networks that produce cortical activation. The reticular formation, located in the brainstem, sends projections into the forebrain via a dorsal pathway to ventromedial, midline, and intralaminar thalamic nuclei. A ventral pathway, more recently recognized, projects to the posterior hypothalamus, subthalamus, and nucleus basalis, and thence diffusely to the cortex and hippocampus. This neural pathway can maintain cortical activation if the reticular formation is lesioned (Jones, 1993). Damage to the ventral pathway can cause insomnia.

Transmitter substances involved in wakefulness include the neurotransmitters NE, DA, ACh, histamine (HIS), glutamate, and the neuropeptides CRH, TRH, VIP, and substance P (SP). The neuropeptides are often co-localized with the neurotransmitters. Deficiency of one or more of these agents could produce somnolence. NE, DA, glutamate, and CRH are reduced in neurosomatic disorders.

Cats with the neocortex and striatum surgically removed have a large decrease in sleeping time, suggesting a role for these structures in sleep induction and maintenance. The anatomic structures involved in slow-wave sleep (SWS) include the caudate nucleus and OFC. When these areas are stimulated, SWS is produced (Penalza-Rojas, Elterman, and Olmos, 1964); when they are lesioned, SWS is disrupted (Villablanca, Marcus, and Olmstead, 1976). A circuit that generates SWS includes the solitary tract nucleus, nonspecific thalamic nuclei, anterior hypothalamus-preoptic area, and the basal forebrain. The raphe nuclei are also involved, especially in SWS induction. The role of serotonin-containing neurons is important in dampening certain sensory input and inhibiting motor output in sleep onset (Jones, 1993). Lesions of the raphe nuclei produce total insomnia. 5-HT acts primarily as a neuromodulator, altering post-synaptic neuronal responses to other transmitters. Transmitters regulating SWS include 5-HT (onset only), GABA, adenosine, opioids, alpha-MSH (melanocyte-stimulating hormone), somatostatin (SOM), prostaglandin D_2, uridine, insulin, CCK (cholecystokinin), and bombesin. Muramyl dipeptides from gut microflora can produce sleep directly as well as stimulating the synthesis and release of sleep-inducing cytokines such as interleukin-1 (IL-1). These neuronal systems also produce neuroendocrine responses during SWS, notably the release of growth hormone (GH). If SWS is interrupted by alpha-wave intrusion, as has been reported in CFS and FMS (Moldofsky, 1989), or if SWS is otherwise deficient because of functional lesions in the caudate nucleus and OFC, as may exist in neurosomatic disorders, GH secretion could be reduced, as has been postulated by Bennett et al. (1992).

The solitary tract nucleus receives direct projections from the PFC, which also supplies input to the preoptic area, hypothalamus, and pontine parabrachial nuclei (Van der Kooy et al., 1984). These regions may form a complex visceral regulatory system involved in sleep generation, which does not occur solely because the reticular nucleus inhibits thalamocortical neurotransmission. There are also sleep-active neurons in the basal forebrain that antagonize ascending reticular activity (Szymusiak and McGinty, 1986). No one brain structure is uniquely involved with the control of a single sleep or waking state. Different densities of sleep or wake-active cells occur in each region.

Slow-wave sleep can be distinguished from wakefulness and rapid eye movement (REM) sleep by high amplitude and synchronous EEG rhythms. Synchronization occurs when one or more neuronal networks, usually responding to the same transmitter(s), fire together in a rhythmic manner. Desynchronization of the EEG replaces large, fairly regularly occurring waves with fast rhythms of low amplitude. This state is associated with activation, which occurs internally rather than behaviorally in REM sleep because physical movements, as well as wakefulness, are inhibited. "Activation" implies vigilance, and readiness of neural networks to receive information and produce a rapid response. The neurotransmitters and some of the neuropeptides associated with arousal produce cortical desynchronization. As previously mentioned, much activation occurs by a global blockade of thalamic inhibitory effects by GABA at the level of the reticular nucleus. Inhibitory neurons among all major thalamic nuclei block some information transmission locally to provide better receptive field specificity and response selectivity (Steriade et al., 1993).

The major sensorimotor thalamic nuclei receive about 90 percent of their innervation from brainstem cholinergic reticular afferents. In contrast, the associational and diffusely projecting thalamic nuclei, which are more involved with neurosomatic disorders, receive noncholinergic brainstem projections, but the transmitters in these afferents have yet to be identified (Steriade et al., 1988). NE is a leading candidate.

Despite the importance of the thalamus in activation, "the majority of neurons that form the arousal system project to the cerebral cortex" (Marrocco, Witte, and Davidson, 1994). Their neurotransmitters, neuropeptides, and neuromodulators have been listed above. Recall that noradrenergic projections are more dense in the right hemisphere than the left. The opposite is true for DA and ACh. Thus problems with signal-to-noise extraction might be more common in right hemispheric disorders, as some neurosomatic illnesses might be.

Neurochemical arousal systems alter cellular activity by blocking potassium conductance and cause dysynchronization of neuronal activity. The arousal systems interact, probably by presynaptic heteroceptors. An autoreceptor modulates neuronal activity by sensing the same transmitter its neuron secretes. A heteroceptor alters neuronal activity presynaptically by sensing a different receptor than its neuron secretes. For example, NE can facilitate ACh-mediated attentional movements in monkeys (Marrocco, Witte, and Davidson, 1994). It has been proposed that a decrease in NE function increases distractibility (seen in CFS), that impairment of mesolimbic dopamine output increases response latency (seen in depression), that destruction of the cholinergic basal forebrain reduces discrimination accuracy (perhaps found in neurosomatic disorders), and that lesions of forebrain serotonergic cells increase impulsivity (seen in OFC lesions) (Robbins and Everett, 1993). Neurosomatic patients rarely have impulse-control disorders, an observation that suggests that 5-HT deficiency is not important in their pathophysiology (Hollander and Wong, 1995a,b).

Although many neurosomatic patients state that their symptoms are worsened by ingestion of simple sugars, there is good evidence that increasing blood glucose enhances certain forms of animal and human memory. This effect is not related to basal glucose levels. It has been suggested that the memory improvement is a result of increasing acetyl CoA (coenzyme A), a substrate for ACh (Benton and Owens, 1993).

This phenomenon has been studied in rats, in which i.c.v. (intracerebroventricular) administration of glucose improved retention (Lee, Graham, and Gold, 1988). Scopolamine, a well-known anticholinergic agent used in the diagnosis of Alzheimer's disease, produces task deficits that can be attenuated by i.c.v. glucose. Insulin can decrease post-training scopolamine-induced amnesia in rats (Messier and Destrade, 1994). Since insulin is released by glucose injections, it is possible that the glucose attenuation of scopolamine-induced amnesia is produced by insulin release, rather than by augmentation of ACh biosynthesis. Both ACh and insulin can produce cortical activation.

Insulin neuronal receptors are very dense in limbic structures, although their function is not well understood. Insulin is one of the substances involved in brain arousal. It stimulates choline acetyltransferase in cultured embryonic chicken retina neurons (Kyrakis, Hausman, and Peterson, 1987), and induces the release of DA and NE from hypothalamic slices (Pavcovich et al., 1990). It is possible that these mechanisms could be dysregulated in neurosomatic patients.

Impulsive disorders, which include borderline personality disorder and antisocial personality disorder, have been grouped into a large number of "obsessive-compulsive spectrum disorders." These include somatoform disorders (especially hypochondriasis and body dysmorphic disorder), dissociative disorders and depersonalization, tic disorders, personality disorders, "schizo-obsessive" spectrum disorders, and a wide range of neurologic disorders, including epilepsy, autism, and several basal ganglia disorders, e.g., Tourette's syndrome (see Figure 24, illustration section).

All of these illnesses are characterized by response to serotonin reuptake inhibitors (Hollander and Wong, 1995a,b). Almost all of the obsessive-compulsive spectrum disorders are uncommon in neurosomatic medicine. I administered the Yale-Brown Obsessive-Compulsive Scale (Y-BOCS) to 100 consecutive CFS patients. Only two scored in the clinically significant range, a lower rate than the 3 percent expected in the general population. When neurosomatic patients with obsessive-compulsive spectrum disorders respond to an agent on my protocol, they exhibit significant anxiolysis and a marked reduction in their obsessive-compulsive symptoms. Serotonin reuptake inhibitors are thus often not necessary.

Irritable Bowel Syndrome

Within me is a hell.

—William Shakespeare
King John, V, vii, 46

Although the most common disorder for which patients consult gastroenterologists, irritable bowel syndrome (IBS) is still poorly understood and inadequately managed. It is variously considered a disorder of smooth muscle function, an enteric neuropathy, or an abnormality in visceral nociception. The role of chronic stress in IBS is not well defined and is "controversial" (Talley, 1994; Gorard and Farthing, 1994; McIntyre and Pemberton, 1994).

CNS function has not been well studied in IBS. There are no published reports of functional brain imaging in the disorder, for example, and electrophysiologic investigations of the brain, such as evoked responses, have not been well explored. Problems with lethargy, backache, premature satiety, and urinary frequency can distinguish IBS from organic bowel disease (Maxton, Morris, and Whorwell, 1991). Psychosocial factors in IBS patients such as "neurosis" or adjustment disorders are correlated "as much with health care seeking behavior as with symptom severity," and it is said that the symptom profile can be explained by "hyperventilation syndrome" (Nyhlin et al., 1993). Chest pain of unknown etiology is often grouped among the "functional gastrointestinal disorders because it is presumed to be allotted to esophageal dysmotility" (Richter et al., 1992). The possibility of a thalamic etiology for this pain (Lenz et al., 1994), as well as other types of visceral pain (Davis et al., 1995), has not been considered in the gastroenterologic literature.

Antidepressants are beneficial in IBS, especially for pain management (Heefner, Russell, and Wilson, 1978). Desipramine, a tricyclic antidepressant, was found to be globally superior to an anticholinergic

(Greenbaum et al., 1987). Agents that modulate nociceptive visceral sensation such as ondansetron, a 5-HT$_3$ receptor antagonist used for pain caused by esophageal balloon distension (Stark et al., 1991), and octreotide, a somatostatin analog used to relieve pain from rectal distension (Hasler, Soudah, and Owyang, 1993), are being increasingly prescribed for the IBS population. Levels of somatostatin in the cerebrospinal fluid were measured in patients with schizophrenia, major depression, mania, and schizoaffective disorder. The results were: mania > depression > schizoaffective > schizophrenic (Sharma et al., 1995). Octreotide, occasionally helpful for global neurosomatic symptoms, increases thresholds of colonic visceral perception in IBS patients without modifying muscle tone (Bradette et al., 1994). Octreotide may be effective in fibromyalgia (Hasler, Soudah, and Owyang, 1993), reflex sympathetic dystrophy (Ellis, 1990), dysautonomia and intestinal pseudo-obstruction. I have used octreotide at least fifty times in intractable neurosomatic patients. Only one demonstrated consistent benefit. Perhaps this treatment failure is due to the fact that I try nimodipine first. Nimodipine increases CSF somatostatin levels in certain patient groups (Pazzagalia et al., 1995). Tricyclic antidepressants, in doses less than those used for mood disorders, are favored for the treatment of IBS, and help pain more than dysmotility complaints (Clouse, 1994). SRIs, MAOIs, bupropion, or venlafaxine have not been systematically investigated. Anxiolytic drugs such as benzodiazepines and azaspirones, although widely prescribed, have not been experimentally studied except for alprazolam in one retrospective review (Clouse et al., 1994). My own experience is that IBS symptoms respond quite well to agents on the neurosomatic protocol and that the improvement is not restricted to gastrointestinal symptoms, but is usually widespread over the entire neurosomatic spectrum. The best treatment I have found for intractable IBS is intravenous lidocaine.

For several years, John Mathias and his group have been studying the effects of leuprolide (Lupron), a molecular analog of gonadotropin-releasing hormone, in IBS patients. Reporting on a double-blind placebo-controlled study in premenopausal women, they found a significant decrease in nausea, vomiting, bloating, abdominal pain, and early satiety (Mathias, Clench, Reeves-Darby et al., 1994). When the patients were continued on leuprolide after the 12-week study period, they continued to improve (Mathias, Clench,

Roberts, and Reeves-Darby, 1994). Nonalimentary symptoms were not evaluated. Leuprolide pharmacology could modify the function of the enteric nervous system hormonally or electrophysiologically, or might affect the brain or spinal cord (Wood, 1994). In my experience, nafarelin nasal spray (Synarel), is often effective in selected patients in a week or two.

A pathophysiology compatible with the neurosomatic hypothesis has been described by Mayer and Gebhart (1994). They postulate that central sensitization can occur from visceral afferents to dorsal horn neurons projecting subsequently to the thalamus, resulting in hyperalgesia in different parts of the gut:

> In addition to long lasting, plastic neuronal changes, the sensitivity of visceral sensory pathways can be acutely modulated by neurohormonal mechanisms related to food intake and stress. This acute, transient modulation can occur at the level of the spinal cord, the mesenteric ganglia, or the peripheral terminals. (p. 92)

This model is similar to that of Yunus (1992), discussing fibromyalgia, and Nicolodi et al. (1994), explaining migraine headache as an aspect of visceral hyperalgesia.

Mayer and Gebhart (1993) emphasize that gastrointestinal dysmotility has been eliminated as a cause for IBS symptoms. They believe that hypersensitivity of gastrointestinal mechano- and chemoreceptors is an essential part of IBS pathophysiology, and that initial trauma of some sort to these receptors may incite a pathophysiologic cascade that includes descending pain modulatory systems as well as genetic and developmental factors.

I view this praiseworthy synthesis as being of the "bottom-up" variety, in which symptoms originate in the GI tract and produce central changes. My approach is more "top-down." The evidence from brain functional imaging (see the next paragraph), as well as global symptom response to treatment, argues for the basic problem being one of impaired central gating of normal sensory input in most cases. Thalamic and dorsal horn dysregulation in IBS would stem from prefrontal cortical dysfunction in this paradigm. There is no heuristic reason to complicate matters by invoking some peripheral lesion, although such may occur, just as primary immune dysfunction may occasionally cause CFS, and a post-traumatic myofascial pain syndrome may produce fibromyalgia.

Functional bowel disease (FBD) was found to occur in 72 percent of patients with CFS using a validated bowel symptom questionnaire developed by N.J. Talley (Diehl, Fullerton, and Mayer, 1995). I compared brain SPECT results from 21 CFS patients positive for FBD on the Talley questionnaire to 11 CFS patients who were FBD-negative. There was no difference between the two groups in regional cerebral blood flow. FBD-positive CFS patients had more severe hypoperfusion than FBD-negative CFS patients (Goldstein and Mena, 1995). These results are similar to those for CFS patients with and without fibromyalgia (Goldstein, Mena, and Yunus, 1993), and suggest a common central etiology for neurosomatic disorders, which is the thesis of this book.

Receptor Desensitization
and Drug Tolerance

Now remains that we find out the cause of this effect, or rather
say the cause of this defect, for this effect defective comes by
the cause.

–William Shakespeare
Hamlet, II, ii, 101

A significant problem in treating neurosomatic patients is the
development of tolerance to a previously effective rapidly acting
agent on the treatment protocol. Tolerance can even occur after one
dose of a medication. In the usual clinical setting it would be impos-
sible to distinguish this response from a very short-acting placebo
effect.

Case Report

A 29-year-old single Caucasian female teacher fell ill with acute
mononucleosis five years previously while at Harvard, but recovered. Three years before seeing me she developed an acute viral
illness and could not get out of bed. She tried to continue teaching
but required 15 hours of rest per day and was often too fatigued to
travel to her school at all. She had significant memory disturbances,
at times forgetting her phone number and her address. She had
diffuse pain and fibromyalgia tender points, and felt as if she had the
flu all the time. She had not improved on numerous treatment trials
prior to consulting me. She did not respond to fluoxetine, intravenous immunoglobulin, bupropion, kutapressin, phenelzine, sertraline, nimodipine, and ranitidine. She had severe vertigo and was
unable to read for more than 20 minutes. All symptoms were exacer-

bated by even mild exertion. Two minutes after taking 0.04 mg of sublingual nitroglycerin almost all her pain was gone and she felt fairly energetic. Her vertigo completely resolved, as did her "brain fog." She was able to swim in the ocean. This beneficial effect gradually decreased over the next week until nitroglycerin was ineffective. The patient subsequently tried virtually every medication discussed in this book as well as quite a few others. Sadly, she had no response to any of them and is still disabled.

It appears that rapid responses to neurosomatic agents are alpha-1 adrenergically mediated, since they are associated with diffuse cerebral vasoconstriction. Beta receptors may also be stimulated by increasing noradrenergic transmission. This postulate is difficult to dissect pharmacologically, since neurosomatic patients do not respond in any predictable fashion to alpha and beta receptor agonists or antagonists. Noradrenergic co-transmitters such as neuropeptide Y (NPY), modulators released from second-order neurons such as oxytocin, or vasoactive agents released from the endothelium as a result of vasoconstriction, such as nitric oxide, may all play a role.

In the last 15 years much has been learned about molecular mechanisms of adrenergic (particularly beta-adrenergic) receptor desensitization (Lohse, 1993). Just as the brain and neuroendocrine systems have complex feedforward and feedback loops, so do individual cells. These loops regulate signalling within the cell, particularly those of "second messengers," i.e., signals generated in response to occupation of a membrane-bound receptor by a ligand. Second, third, and fourth messenger regulatory systems are extremely complex and an in-depth discussion of their function is beyond the scope of this book. Textbooks of neurobiology provide a good overview of this topic (e.g., Kennedy, 1992), which has recently been reviewed for the clinician (Duman, Heninger, and Nestler, 1994).

Intracellular regulatory systems are activated by occupation of a receptor by a ligand and usually serve to decrease the response to receptor stimulation, a process called "desensitization." Inhibitory neurotransmitters are not desensitized as readily as stimulatory ones. Desensitization can be very rapid, occurring within minutes. It occurs by two basic mechanisms: "uncoupling," a loss of receptor signalling function, and "downregulation," a loss of receptor number.

THE MODE OF ACTION
OF DESENSITIZATION

Desensitization has been best characterized in the beta-adrenergic receptor, which is coupled to the stimulatory G-protein G_s, and thence stimulates the production of cyclic AMP (cAMP). Receptors can rapidly lose function by being phosphorylated. There are specific beta-adrenergic receptor kinases (BARKs) that phosphorylate only agonist-occupied, active receptors. After phosphorylation occurs the affinity of the receptors for the inhibitor protein beta-arrestin greatly increases, and this binding *uncouples* the beta receptor from the G_s protein (Lohse et al., 1992). This type of desensitization is called "homologous" because it occurs at a specific receptor. It requires four components: receptor, receptor specific kinase, arrestin protein, and G-protein.

Many G-protein coupled receptors are phosphorylated by their own effector kinases, such as protein kinases A and C (PKA, PKC). Since this desensitization pathway is not receptor specific, it is termed "heterologous." Heterologous desensitization occurs more slowly than homologous desensitization. I have discussed the possible roles of PKA and PKC in chronic fatigue syndrome in previous works (Goldstein, 1990; 1993).

Receptor sequestration and downregulation are more familiar phenomena to most physicians who had long since left medical school when G-proteins were discovered in the 1980s. Receptors can be translocated to intracellular sites after they are occupied by an agonist. The signals involved in receptor sequestration are unknown (Lohse, 1993).

Receptor number can decrease, or be "downregulated." This process occurs more slowly than those thus far described, and can take up to 24 hours in experimental preparations. Receptors can be more rapidly degraded or less rapidly manufactured, both of which can result in downregulation. Reduction in beta-2 receptor mRNA occurs as a result of its destabilization, since it occurs after administration of actinomycin D (Hadcock, Wang, and Malbon, 1989). Desensitization can also occur by G-protein phosphorylation, particularly of the alpha subunit (Hausdorff et al., 1992).

The alpha-1 receptor functions differently than the beta receptor.

Its G protein is coupled to phospholipase C, and thence to phosphatidyl inositol, which is metabolized to inositol triphosphate (IP_3) and diacylglycerol (DAG) (Lefkowitz, Hoffman, and Taylor, 1990). The alpha-1 receptor is also coupled to the effectors phospholipase A_2 and phospholipase C (Lomasney and Allen, 1993). There are four subtypes of alpha-1 receptor (A→D), but their functional differences are not yet understood. The principles of the desensitization of the alpha-1 receptor are not well characterized. IP_3 stimulates release of calcium from intracellular stores and DAG stimulates PKC, which may mediate phosphorylation reactions (Sibley et al., 1987). The physiology of inositol phospholipids and phosphates is complex (Hughes and Michell, 1993).

There are few current therapies that modulate second, third, and fourth messengers. A major advance in the near future of pharmacology will be the development of such agents. It may be possible to stimulate IP_3 by giving large doses of exogenous inositol in the treatment of depression. Inositol took about two weeks to have an antidepressant effect in a dosage of 6 grams per day in an open study of treatment-resistant patients (Levine et al., 1993). A double-blind study using 12 gram per day of inositol was efficacious in the treatment of depression (Levine et al., 1995). Inositol is also an effective treatment for panic disorder (Benjamin et al., 1995).

Lithium inhibits inositol monophosphatase noncompetitively, which recycles inositol from inositol phosphates. This mechanism has been used to explain the effectiveness of lithium in alleviating bipolar affective disorder. Lithium decreased CSF inositol monophosphatase activity in a double-blind study of normal human volunteers (Molchan, Atack, and Sunderland, 1994). Lithium also blocked the stimulus-induced release of NE from rat brain slices (Cooper, Bloom, and Roth, 1982). One might think that high-dose inositol (the substance penetrates the blood-brain barrier poorly) might act in a fashion opposite to lithium (a drug that is quite ineffective in ameliorating neurosomatic symptomatology), although it theoretically should decrease tachyphylaxis by its inhibition of PKA (Lomasney and Allen, 1993). Phosphatidyl inositol (lecithin) is more lipophilic, but has not been tested in this paradigm.

Similarly, agents could be used to stimulate PKC. Overstimulation of PKC may cause CFS (Goldstein, 1990) when vapors are inhaled while applying the sealant tung oil. The dosage of whatever phorbol ester (the main component of tung oil) is selected to modulate the kinase should be carefully titrated. A currently available medication, acetyl-L-carnitine, is a PKC activator (Pascale et al., 1994). Its effects may be mediated by the cholinergic system. PKC activation by phorbol esters also enhances calcium-dependent glutamate release (Terrian, 1995), which could be beneficial in neurosomatic disorders, but neurotoxic if glutamate is excessively secreted. Specific PKC inhibitors exist (Mathis, Lehmann, and Ungerer, 1992), but have not been used clinically. They can cause amnesia in rats by blocking LTP (Jerusalinsky et al., 1994).

Case Report

A 16-year-old Caucasian female consulted me for symptoms of chronic fatigue syndrome experienced for two years, which resulted in her being homebound. She was too cognitively impaired to receive home schooling, although she had been an "A" student prior to her illness. Her mother and a 14-year-old sister had milder forms of the illness. She initially had excellent responses to ranitidine, naphazoline, nimodipine, oxytocin, and several antidepressants, but the benefit was always short-lived. After taking one gram of inositol she felt considerably better and was encouraged to resume agents to which she had developed tolerance. As long as she continued to take inositol one gram QID, these medications were again effective. She has returned to high school and will be graduating shortly.

Finally, most neurosomatic treatments discussed in this book appear to act at the level of the sympathetic ganglia, locus ceruleus, or brainstem noradrenergic nuclei. Perhaps tolerance occurs more easily in such structures than it would in areas that would *regulate* autonomic function, such as the PFC via glutamatergic afferents. More effective future treatments may modulate sympathetic neuronal function rather than directly stimulating it.

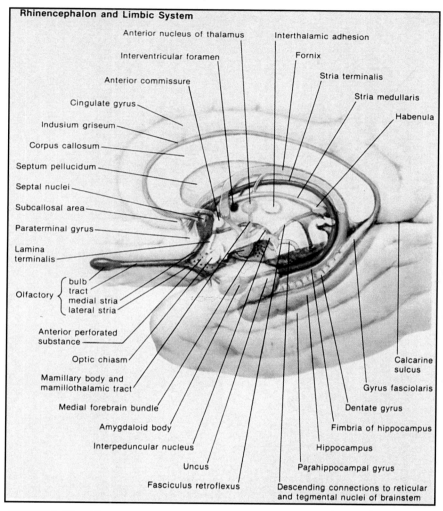

Rhinencephalon and Limbic System

Anterior nucleus of thalamus

Interthalamic adhesion

Interventricular foramen

Fornix

Anterior commissure

Stria terminalis

Stria medullaris

Cingulate gyrus

Habenula

Indusium griseum

Corpus callosum

Septum pellucidum

Septal nuclei

Subcallosal area

Paraterminal gyrus

Lamina terminalis

Olfactory
- bulb
- tract
- medial stria
- lateral stria

Anterior perforated substance

Optic chiasm

Calcarine sulcus

Mamillary body and mamillothalamic tract

Gyrus fasciolaris

Medial forebrain bundle

Dentate gyrus

Amygdaloid body

Fimbria of hippocampus

Interpeduncular nucleus

Hippocampus

Uncus

Parahippocampal gyrus

Fasciculus retroflexus

Descending connections to reticular and tegmental nuclei of brainstem

FIGURE 1. The olfactory tract synapses directly with the limbic system without a thalamic intermediary, perhaps accounting for cacosmia.

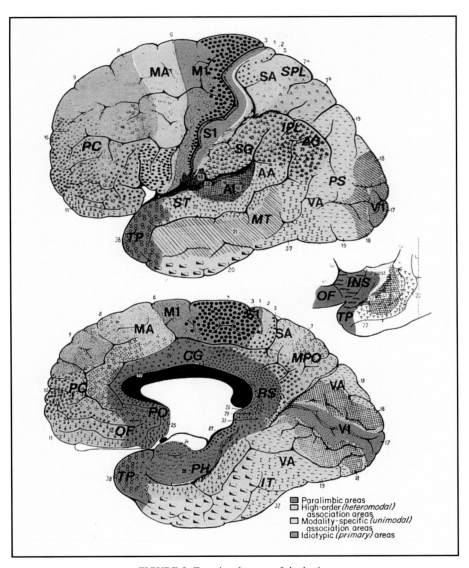

FIGURE 2. Functional zones of the brain.

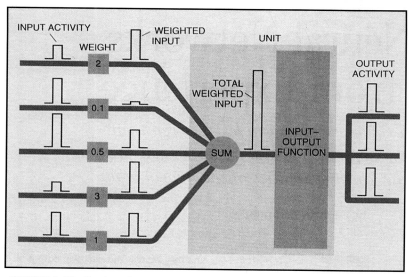

FIGURE 3. Idealization of neuron processing activities, or signals. Each input activity is multiplied by a number called the weight. The "unit" adds together the weighted inputs. It then computes the output activity using an input-output function.

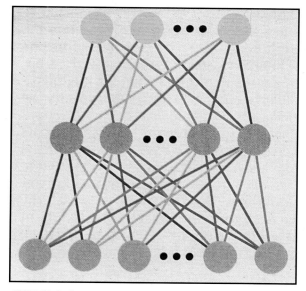

FIGURE 4. Common neural network consists of three layers of units that are fully connected. Activity passes from the input units (green) to the hidden units (gray) and finally to the output units (yellow). The reds and blues of the connections represent different weights.

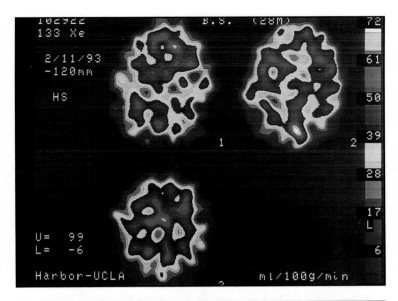

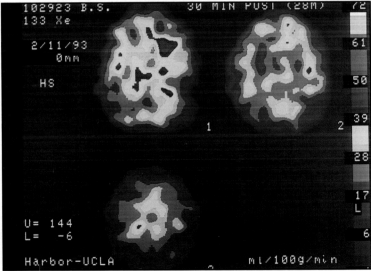

FIGURE 5. A typical pre- and post-exercise or pre- and post-treatment ^{133}Xenon Brain SPECT in a CFS patient, demonstrating frontotemporal hypoperfusion at baseline, and increased global hypoperfusion after the intervention. Hypoperfusion after exercise may be related to endothelin, and after treatment to norepinephrine and neuropeptide Y.

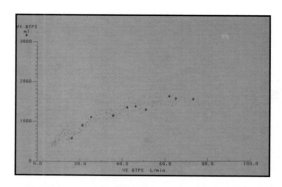

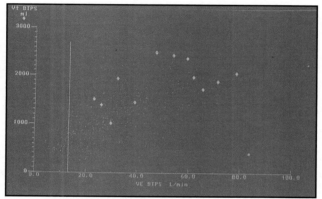

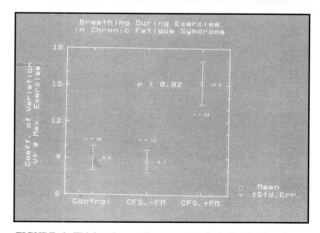

FIGURE 6. Tidal volume, the amount of air inspired and expired, should increase with exercise in a linear manner and then plateau when maximal tidal volume is attained. Automatic respiration, regulated by the prefrontal cortex and limbic system, is dysregulated in CFS, and demonstrates marked variability, especially in those CFS patients with concomitant FMS.

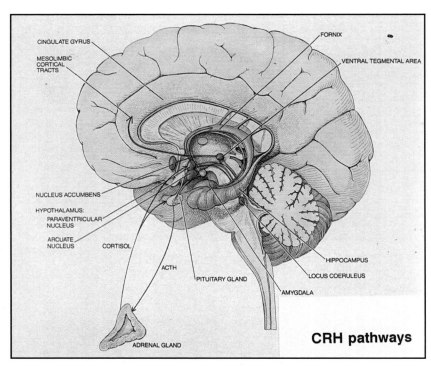

FIGURE 7. Corticotropin releasing hormone (CRH) regulates ACTH secretion and hence cortisol secretion. It also regulates the function of the prefrontal cortex and the locus ceruleus, where much of the norepinephrine in the brain is manufactured. CRH secretion is decreased in CFS/FMS.

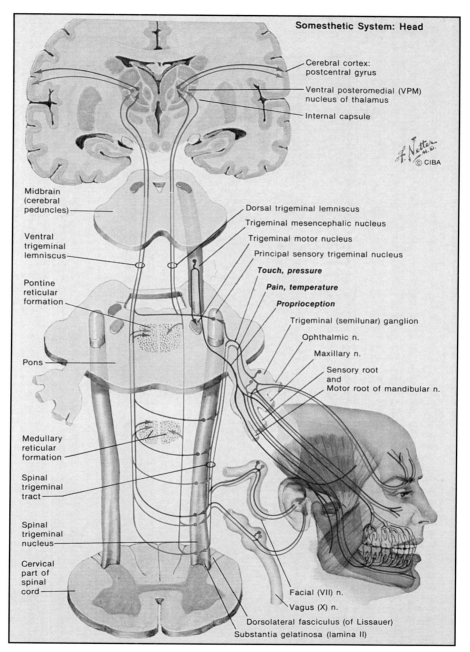

Somesthetic System: Head

Cerebral cortex: postcentral gyrus

Ventral posteromedial (VPM) nucleus of thalamus

Internal capsule

Midbrain (cerebral peduncles)

Ventral trigeminal lemniscus

Pontine reticular formation

Pons

Medullary reticular formation

Spinal trigeminal tract

Spinal trigeminal nucleus

Cervical part of spinal cord

Dorsal trigeminal lemniscus

Trigeminal mesencephalic nucleus

Trigeminal motor nucleus

Principal sensory trigeminal nucleus

Touch, pressure

Pain, temperature

Proprioception

Trigeminal (semilunar) ganglion

Ophthalmic n.

Maxillary n.

Sensory root and Motor root of mandibular n.

Facial (VII) n.

Vagus (X) n.

Dorsolateral fasciculus (of Lissauer)

Substantia gelatinosa (lamina II)

FIGURE 8. V$_1$ synapses in the reticular formation and in the thalamus. Both structures modulate how the brain interprets sensory information.

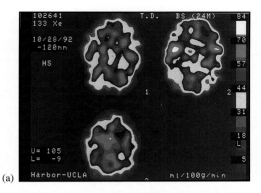

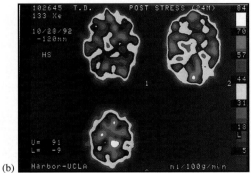

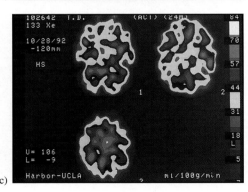

FIGURE 9. Some patients do not fatigue with exercise, but feel exhausted after intellectual exertion. This patient (a) could run marathons (b), but had to drop out of Cambridge after becoming ill because doing calculations made him feel much worse (c).

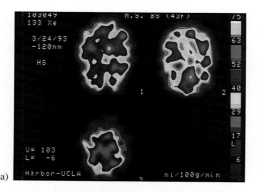

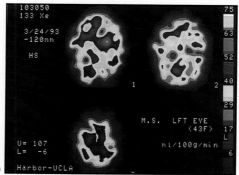

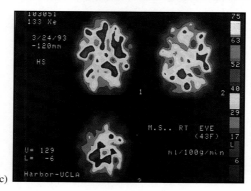

FIGURE 10. A CFS patient, scanned at baseline (a), felt moderately improved after naphazoline was instilled into one eye (b), and much better after both eyes were instilled (c). Note the progression of global hypoperfusion, which is not ipsilateral as it would be if the trigeminovascular system were being affected.

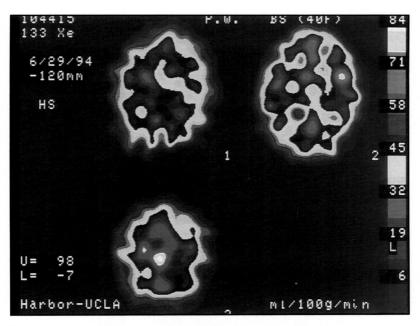

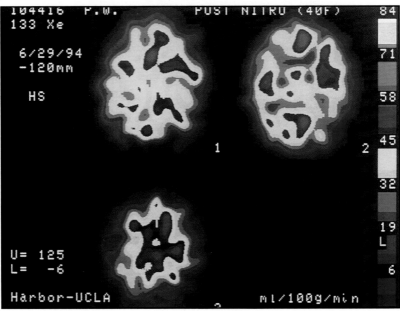

FIGURE 11. Nitroglycerin, a vasodilator by virtue of its metabolism into nitric oxide, produces global cerebral hypoperfusion when the CFS patient has symptomatic improvement.

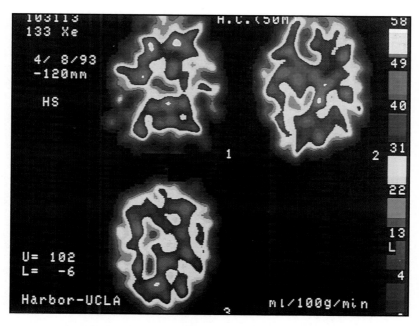

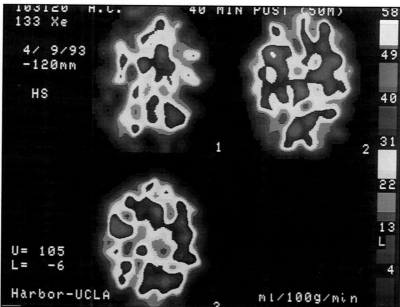

FIGURE 12. Nimodipine, a centrally-acting dihydropyridine calcium channel blocker used to treat vasospasm of subarachnoid hemorrhage, also produces global cerebral hypoperfusion when effective.

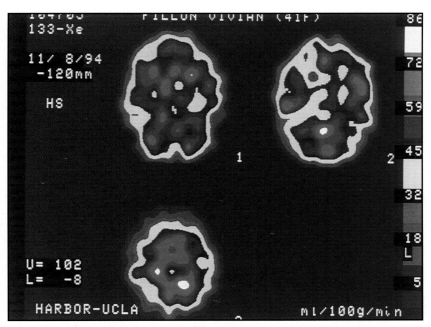

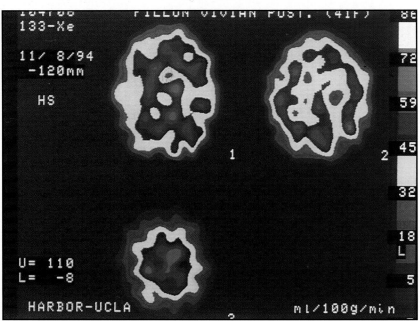

FIGURE 13. Acetazolamide (Diamox) is used as a cerebral vasodilator in nuclear medicine. When it improves CFS symptoms, it produces global hypoperfusion.

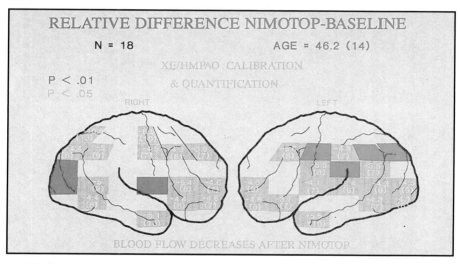

FIGURE 14. A statistical analysis of the decrease in cerebral blood flow in eighteen CFS responders to nimodipine.

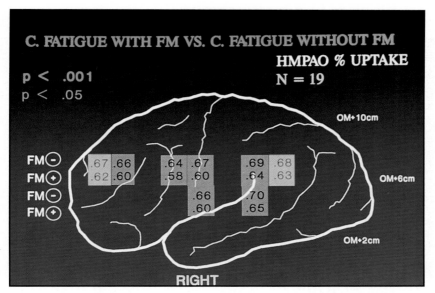

FIGURE 15. Chronic Fatigue Syndrome patients with and without fibromyalgia tender points have the same areas of regional hypoperfusion. The perfusion of patients with fibromyalgia is slightly more decreased.

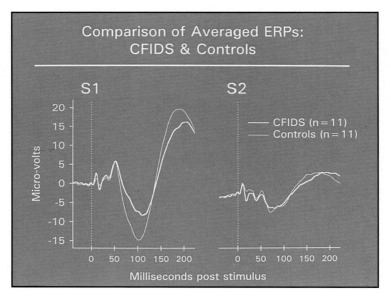

FIGURE 16. Patients with Chronic Fatigue Syndrome have a decreased amplitude of the N-100 wave on auditory evoked response testing. There are no abnormalities in prepulse inhibition, i.e., the amplitude of the second p50 wave decreases appropriately after the second auditory stimulus, 500 milliseconds after the first.

PATIENT / TESTS	KB	SB*	B	D	R
F REC	9	5	7	8	6
P ASSOC	11	8	3	3	8
REC	11	8	10	12	9
MET EST	7	6	10	12	10
MET RAT	.8	1.2	1.4	1.5	1.7
ERROR	3	0	9	3	1
PI ER	3	0	6	0	1
Y SLP (ERRORS)	126 (3,1,1)	159 (1,1,2)	60 (1,1,2)	605 (4,6,11)	72 (2,1,2)
Y INT	403	834	481	388	1044
N SLP (ERROR)	75 (2,1,0)	260 (2,0,0)	28 (2,0,0)	-945 (5,11,12)	242 (1,0,4)
N INT	606	963	684	3108	788
F REC	11	11	11	12	10
P ASSOC	12	9	7	9	10
REC	12	6	12	8	10
MET EST	8	6	10	11	8
MET RAT	.7	.5	.9	.9	.8
ERROR	2	0	0	0	0
PI ER	2	0	0	0	0
Y SLP (ERROR)	86 (1,1,0)	81 (1,2,0)	49 (2,1,2)	219 (2,2,8)	0 (1,1,0)
Y INT	462	586	425	699	759
N SLP (ERROR)	65 (2,0,0)	26 (1,0,0)	68 (1,0,0)	847 (7,5,10)	255 (1,0,2)
N INT	598	695	438	270	519

FIGURE 17. Many patients with CFS cognitive dysfunction can virtually normalize their performance on neuropsychological testing repeated one hour after treatment.

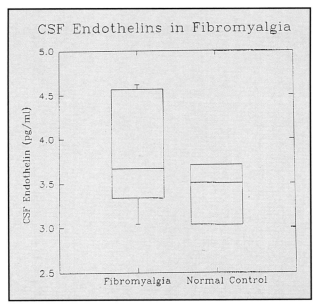

FIGURE 18. Endothelin levels in the cerebrospinal fluid of FMS patients are slightly elevated.

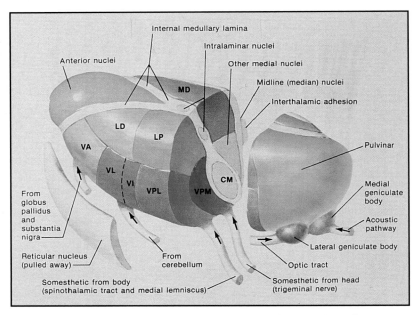

FIGURE 19. Anatomy of the thalamus and location of the reticular nucleus.

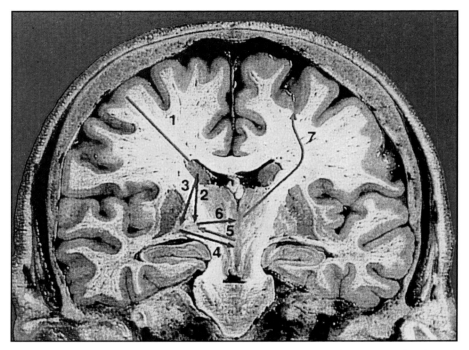

FIGURE 20. The cortico-striatal-thalamo-cortical neural network. A pallidotomy would be located between the arrowheads #2 and #3. Red arrows are excitatory, and blue arrows are inhibitory. Note that the only striatal-thalamo-cortical excitation comes from the subthalamic nucleus (arrow #5). Other excitation must occur by inhibitory neurons. Arrow #7 is shown returning to the contralateral cortex for the purposes of illustration only.

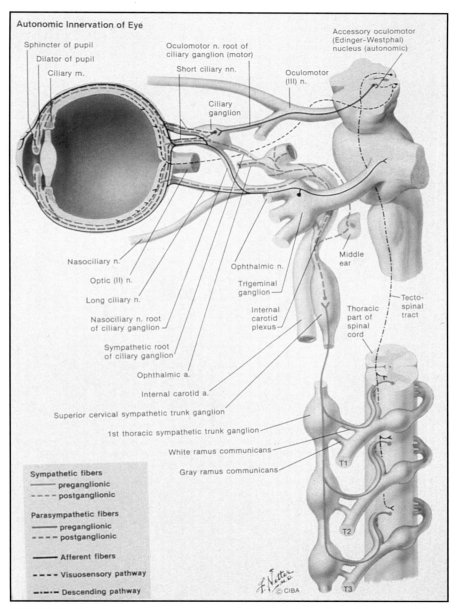

Autonomic Innervation of Eye

Sphincter of pupil

Dilator of pupil

Ciliary m.

Oculomotor n. root of
ciliary ganglion (motor)

Short ciliary nn.

Ciliary
ganglion

Accessory oculomotor
(Edinger-Westphal)
nucleus (autonomic)

Oculomotor
(III) n.

Nasociliary n.

Optic (II) n.

Long ciliary n.

Nasociliary n. root
of ciliary ganglion

Sympathetic root
of ciliary ganglion

Ophthalmic a.

Internal carotid a.

Superior cervical sympathetic trunk ganglion

1st thoracic sympathetic trunk ganglion

White ramus communicans

Gray ramus communicans

Ophthalmic n.

Trigeminal
ganglion

Internal
carotid
plexus

Middle
ear

Thoracic
part of
spinal
cord

Tecto-
spinal
tract

T1

T2

T3

Sympathetic fibers

——— preganglionic

- - - - postganglionic

Parasympathetic fibers

——— preganglionic

- - - - postganglionic

——— Afferent fibers

- - - - Visuosensory pathway

-··-··- Descending pathway

FIGURE 21. There is noradrenergic receptor upregulation on the surface of the eye resulting in hypersensitivity to topical alpha agonists.

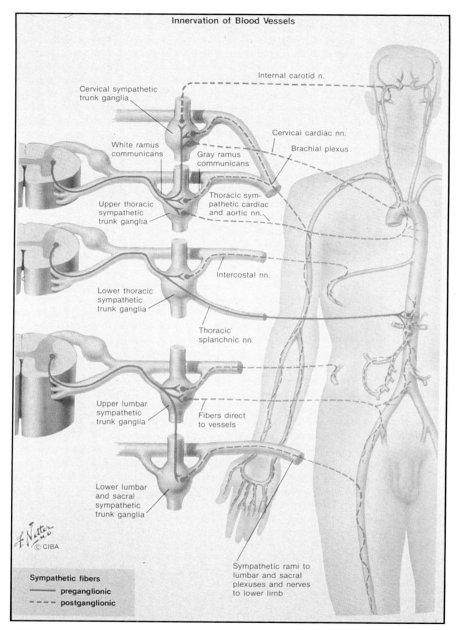

Innervation of Blood Vessels

Internal carotid n.

Cervical sympathetic trunk ganglia

Cervical cardiac nn.

White ramus communicans

Brachial plexus

Gray ramus communicans

Upper thoracic sympathetic trunk ganglia

Thoracic sympathetic cardiac and aortic nn.

Intercostal nn.

Lower thoracic sympathetic trunk ganglia

Thoracic splanchnic nn.

Upper lumbar sympathetic trunk ganglia

Fibers direct to vessels

Lower lumbar and sacral sympathetic trunk ganglia

Sympathetic rami to lumbar and sacral plexuses and nerves to lower limb

© CIBA

Sympathetic fibers
— preganglionic
- - - postganglionic

FIGURE 22. Dysautonomia in neurosomatic disorders is manifested by low blood pressure, Raynaud's phenomenon, rapid heart rate, thermoregulatory dysfunction, and livedo reticularis. The autonomic ganglia are dysregulated from supraspinal centers.

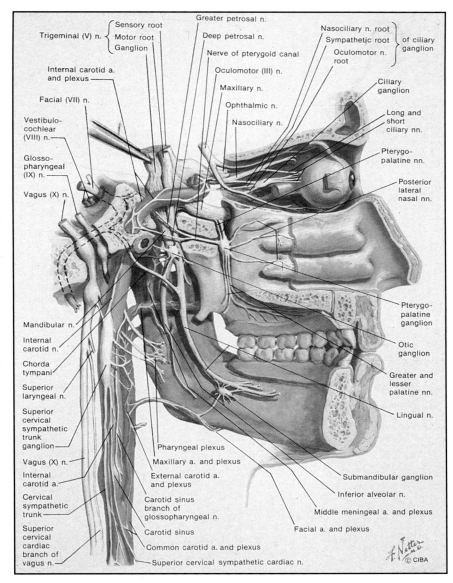

Trigeminal (V) n. { Sensory root, Motor root, Ganglion

Internal carotid a. and plexus

Facial (VII) n.

Vestibulo-cochlear (VIII) n.

Glosso-pharyngeal (IX) n.

Vagus (X) n.

Greater petrosal n.

Deep petrosal n.

Nerve of pterygoid canal

Oculomotor (III) n.

Maxillary n.

Ophthalmic n.

Nasociliary n.

Nasociliary n. root, Sympathetic root, Oculomotor n. root } of ciliary ganglion

Ciliary ganglion

Long and short ciliary nn.

Pterygo-palatine nn.

Posterior lateral nasal nn.

Pterygo-palatine ganglion

Otic ganglion

Greater and lesser palatine nn.

Lingual n.

Mandibular n.

Internal carotid n.

Chorda tympani

Superior laryngeal n.

Superior cervical sympathetic trunk ganglion

Vagus (X) n.

Internal carotid a.

Cervical sympathetic trunk

Superior cervical cardiac branch of vagus n.

Pharyngeal plexus

Maxillary a. and plexus

External carotid a. and plexus

Carotid sinus branch of glossopharyngeal n.

Carotid sinus

Common carotid a. and plexus

Superior cervical sympathetic cardiac n.

Submandibular ganglion

Inferior alveolar n.

Middle meningeal a. and plexus

Facial a. and plexus

FIGURE 23. Relationships of autonomic nerves and ganglia in the head and neck. Note the location of the superior cervical sympathetic trunk ganglion (superior cervical ganglion), which innervates the middle cerebral artery and its branches.

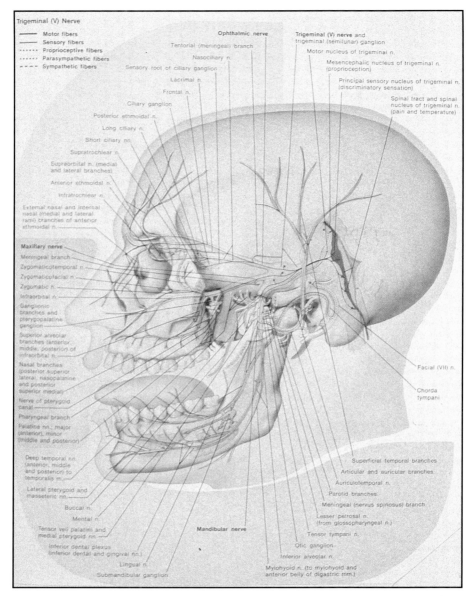

Trigeminal (V) Nerve

Motor fibers
Sensory fibers
Proprioceptive fibers
Parasympathetic fibers
Sympathetic fibers

Ophthalmic nerve

Tentorial (meningeal) branch

Nasociliary n.

Sensory root of ciliary ganglion

Lacrimal n.

Frontal n.

Ciliary ganglion

Posterior ethmoidal n.

Long ciliary n.

Short ciliary nn.

Supratrochlear n.

Supraorbital n. (medial and lateral branches)

Anterior ethmoidal n.

Infratrochlear n.

External nasal and internal nasal (medial and lateral rami) branches of anterior ethmoidal n.

Maxillary nerve

Meningeal branch

Zygomaticotemporal n.

Zygomaticofacial n.

Zygomatic n.

Infraorbital n.

Ganglionic branches and pterygopalatine ganglion

Superior alveolar branches (anterior, middle, posterior of infraorbital n.)

Nasal branches (posterior superior lateral, nasopalatine and posterior superior medial)

Nerve of pterygoid canal

Pharyngeal branch

Palatine nn.: major (anterior), minor (middle and posterior)

Deep temporal nn. (anterior, middle and posterior to temporalis m.)

Lateral pterygoid and masseteric nn.

Buccal n.

Mental n.

Tensor veli palatini and medial pterygoid nn.

Inferior dental plexus (inferior dental and gingival nn.)

Lingual n.

Submandibular ganglion

Trigeminal (V) nerve and trigeminal (semilunar) ganglion

Motor nucleus of trigeminal n.

Mesencephalic nucleus of trigeminal n. (proprioception)

Principal sensory nucleus of trigeminal n. (discriminatory sensation)

Spinal tract and spinal nucleus of trigeminal n. (pain and temperature)

Facial (VII) n.

Chorda tympani

Mandibular nerve

Superficial temporal branches

Articular and auricular branches

Auriculotemporal n.

Parotid branches

Meningeal (nervus spinosus) branch

Lesser petrosal n. (from glossopharyngeal n.)

Tensor tympani n.

Otic ganglion

Inferior alveolar n.

Mylohyoid n. (to mylohyoid and anterior belly of digastric mm.)

FIGURE 24. The first division of the trigeminal nerve (V_2) (from the eye) regulates the mesen-cephalic tract of the trigeminal nerve (in blue) in the brainstem.

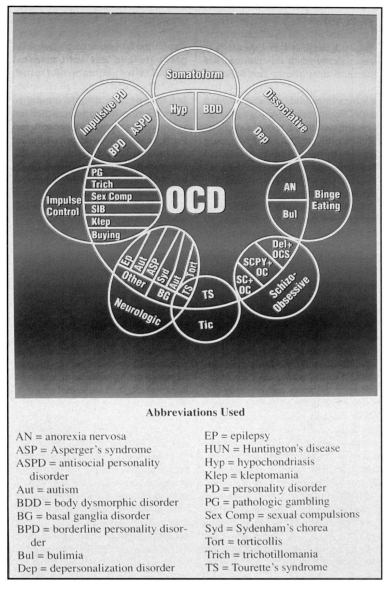

Abbreviations Used

AN = anorexia nervosa
ASP = Asperger's syndrome
ASPD = antisocial personality
   disorder
Aut = autism
BDD = body dysmorphic disorder
BG = basal ganglia disorder
BPD = borderline personality disor-
   der
Bul = bulimia
Dep = depersonalization disorder

EP = epilepsy
HUN = Huntington's disease
Hyp = hypochondriasis
Klep = kleptomania
PD = personality disorder
PG = pathologic gambling
Sex Comp = sexual compulsions
Syd = Sydenham's chorea
Tort = torticollis
Trich = trichotillomania
TS = Tourette's syndrome

FIGURE 25. Obsessive-compulsive spectrum disorders are infrequently encountered in the CFS patient. The functional neuroanatomy of CFS is in some respects the opposite of OCD.

FIGURE 26. Desensitization (through receptor-G protein uncoupling) mediated by receptor-specific kinases (e.g., ßARK) is enhanced by an additional protein, ß-arrestin. These regulatory components have been described for other members of the G protein-coupled receptor superfamily (e.g., rhodopsin, M_2 muscarinic acetylcholine receptors and $ß_2$-adrenoreceptors).

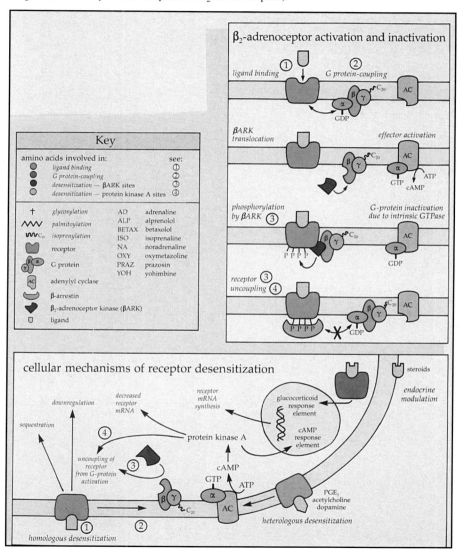

FIGURE 27. Desensitization also occurs via phosphorylation by protein kinase A and serves as a means of negative feedback, which is also responsible for the clinically important phenomenon of tachyphylaxis.

EXERCISE NEUROENDOCRINE FINDINGS IN CHRONIC FATIGUE SYNDROME		
	NORMAL	CFS
Cortisol	↑	→
Growth Hormone	↑	→ or ↓
Somatostatin	↑	→
Beta Endorphin	↑	→
IL-1	↑	variable
IL-1ra	↑	↑
IL-6	↑	→
Catecholamines	↑	→
Temperature	↑	→ or ↓
Regional Cerebral Blood Flow	↑	↓

FIGURE 28. Exercise should increase levels of IL-1 beta, CRH, and norepinephrine. If this increase does not occur appropriately, and if elevated baseline concentrations of central substance P are augmented, post-exercise exacerbation of sensory input dysfunction and neuroendocrine dysregulation may occur.

Treatments

Surely every medicine is an innovation, and he that would not apply new remedies, has to expect new evils.

—Francis Bacon

It should be apparent by now that patients with chronic fatigue syndrome (CFS) and other neurosomatic disorders (e.g., fibromyalgia, irritable bowel syndrome, premenstrual syndrome) do not all respond to any one treatment. Many of these individuals could be described as "treatment resistant," since they may not have been helped by the usual medical interventions such as antidepressants, anxiolytics, and analgesics. Since there is much evidence that the mechanism for symptom production in CFS is an interplay between a genetic predisposition and the effect of multiple environmental triggers, it is not surprising that there should be a heterogeneity in treatment response.

Several medications have been released recently that can improve the symptoms of certain CFS patients, and long-existing medications may be adapted for new uses. Since it is still not possible for me to tell which individual will respond to what medication, I have been prescribing treatment trials of the following medications about 45 minutes apart. All of these drugs are fairly safe, and almost all of them work rapidly, so that one trial should be sufficient if I am seeing the patient on a symptomatic day. With such a profusion of potential treatments, most patients can significantly improve.

ACETAZOLAMIDE (DIAMOX)

Patients with neurosomatic disorders will occasionally have a reduction in symptomatology with acetazolamide. This drug, a carbonic anhydrase (CA) inhibitor, is primarily used to lower intraocular pressure in glaucoma and to treat high altitude sickness. It has recently been recommended as a possible treatment for bipolar disorders (Hayes, 1993).

Inhibitors of CA alter respiratory responses as well as inhibiting neural responses to CO_2 (carbon dioxide), causing intracellular acidification. Acetazolamide is routinely used as a cerebral vasodilator in nuclear medicine. The acetazolamide (Diamox) challenge paradigm characterizes the vascular reserve of brain tissue in patients with decreased regional cerebral blood flow (rCBF), i.e., whether a patient can increase his or her rCBF if necessary. Patients with poor vascular reserve respond with little or no increase in flow after acetazolamide. In contrast, those with deafferentation show normal or augmented responses compared to controls. Cocaine abusers, for example, have a robust response in rCBF to acetazolamide (Bell et al., 1994), markedly increasing cerebral perfusion after it is administered.

The most common adverse reaction to acetazolamide is paresthesias. Tingling of the tongue when drinking carbonated beverages is due to CO_2 in the drink, which acidifies the lingual nerve by conversion to carbonic acid (H_2CO_3).

Acetazolamide inhibits responses of the lingual nerve (a branch of the trigeminal nerve) to CO_2 (Komai and Bryant, 1993). The inhibition of the lingual nerve by acetazolamide is specific to CO_2, and affects no other mediators. CA is located in many neurons and glia and may participate in a process of rapid acidification (Neubauer, 1991). This acidification is responsible for cerebral vasodilation when acetazolamide is administered. Decreased pH also may cause cutaneous nociception, which can be inhibited by acetazolamide (Steen et al., 1992).

Neurons that are excited by CO_2 are common in the nervous system; most are suppressed by increased levels of CO_2 (Carpenter et al., 1972). CA, in proximity to pH-sensitive neural structures in conjunction with proton-sensitive K channels, could produce CO_2-induced membrane depolarization and generation of action potentials (Komai and Bryant, 1993), much like other medications effective in neurosomatic disorders. These action potentials produce the paresthesias associated with acetazolamide.

Case Report

A 41-year-old married Caucasian female graphic artist was well until 1988, when she was in a motor vehicle accident and developed post-traumatic fibromyalgia, which had persisted for six years when I first saw her. She could be active only until noon and had to rest for the remainder of the day. Multiple specialist consultations and many medication trials had been to no avail. Her symptoms included diffuse pain, fatigue, cognitive dysfunction, exercise intolerance, sleep disorder, blurred vision, paresthesias, dysequilibrium, weakness, dysarthria, photophobia, decreased libido, nonrestorative sleep, irritable bowel syndrome, night sweats, PMS, chest pain, cold hands and feet, and heat and cold intolerance. Interestingly, her husband also had posttraumatic fibromyalgia from a different motor vehicle accident.

She had a marked improvement (60 to 80 percent per patient report) with naphazoline eyedrops. Her pain and tenderness decreased and her range of motion increased. After taking nimodipine and hydralazine, she was able to walk up and down the stairs in my office building several times. Unfortunately, she developed adverse reactions (headaches) to nimodipine and hydralazine and they were discontinued. Naphazoline was still effective, but tolerance was developing. Acetazolamide 250 mg eliminated her pain, helped her to feel very relaxed, and markedly reduced her other symptoms. On pre- and post-treatment brain SPECT there was marked diminution of global CBF with acetazolamide, which she continues to take with good results. Occasional recrudescence of pain is managed nicely p.r.n. (as needed) by baclofen, a $GABA_B$ agonist.

ASCORBIC ACID

Recent research into the role of ascorbic acid in the brain (which has the highest concentrations of this substance in the entire body) has shown that this agent may be beneficial in certain patients with CFS. Some studies indicate that in order to obtain a dose that will produce adequate results, ascorbic acid must be administered intravenously. Trials of high-dose oral ascorbic acid have been generally disappointing. Despite the marked success in treating CFS with oral agents, there are still 5 to 10 percent of patients who do not respond to them. Ascorbic acid may benefit these individuals by modulating the effects of two important neurotransmitters, glutamate and dopamine.

Originally, I hypothesized that IV ascorbic acid was working in CFS as a free radical scavenger in the brain, which has regional hypoperfusion, perhaps to the point of ischemia, and in the immune system, which was activated in many CFS patients. Cerebral antioxidants include water- and fat-soluble molecules as well as enzyme systems that quench "free radicals," which can be destructive to tissues in the brain and elsewhere. The two principal water-soluble antioxidants are ascorbate (ascorbic acid) and glutathione (GSH). Both can scavenge free radicals and prevent the oxidation of lipid-soluble Vitamin E (alpha-tocopherol), which in turn protects cell membranes from lipid peroxidation (Rice, Perez-Pinon, and Lee, 1994). Thus ascorbate has been found to be neuroprotective, particularly by inhibiting a redox site on the NMDA receptor and diminishing calcium influx. Ascorbate, therefore, may be considered to be an NMDA antagonist. NMDA antagonists are being investigated as treatments for depression, since a common mode of action of antidepressants in use today appears to be desensitization of the NMDA receptor (Nowak et al., 1993; Papp and Moryl, 1994). Furthermore, ascorbic acid with EDTA (ethylenediaminetetraacetic acid) had been shown to be an effective treatment for depression (as effective as amitriptylene) in a double-blind experiment published in 1984 (Kay et al., 1984). Depression, commonly experienced by CFS patients, is primarily a disorder of limbic function. The limbic system is a neural network in the brain that regulates mood, memory, anxiety, eating, temperature, activity, and numerous other functions (Goldstein, 1993).

Adding magnesium sulfate is recommended because ascorbic acid can cause magnesium shifts from extracellular to intracellular compartments. Responders to IV ascorbic acid generally feel considerably better in most respects the day after treatment. Administration of ascorbic acid is done in doses of 25 to 50 grams diluted in half-normal saline or Ringer's lactate over a period of about 90 minutes. It is beneficial to add 500 mg of calcium gluconate since ascorbic acid is a calcium chelator and could possibly lower serum calcium. Adverse effects are uncommon. They are usually mild and consist of some dysphoria for a day or so. If the ascorbic acid solution is not administered directly into the vein, it can cause local tissue irritation. Concentrated ascorbic acid can inflame the vein into which it is infused; diluting it obviates this problem. Since ascorbic acid is not tolerated well in patients with an unusual disorder called glucose-6-phosphate dehydrogenase deficiency, measuring the levels of this enzyme with a blood test before initiating intravenous therapy is recommended.

The brain is known to have high levels of ascorbate that protect it from oxidative stress (Rose, 1993). There may be a deficiency in regional glutamatergic neurotransmission in CFS (Goldstein, 1993), and ascorbate is often colocalized with glutamate in cortico-neostriatal neurons. Glutamate antagonists decrease brain ascorbate (Pierce and Rebec, 1993), an action that has been known since at least 1979 (Tolbert et al., 1979) to have behavioral effects. Ascorbate is thought to modulate dopamine-induced behavioral activation, and also modulates nondopaminergic (glutamatergic) behavioral activation.

Amphetamine and other dopaminergic agonists release ascorbate by indirectly activating glutamatergic cortico-neostriatal neurons via a multisynaptic pathway that includes the substantia nigra reticulata and ventromedial thalamus (Rebec, 1994). Neostriatal glutamate release is potentiated by increases in extracellular ascorbate levels, which also modulate the behavioral effects of amphetamine and behavioral response to haloperidol, an antipsychotic drug and dopaminergic antagonist. Increases in extracellular ascorbate have been shown to have neuroleptic effects (Pierce et al., 1994; deAngelis, 1995). Large doses must be used to potentiate haloperidol in phencyclidine psychosis (Giannini et al., 1987) and acute schizophrenia (Beauclair et al., 1987). Haloperidol, amphetamine, and ascorbate itself at least double neostriatal ascorbate concentrations. It has been hypothesized that, rather than being an NMDA antagonist, ascorbate enhances glutamatergic neurotransmission (Pierce et al., 1994).

Systemic administration of ethanol induces the release of brain extracellular ascorbate. CPP, a competitive NMDA antagonist, completely reverses the ethanol-evoked ascorbate release (Wu, 1993). Ethanol exposure, acute and chronic, enhances brain glutamate release (McBride et al., 1986), and glutamate stimulates the release of ascorbate from synaptosomes (Grunewald and Fillenz, 1984). Therefore, glutamate and ascorbate transport to intracellular compartments may be coupled (Wu, 1994; Mielle, Boutelle, and Fillenz, 1994). There is data that ascorbic acid may reduce the toxic effects of alcohol, and it is well established that chronic alcoholics have low plasma and white cell ascorbic acid levels. "It is common practice to administer ascorbic acid intravenously to such patients during conventional detoxification therapy" (Wickramsinghe and Hasan, 1994).

Peptide amidation is an ascorbate-requiring process that synthesizes active hormones from inactive precursors. Peptidylglycine alpha-hydroxylating monooxygenase is a rate-limiting enzyme involved in peptide amidation that requires ascorbate (Mains, 1993). Several neuropeptides may be hyposecreted in patients with CFS and related disorders (Demitrack et al., 1991; Goldstein, 1992).

Ascorbate is an essential cofactor as a source of electrons for the action of dopamine-beta-hydroxylase, the enzyme that metabolizes dopamine to norepinephrine. Abnormalities in biogenic amines are a standard concept in the etiology of psychophysiologic disorders.

Some studies have found that ascorbate can inhibit binding of D_1 and D_2 agonists (Tolbert et al., 1992; Rebec, 1994), and can act as a dopamine neuromodulator. It may work in such a fashion to inhibit opioid withdrawal (Johnson and Chahl, 1992). It is required for release of acetylcholine and norepinephrine from synaptic vesicles (Hata et al., 1976; Kuo et al., 1979). Ascorbate can alter membrane fluidity and thereby decrease reuptake of dopamine and serotonin, as some antidepressants do (Ramassamy et al., 1993). Hyperbaric oxygen therapy increases release of brain ascorbate (Narkowicz, Vial, and McCartney, 1993). We have planned a study of hyperbaric oxygen therapy for CFS (Wallace et al., 1995).

Ascorbate enhances survival of cultured brain neurons (Saito, Saito, and Katsuki, 1993), and has an immunomodulatory effect in HTLV-1 associated myelopathy (Kataoka et al., 1993). Furthermore, ascorbic acid enhances natural killer cell function (Vojdani and Ghoneum, 1993), often quite low in CFS, both in normal subjects and in CFS patients (Vojdani and Goldstein, 1992).

From my patients' observations, the effect of ascorbate is usually fairly rapid in onset, suggesting an effect on neurotransmitter modulation. I presented a compilation of data at conferences in 1989 and 1990 that IV ascorbate is a successful treatment.

Intravenous ascorbic acid is a controversial therapy and is considered to be quackery by many physicians. Recent research, however, indicates its efficacy. Based on this research, it would be in the best interest of patients who have not responded well to other agents to be offered this treatment.

BACLOFEN

One of the most effective treatments for neurosomatic disorders is baclofen, an oral $GABA_B$ agonist. Activation of the $GABA_B$ receptor diminishes evoked release of neurotransmitter peripherally and decreases central release of amines, excitatory amino acids (EAAs), neuropeptides, hormones, and GABA itself (via autoreceptors) (Bowery, 1990). Postsynaptic $GABA_B$ receptors also have a physiologic role in the mediation of the inhibitory post-synaptic potentials (IPSPs) produced in the hippocampus after stimulation of the striatum radiatum (Dutar and Nicoll, 1988). $GABA_B$ receptors function in a similar manner in the thalamus (Soltesz et al., 1988). There may be subtypes of the $GABA_B$ receptor, but they have not been well characterized (Ong et al., 1994). $GABA_B$ antagonists, such as phaclofen, are not available for clinical use, but have potential therapeutic applications in enhancing cognitive function, in treating absence epilepsy, and as antidepressants (Bittiger et al., 1993).

Numerous centrally mediated actions have been attributed to $GABA_B$ receptors. Those relevant to neurosomatic disorders include supraspinal analgesia (Giuliani et al., 1988; Smith et al., 1994), stimulation of brown fat thermogenesis (Horton et al., 1988), inhibition of the release of corticotropin-releasing hormone (Calogero et al., 1988), suppression of panic attacks (Breslow et al., 1989), and hyperpolarization of sympathetic ganglia (Newberry and Gilbert, 1989). Activation of $GABA_B$ receptors in the CNS of anesthetized rats stimulates the sympathetic nervous system but not the adrenal medullary response (Nonogaki et al., 1994).

Baclofen is also an anticonvulsant, decreasing amygdala kindling (Wurpel, 1994). It inhibits bronchial hyperresponsiveness and may be useful in asthma (Dicpinigaitis et al., 1994), is a respiratory depressant that decreases hyperventilation (Hey et al., 1995), and is a myorelaxant in rats when injected into the medial nucleus accumbens (Lorenc-Koci et al., 1994). Injection of baclofen into the ventral tegmental area (VTA), the cell body site of the mesolimbic dopamine system, causes a decrease in the dopamine metabolite, DOPAC, in the nucleus accumbens, thought to be due to stimulation of the VTA dopamine autoreceptor (Yoshida et al., 1994). Baclofen inhibits voltage-gated calcium currents in the rat hippocampus (Toselli and Taglietti, 1993) and hyperpolarizes VTA neurons stimulated by glutamate by increasing potassium conductance (Seutin, Johnson, and North, 1994).

Baclofen stimulates growth hormone release, thereby increasing insulin-like growth factor-1 (Bauman et al., 1994). It may improve idiopathic dystonia as well as secondary dystonias (Greene, 1992) by inhibiting dopamine release. Baclofen suppresses afferent fiber transmission in the piriform (olfactory) cortex (Tang and Hasselmo, 1994), and thus may reduce cacosmia and multiple chemical sensitivity (Goldstein, 1993). GABA$_B$ receptors are present pre- and post-synaptically in many brain regions, including the frontal cortex, striatal afferents, and the dendrites (only) of hippocampal pyramidal cells (Bowery, 1990).

In neurosomatic patients, baclofen has its most success in treating central pain. This central pain may manifest itself as fibromyalgia, headache, low back pain, or other regional pain syndromes. It is often quite useful as an anxiolytic, and sometimes increases alertness, perhaps by increasing limbic DOPAC. Tolerance to this latter effect, however, is quick to develop. The drug is usually given in doses of 10 to 20 mg TID (higher doses rarely confer additional benefit) and is well tolerated, the main adverse reaction being sedation. Its onset of action is about 30 minutes. Baclofen occasionally makes patients feel worse, perhaps by reducing CRH secretion or by inhibiting hippocampal function. Impairment of memory, reported in rats receiving baclofen, has not occurred in my patients. Baclofen has not been reported to be an effective antidepressant (Breslow et al., 1989), yet an occasional patient of mine with treatment-resistant depression has had some relief with the medication. Therapy with GABA$_B$ agonists and antagonists has been reviewed recently (Malcongio and Bowery, 1995).

Case Report

Four years prior to consulting me a 48-year-old married Caucasian male construction worker injured his lower back while working. An attempt to return to work the next year was unsuccessful due to exacerbation of his low back pain. He had a right nephrectomy that same year for renal cell carcinoma and subsequently developed symptoms of CFS. His physician diagnosed him as being anxious and depressed, but he did not respond to anxiolytics or antidepressants. The etiology of his back pain was uncertain. An MRI scan was nondiagnostic, and epidural steroid injections were unsuccessful. He complained of chronic right testicular pain as well as the usual CFS symptoms. He walked with a cane. Like many CFS patients, multiple medications were required to treat him. Gabapentin helped him to feel more relaxed, mexilitene eliminated his testalgia, and baclofen greatly reduced his diffuse pain as well as his low back pain, which was then completely relieved with lidocaine trigger point injections into the lumbosacral triangles. Stretching exercises were demonstrated to him, and he left the office stating he was feeling fairly normal for the first time in years. He did well for three months and then was lost to follow-up.

Case Report

A 58-year-old married Caucasian male sales executive had been well except for mild chronic pericarditis treated with low-dose prednisone until he developed sepsis eight months prior to seeing me. After discharge from the hospital he developed severe fatigue, cognitive dysfunction, and diffuse pain. He had chronic lower back pain, which was his most disabling symptom. He had some improvement with sertraline and gabapentin, but after a month of treatment he still did not feel well enough to return to work. He was quite anxious and had panic attacks despite his medication regimen. Thirty minutes after taking baclofen 10 mg he reported that his back pain and anxiety were completely gone, and that he felt much more alert and more energetic. This improvement has persisted for several months.

CANNABINOIDS

Many of my CFS patients over the years have spontaneously reported to me that they have symptomatic improvement when they smoke marijuana. What might be the neuropharmacology of this effect?

The main psychoactive ingredient in marijuana is delta-9 tetrahydrocannabinol (THC), which has been reported to have numerous neuroendocrine effects (Dewey, 1986). Prolactin levels are decreased in animals by THC administration, which increases both serotonergic and dopaminergic neurotransmission (Fernandez-Ruiz et al., 1992). Growth hormone levels are decreased and ACTH and corticosterone levels are increased by administering THC to rats (Dalterio et al., 1981; Puder et al., 1982). The dopaminergic prolactin inhibitory effect is found in females to the greatest extent when THC is administered on the morning of estrus, while males exhibit it continually (Bonnin et al., 1993). This effect appears to be estrogen-related and possibly occurs as a result of THC-induced down-regulation of anterior pituitary dopamine D_2 receptors. Thus THC interacts with gonadal steroids, perhaps as an estrogen receptor antagonist (Murphy et al., 1991). Tamoxifen, an antiestrogen, attenuates the effects of THC on D_2 receptors (Bonnin et al., 1993). It is also possible that endogenous cannabinoid binding sites (Howlett et al., 1990) may fluctuate during the estrus cycle. These binding sites are highly concentrated in the hypothalamus. An endogenous cannabimimetic compound, anandamide, has been identified in the brain (Devane et al., 1992). It inhibits cAMP production, and is a partial agonist at N-type calcium channels in N18 neuroblastoma cells. In calf brain, anandamide synthase levels are highest in the hippocampus, followed by cortex > thalamus, striatum, pons > cerebellum > medulla (Devane and Axelrod, 1994). THC receptors are also quite dense in the amygdala and the paraventricular nucleus of the hypothalamus in the rat (Herkenham et al., 1991).

THC and anandamide given i.c.v. also elevate ACTH and corticosterone levels, via mediation of a central mechanism that increases the secretion of CRH (Weidenfeld, Feldman, and Mechoulan, 1994). Central vasopressin levels in CFS are either normal (Crofford et al., 1994) or low (Bakheit et al., 1993), and central oxytocin levels are low (Russell, personal communication, 1995). Both neuropeptides are secretagogues for CRH and ACTH, but desamino–D–arginine vasopressin (in the form of DDAVP) is ineffective in the treatment of CFS (Goldstein, 1993). Cannabinoid receptor agonists may be helpful neurosomatic therapeutic agents on the basis of their dopaminergic and serotonergic agonist properties, as well as by enhancing CRH secretion.

A nonpsychoactive cannabinoid, HU-211, is an antagonist at the NMDA receptor, where it also blocks calcium uptake. The NMDA receptor when occupied conducts monovalent cations and calcium ions. This conductance is markedly enhanced in an allosteric manner by glycine, which binds to its own site on the receptor and increases the frequency of channel opening (Nadler, Mechoulan, and Sokolovsky, 1993). HU-211 acts at a site distinct from glutamate, glycine, or noncompetitive NMDA antagonists such as MK-801. MK-801 stimulates CRH secretion in the parvocellular paraventricular nucleus of the rat hypothalamus (Lee, Rivier, and Torres, 1994). Thus, cannabinoids are also NMDA antagonists, a property that may benefit a subset of neurosomatic patients, particularly those who do not respond to high-dose (up to 30 grams per day) oral glycine, or low-dose (5 to 50 mg per day) cycloserine, NMDA agonists.

THC has been well studied in humans and its pharmacological effects are reviewed in standard textbooks (Jaffe, 1990). Properties of interest in the THC treatment of neurosomatic disorders are an increase in heart rate, increased supine blood pressure, and reddening of the conjunctivae. These effects can be blocked by propanolol and clonidine, which have no effect on the psychoactive responses of THC. Perhaps the increase in CRH stimulates noradrenergic neurotransmission. In high chronic doses, THC may have adverse effects on the endocrine system, may alter behavior and cognition, may cause dysphoria and depersonalization, and may exacerbate schizophrenia. There may be a mild withdrawal syndrome when volunteers take high doses of THC every few hours for several weeks. Cannabinoids may be useful as analgesics or anticonvulsants (Beal et al., 1995), and delta-9-THC (dronabinol) is approved for use for appetite stimulation in the treatment of AIDS-related anorexia, and as an antiemetic for chemotherapy-induced emesis. Per the PDR, suggested doses are 2.5 mg BID one hour before lunch and supper. Taking THC in the morning results in a higher incidence of adverse reactions. Side effects at this dosage were primarily confined to feeling high, dizziness, confusion, and somnolence, occurred in 18 percent of studied patients (*Physician's Desk Reference*, 1994, p. 2020-2022), and often responded to reduction of dosage to 2.5 mg per day.

There are numerous precautions to be considered when prescribing THC, particularly in patients with a history of depression, substance abuse, mania, schizophrenia, or heart disease. A nonpsychoactive cannabinoid (there are 60 cannabinoids in marijuana) would be advantageous. The use of dronabinol in neurosomatic disorders should be restricted to rare, severe, treatment-resistant disabling conditions. It has not been studied in the pediatric or geriatric population. Another cannabinoid, cannabidiol, has been reported to have an atypical antipsychotic effect (Zuardi et al., 1995).

ERGOLOID MESYLATES (HYDERGINE)

Hydergine is approved for use in Alzheimer's disease by the Food and Drug Administration, but evidence is lacking that the medication is effective for this indication. The drug does, however, alter dopaminergic and cholinergic transmission in a manner that is sometimes beneficial in those patients with neurosomatic disorders, as well as Parkinson's disease.

Hydergine, thought to modulate dopamine neurotransmission, was compared to selective D_1 and D_2 agonists in its effect on acetylcholine release in the hippocampus and the striatum. Hydergine increased hippocampal cholinergic, and decreased striatal cholinergic transmission, mimicking the effect of the D_2 agonist LY 171555 (Imperato and Gessa, 1994). Thus Hydergine has a profile of a selective D_2 agonist, and can augment hippocampal cholinergic function while decreasing striatal cholinergic function, perhaps increasing energy and memory, while decreasing parkinsonian symptomatology.

Cocaine and amphetamine also increase hippocampal acetylcholine secretion, as well as ACh release in the caudate nucleus. Hippocampal ACh increase is produced by a D_2, and enhanced by a D_1, agonist, similar to maximally effective doses of cocaine, morphine, and D-amphetamine. The D_2 agonist increases caudate ACh secretion, but the D_1 agonist decreases it. Thus dopamine, acting at both D_1 and D_2 receptors, may enhance encoding (the making of new memories) in the hippocampus, and a D_2 agonist could enhance caudate cholinergic function (Imperato, 1994).

Unfortunately, dopamine agonists have been of little value in treating neurosomatic disorders. A minority of neurosomatic patients do have a favorable response to psychostimulants, which release both DA and NE. It has not been possible for me thus far to predict which patient will respond to what medication. Methamphetamine (which I rarely prescribe) is the most lipophilic (Mitler, Hadjukovic, and Erman, 1993), and works the best. Thereafter the order of efficacy is dextroamphetamine > methylphenidate > pemoline.

Hydergine is sometimes effective in neurosomatic disorders in a dose of about 9 mg per day, and may be useful in Parkinson's disease in a dose of 15 to 30 mg per day (Iacono, personal communication, 1995). Adverse effects are uncommon.

Case Report

A 42-year-old married Caucasian male landscape architect consulted me with a 20-year history of chronic fatigue syndrome symptoms. He had not been able to exert himself at his job for the past six or seven years. Many workups had been within normal limits, and all trial medications, including serotonin reuptake inhibitors, had not helped him particularly. He had to disassemble his successful company because of decreased energy. He also had a disorder of initiating and maintaining sleep and experienced nonrestorative sleep.

He stated, "My mother always had difficulty sleeping but had a normal polysomnogram." The patient had bruxism and wore a night splint. He also complained of weakness, cognitive dysfunction, palmar dyshidrosis, arthralgias, and feeling tense. Seven years previously, when he became too fatigued to walk upstairs, he had had a treadmill test, which was within normal limits. He complained of dyspnea on exertion, a common symptom of neurosomatic patients. The dyspnea is usually central (Goldstein, 1993), although asthma is fairly frequent in this population and can be comorbid with panic disorder. An anxious asthmatic patient with central air hunger can be difficult to evaluate, since symptoms may persist as airway flow improves.

Past medical history was noncontributory. He had not responded to doxepin, which made him feel groggy. Physical examination was unremarkable. He had no response to naphazoline or nitroglycerin. He felt much more alert after taking nimodipine but there was no alteration in his diffuse pain. However, after taking hydralazine 25 mg he stated he was able to read a book and retain its basic facts, which he had not been able to do for years, and had much less pain. He thought perhaps he could even do some physical labor.

At one-week follow-up, he stated, "I haven't felt this good in years." He was able to discontinue nonsteroidal antiinflammatory drugs and was able to be physically active in his work.

At six-months follow-up, he reported that he was still feeling fairly well but had some weakness in his arms, a new symptom. His vision was clearer, he was more alert, his cognition had improved, and he believed that the hydralazine had ameliorated a previously diagnosed developmental reading disorder. He still complained of dyspnea on exertion, air hunger, allergic rhinitis, and frequent headaches, and still had some arthralgia. He was continuing to take nimodipine four times a day. He had no response to mexiletine or pyridostigmine, but after 2 mg of Hydergine he felt more alert.

The Hydergine worked so well that over the next year or so he was able to discontinue much of his other medication. He was seen 18 months later when he had inadvertently run out of his Hydergine and complained, "This is the worst I've felt in a long time." He complained of having weak arms, headache, and exhaustion despite taking nimodipine, aspirin, and hydralazine. He had not had any Hydergine for two weeks and had begun to develop paroxysmal limb movements during sleep, despite taking zolpidem h.s. (at bedtime). One-half hour after taking 2 mg of Hydergine he stated, "I feel fine." He continues on Hydergine 1 mg TID.

At his most recent visit, two years after his initial consultation, he remarked, "I'm still doing fine; if I don't take my medication I can't get any rest." He noted that his legs twitched and that they felt "uneasy" and fatigued if he did not take Hydergine. He stated, "The medication helps me a lot. I can tell when I forget to take it."

FELBAMATE (FELBATOL)

Felbamate is a unique compound in clinical medicine at this time. Marketed as an anticonvulsant, it may also be useful in mood disorders and as an analgesic. Some CFS patients decrease all their symptoms after taking it. Felbamate is an antagonist at the glycine coagonist site of the NMDA (N-methyl-D-aspartate) receptor. For those of you who follow my work, I have previously suggested that some CFS patients have deficiencies in excitatory amino acid neurotransmission (especially involving the amino acid glutamate), resulting in impaired production of nitric oxide, an important integrative transmitter substance in the brain. There may, however, be some patients who overproduce glutamate, regionally or globally, and may thus release too much nitric oxide in the brain. Such patients may respond to nitric oxide synthase inhibitors. The situation is further complicated by the finding that nitric oxide may change to the nitrosonium ion, which binds to a redox modulatory site on the NMDA receptor, resulting in decreased activity of the NMDA receptor (Lipton and Rosenberg, 1994). Nitric oxide may also generate free radicals and thus enhance the secretion of excitatory amino acids without necessarily acting as a retrograde messenger (Huie and Padmaja, 1993). I have not been impressed with available nitric oxide synthase inhibitors: niacinamide and ethacrynic acid. More specific inhibitors are being studied and should be released in the next few years. CFS patients are also less likely than the normal population to have generalized seizures. I surveyed four CFS practices with a total of 4,000 patients. Only two CFS patients had a generalized seizure disorder. Such a decreased incidence may be due in part to glutamate deficiency.

Blocking the function of the NMDA receptor at various sites will result in decreased activity. There are several sites that may be antagonized. Directly blocking NMDA glutamate receptors apparently causes too much toxicity for use in humans, but since blocking the glycine co-agonist site is well tolerated, such an intervention is practicable. Felbamate is a useful agent, and I continue it if it is effective. A glycine site antagonist has been reported to impair working memory performance in rats (Ohno, Yamamoto, and Watanabe, 1994), but I have not seen this effect with felbamate in my patients. Felbamate also potentiates hippocampal $GABA_A$ receptor chloride currents (Rho, Donevan, and Rogowski, 1994). $GABA_A$ agonists may be useful in treating central pain conditions, which include fibromyalgia, by modulating thalamocortical neurotransmission (Goldstein, 1993). Felbamate additionally enhances the function of $GABA_A$ receptors under conditions in which GABA-ergic transmission is reduced, and potentiates the activity of diazepam at the $GABA_A$ receptor (Serra et al., 1994). The use of felbamate has been associated with secondary mania (Hill, Stagno, and Tesar, 1995). Felbamate and gabapentin may synergize in the neurosomatic patient.

Although felbamate has few adverse reactions, it has recently been linked with aplastic anemia in 31 patients worldwide, ten of whom died. No cases have been reported in the 14 months since the manufacturer recommended routine hematologic monitoring. It can cause weight loss and is being investigated as an appetite suppressant (Bergen et al., 1995). It should be used only if the benefits clearly outweigh the risks.

GABAPENTIN AND LAMOTRIGINE

Gabapentin (GBP), an antiepileptic drug (AED) with a novel mechanism of action, has become one of my five favorite medications (the others are oxytocin, nimodipine, baclofen, and intravenous lidocaine) to treat neurosomatic disorders. It is a very safe medication and is excreted unmetabolized. The most common adverse effects are somnolence, dizziness, and fatigue. GBP is approved for refractory partial seizures and is recommended as an "add-on" drug. I prescribe it in doses of 100 to 300 mg three times a day. Many patients report a marked increase in energy after the first dose, and GBP is a remarkably effective anxiolytic in certain patients. It also appears to have antidepressant effects in a few individuals, and may have a beneficial effect on the entire spectrum of neurosomatic disorders.

Originally thought to be a GABA-mimetic agent, the mode of action of GBP in epilepsy is currently unclear. It may enhance the releasable pool of GABA in the CNS (Kocsis and Honmou, 1994; Loscher, Honack, and Taylor, 1994), and this mode of action may be the most relevant for neurosomatic disorders although not necessarily for epilepsy (Taylor, 1994), since it may enhance the function of the thalamic reticular nucleus. GBP increases the release of GABA from brain slices in vitro by an indirect method (Gotz et al., 1993) in a concentration range not thought to be relevant for antiepileptic effect. Its anticonvulsant action may occur by inhibiting the metabolism of L-leucine and other branched chain amino acids to glutamate. GBP apparently has this action as a result of competitively inhibiting branched-chain amino acid amino transferase (BCAT) (Taylor, 1994). It also enhances the action of glutamate dehydrogenase and is a weak inhibitor of GABA-transaminase (GABA-T), which degrades GABA into other amino acids.

The AED vigabatrin (VIG) acts solely by irreversibly inhibiting GABA-T and is anxiolytic in animal models (Sherif and Oreland, 1994). It has also caused depression in 4 to 9 percent of patients when used as an AED (Grunewald et al., 1994). It might be effective in neurosomatic disorders if it increases GABA concentrations in the reticular nucleus of the thalamus. The weak GABA-T inhibition of GBP does not seem relevant to its clinical action. GBP has no affinity for any known receptor or ion channel, supporting a claim for a novel mechanism of action. It may bind on neuronal cell bodies to the "system L" neutral amino acid transporter, a binding not affected by NMDA agonists or antagonists, or by other anticonvulsants. The anticonvulsant action of GBP occurs substantially beyond its attaining peak plasma values, suggesting a need for delayed biochemical changes or prolonged attachment to an extracellular receptor (Welty et al., 1993). Since the clinical effect of GBP in patients with neurosomatic disorders is fairly rapid, occurring in about 30 minutes, its anticonvulsant action may not be relevant to this group of individuals.

GBP resembles phenytoin and carbamazepine in depressing segmental and reticular excitatory mechanisms (Fromm, 1994), and this mode of action may be relevant to those neurosomatic patients who are overly activated neurobiologically, even though they do not manifest behavioral hyperactivity. Indeed, certain patients become extremely stimulated by very low doses of GBP.

Case Report

A 48-year-old married Caucasian male novelist was "sickly" since childhood, experiencing ongoing problems with headaches, insomnia, anxiety, and dyspepsia. Nevertheless, he was a national champion in equestrian sports until he developed a flulike onset of illness with severe fatigue about 18 months before consulting me. He also developed debilitating nausea as well as intermittent diplopia, paresthesias, and diarrhea. He became very weak and complained of short-term memory problems. He had seen many physicians without benefit. He had a prompt response to nitroglycerin, nimodipine, and hydralazine, but unfortunately developed tolerance to all of them. GBP 100 mg made him feel "jet-propelled," so much so that he needed to take only about 50 mg twice a day; higher doses made him feel agitated. He continues on GBP and has resumed his premorbid level of functioning. In this case, I would assume that increased GABA was inhibiting an inhibitory system, resulting in excitation. As seen on electron microscopy, axonal terminals of reticular thalamic neurons contact local circuit short-axoned neurons (Montero and Singer, 1985). Both sets of neurons are inhibitory, and both are GABAergic. Thus local circuit GABAergic cells could be disinhibited if disconnected from the reticular nucleus (Steriade et al., 1985).

Case Report

A 44-year-old married Caucasian housewife developed symptoms of malaise, diffuse pain, fatigue, chest pain, cognitive dysfunction and many other neurosomatic symptoms one year before first seeing me. The onset of her illness was coincident with an episode of cystitis. As many patients do, she was able to give the exact date of the onset of her symptoms. She had seen many physicians and said "I've been from doctor to doctor to doctor."

Thirty minutes after taking gabapentin 300 mg she felt "normal." Over the next few months she felt so well that she stopped her gabapentin. She started phentermine and fenfluramine from another physician to lose weight and had been taking DHEA 50 mg per day when she returned to my office complaining of a "total relapse" 2 weeks previously. She felt anxious but denied situational stress. "I'm very happy except that I'm in so much damn pain." Gabapentin 300 mg relieved almost all symptoms, and an additional 300 mg made her feel "as good as I was before I got sick."

Some patients require doses of up to 4000 mg per day of gabapentin to achieve maximum benefit.

Case Report

A 38-year-old divorced Caucasian female marketing specialist first consulted me five years ago, citing a ten-year history of fatigue, exercise intolerance, malaise, arthralgias, myalgias, weakness, sore throat, allergic rhinitis, low-grade fevers, heart palpitations, hair loss, cold hands and feet, and cognitive dysfunction ever since having mononucleosis. She had some response to intravenous immunoglobulin and intravenous ascorbic acid but these agents had to be given very frequently and were expensive. She also had severe headaches and had developed osteoarthritis of her temporomandibular joints, which required reconstructive surgery.

She had tried all medications on the neurosomatic protocol without response until taking gabapentin shortly after it was released.

A brain SPECT had shown left frontotemporal hypoperfusion. She had not been able to work during the five years since I had first seen her, and she had subsequently been told that she had post-rubella syndrome from a vaccination. She continued to receive intravenous immunoglobulin and intravenous ascorbic acid from her personal physician, which enabled her to function well enough to take care of her child. She was still quite fatigued, however, until she took gabapentin 100 mg. Thirty minutes later, she stated that all of her symptoms had resolved and that she felt normal for the first time in 14 years. She felt clear, alert, and productive. She was able to utilize a greater vocabulary, had a better sense of humor, increased energy, and much improved problem-solving abilities, was much less sensitive to stress, had increased appetite (she was quite thin) and no further headaches (she had had a constant daily headache), thought that she would be able to ride a bicycle, and was able to enjoy life.

This improvement has persisted for several months at the time of this writing. The patient is dealing with the problem of having to completely restructure her life from one of semi-invalidism.

Another new AED that may be useful in neurosomatic disorders is lamotrigine (LTG). This agent decreases presynaptic excitatory amino acid release by blocking voltage-sensitive sodium channels, thus attenuating neuronal excitation (Messenheimer, 1994). LTG in a dose of 50 mg per day may improve alertness in neurosomatic patients. Rash is more common in my patients than the 2 percent incidence reported in clinical trials. Dizziness, ataxia, somnolence, and nausea have also been reported as adverse reactions, but are not common in my patient population at the 50 mg dose. LTG has been anecdotally reported to have mood-elevating effects and VIG and LTG can be safely combined (Stolarek et al., 1994). I have observed a similar synergistic effect in my neurosomatic patients with GBP and phenytoin, which is also a sodium channel blocker. As with GBP, phenytoin needs only to be administered in low 100 mg doses, dissociating its AED effects from its other neuroregulatory properties. Phenytoin is also a class I_B antiarrhythmic drug like lidocaine, tocainide, and mexiletine.

Loreclezole, another new AED, is an allosteric modulator at the $GABA_A$ receptor beta subunit. It strongly potentiates GABA-mediated chloride channels and acts at a site distinct from the benzodiazepine, barbiturate, and steroid receptor sites. It should be anxiolytic as well, and may be additive in its effect to compounds that stimulate other regions of the GABA receptor (Wafford et al., 1994). Of course, various neurosteroids should have value in treating neurosomatic disorders, as I have discussed in a previous volume (Goldstein, 1993) and has been elsewhere reviewed (Myslobodsky, 1993).

GLYCINE

Case Report

A 53-year-old Caucasian male real estate developer was in good health and earning a high six figure income until 1987 when he had a coronary angioplasty on two arteries. During that hospitalization he was noted to have thrombocytopenia. In 1988 he developed weakness and fatigue, had a positive Tensilon test, and had an EMG consistent with a neuropathic process. He had elevated CPKs. Subsequently he developed cognitive and attentional deficits to the point of eventually being diagnosed as being demented by neuropsychological testing. A brain SPECT in 1990 showed bilateral temporal hypoperfusion. A repeat SPECT was done in 1991 after a motor vehicle accident without loss of consciousness produced increased cognitive dysfunction, and showed bilateral frontotemporal hypoperfusion. He became too cognitively impaired to work and his conversations were tangential and circumlocutory. It took him two hours to shower and dress. A 15 minute office visit for anyone else took an hour for him. Executive functions were significantly impaired. He developed a severe chronic daily headache. Muscle biopsy in 1991 was consistent with denervation. It was concluded that he had an autoimmune polyneuropathy. None of a panoply of medications produced dramatic improvement.

The patient's condition continued to deteriorate and he had to declare bankruptcy. High-dose oral glycine was begun. There was no change in his status until he reached 15 gm per day, at which time his headache decreased somewhat. At a dose of 20 gm per day, he had a moderate improvement in energy and he was able to take walks and go bicycle riding for the first time in seven years. He stopped taking pyridostigmine, which had been helping his weakness somewhat. His headache disappeared and he was able to organize and complete paperwork. Conversations with him were much more focused. He is currently titrating his glycine dosage to optimum levels. He weighs 80 kg (176 lb). He has had almost complete relief of his symptoms at a dose of 0.4 mg/kg per day. Increasing the glycine to 40 gm per day did not confer any additional benefit and gave him a headache.

Glycine crosses the blood-brain barrier poorly and undergoes peripheral metabolism. For this reason, it must be taken in very high doses. Glycine powder mixed with juice is palatable. Serine may also be tried, but the more potent cycloserine, an antituberculous drug when given in doses of 250 mg qd, has exacerbated schizophrenia in one study (Cascella et al., 1994). It was safe in doses of 50 mg per day or less in an elderly population (Mohr et al., 1995), and inhibits the response to dopaminergic transmission in rats by an increase in glutamatergic transmission (Dall'olio, Rimondini, and Gandolfi, 1994). It also enhances social behavior in mice under certain circumstances (McAllister, 1994). Glycine has had no serious adverse reactions in any of my patients thus far, and may be a useful agent, particularly since no effective central glutamate agonists are available. Cycloserine, which I have been prescribing for only a short time, appears to be a significant improvement over glycine in the treatment-resistant patient.

Glycine is also an inhibitory neurotransmitter and is frequently colocalized with GABA in cat spinal motoneurons and brainstem terminals (Taal and Holstege, 1994). Two other small amino acids, glutamate and aspartate, are excitatory. Even glutamate, acting at the metabotropic receptor, and GABA, acting at the $GABA_B$ receptor, have neuromodulatory properties (Hasselmo, 1995). Neurotransmission may be defined as the direct transfer of information in neural structures. Neuromodulators "appear to alter the processing characteristics of cortical structures through influences on physiological phenomena such as synaptic transmission and pyramidal cell adaption" (Hasselmo, 1995). Furthermore, "activation of receptors on a protein structure directly incorporating an ion channel . . . is defined as neurotransmission, while activation of receptors coupled indirectly to channels (e.g., via second messenger pathways) [is] defined as neuromodulation." All other neurotransmitters except the inhibitory adenosine (Wu and Saggau, 1994), may in most cases (Hasselmo, 1995), be viewed as modulating the activity of glycine, GABA, glutamate, and aspartate. The ions Ca^{++}, Mg^{++}, Na^+, and K^+ may also have transmitter functions (especially intracellular Ca^{++}).

Glycine-site NMDA antagonists have behavioral effects and possible wider therapeutic applications. A concern is that they may produce phencyclidine (PCP)-like symptoms ("discriminative stimulus effects"). Many of them do not (Balster, 1994). Glycine is an obligatory co-agonist at a strychnine-insensitive site at the NMDA channel, i.e., the NMDA channel will not open in the presence of glutamate or aspartate if the glycine site is not occupied

(Weber, 1994). Furthermore, glycine is an inhibitory neurotransmitter in the brainstem and spinal cord, separate from its role at the NMDA receptor. It can inhibit noradrenergic transmission at the locus ceruleus, serotonergic transmission in and out of the raphe nuclei, and cholinergic transmission in the pedunculopontine and lateral tegmental nuclei (Fort, Luppi, and Jouvet, 1993). Glycine, acting at strychnine-sensitive receptors, is also a neurotransmitter in the telencephalon, including the substantia nigra, the corpus striatum, the mesolimbic area, and the hippocampus, and its release can be potentiated from human brain cortex synaptosomes by acetylcholine acting at M_4 muscarinic receptors. Thus the cholinergic system may indirectly enhance, through the release of glycine, glutamatergic transmission in the human brain (Russo et al., 1993).

Glycine-site antagonists are being investigated in the treatment of anxiety (Kehne et al., 1993; Palfreyman et al., 1994), as atypical neuroleptics to downregulate dopamine function (Iverson, 1994), as antidepressants (Nowak et al., 1993), and in the treatment of dementia (Parsons and Quack, 1993).

Some available medications that act downstream from, on, or upstream from the NMDA receptor I have found not effective: dipyridamole, ephedrine, phenytoin (Dilantin), dextromethorphan, allopurinol, dantrolene. Others have been marginally effective: magnesium, amantadine. Nimodipine, an L-type calcium channel antagonist that decreases glutamate release, is the most beneficial oral medication I currently use, although it probably acts in CFS by a different mechanism (Goldstein, 1993, 1994a) than by decreasing glutamate.

HISTAMINE-2 RECEPTOR ANTAGONISTS

The first treatments I developed for CFS were cimetidine and ranitidine (Goldstein, 1986a,b). I based this therapy on my successful experience treating acute infectious mononucleosis with cimetidine (Goldstein, 1983). At that time, it was thought that CFS, like mononucleosis, was caused by the Epstein-Barr virus, and I speculated that blocking H_2 receptors on CD8 lymphocytes might decrease the cytokine excess seen in mononucleosis (Linde et al., 1992), and possibly in CFS (Chao et al., 1991). Since NK function in CFS was usually reduced, I reasoned that cimetidine would improve symptoms by blocking the production of histamine-induced suppressor factor inhibition of NK cells, as it does in vitro (Nair, Cilik, and Schwartz, 1986). The rapidity of the response convinced me that the effect was central. I still am not completely sure how H_2 blockers work in CFS.

Histamine is an excitatory neurotransmitter in the CNS. H_1 receptor antagonists that are centrally active cause sedation. H_1 receptor agonists have vasoconstrictive properties (Miyamoto and Nishio, 1993). The H_3 receptor is an autoreceptor. H_3 receptor antagonists, such as thioperamide, increase histamine secretion, and are therefore activating. Thioperamide attenuates stimulant-induced motor activity in the mouse, however (Clapham and Kilpatrick, 1994). H_3 receptors have been found on 5-HT, DA, and ACh neurons in the brain (Suzuki et al., 1994), and striatal H_3 receptors are influenced by tonic dopaminergic inputs (Ryo, Yanai, and Watanabe, 1994). A review of the behavioral effects of histamine and its antagonists (White and Rumbhold, 1988) yields no information about how H_2 blockers could ameliorate CFS symptoms when acting centrally, especially since ranitidine, the most effective of the H_2 blockers in CFS, penetrates the blood-brain barrier poorly. Histamine is, however, found in the rat superior cervical ganglia (Elfvin, Lindh, and Hokfelt, 1993), and modulating its role in autonomic function may affect central processes. If H_2 receptor antagonism in the SCG causes an increase in central noradrenergic neurotransmission, peripheral immunosuppression may occur.

H_2 antagonists have been reported to cause movement disorders including dystonia, postural and action tremor, chorea, blepharospasm, and cranial dystonia. These disorders occur more frequently with cimetidine, which gets into the brain easily, but also occur with ranitidine. H_2 blockers have a central cholinergic effect by cholinesterase inhibition (Davis, Aul et al., 1994; Mochizuki et al., 1994). If H_2 blockers increase preganglionic cholinergic transmission, they can cause increased postganglionic noradrenergic tone. Histamine depletion decreases memory and learning in rats (Kamei, Okumura, and Tasaka, 1993).

Central histamine is activating and enhances NMDA-mediated synaptic transmission in the hippocampus (Bekkers, 1993). Cimetidine has also caused restless leg syndrome and tardive dyskinesia

(O'Sullivan and Greenberg, 1993), suggesting deficiency of GABA, opioids, and dopamine since agonists of these agents are used to treat restless leg syndrome. H_2 blockade inhibits a portion of systemic morphine-induced nociception (Thorburn et al., 1994), and decreases the antinociceptive properties of histamine in inflammatory hyperalgesia (Netti et al., 1994). H_2 receptors are abundant in cortical, basal ganglia and limbic structures (Traiffort et al., 1992), and may increase ACh secretion by modulating the activity of the septohippocampal cholinergic system via histaminergic projections from the tuberomammillary nucleus of the posterior hypothalamus.

H_2 receptors have no effect on release of DA in the restrained rat (Fleckenstein, Lookingland, and Moore, 1994a), or NE in the same experimental paradigm (Fleckenstein, Lookingland, and Moore, 1994b). The H_2 blocker famotidine, however, had beneficial effects on the negative symptoms of schizophrenia in an open study (Deutsch et al., 1993), although the mechanism of action was unclear. Cimetidine can cause seizures in humans, even at normal doses (Autret, Mercier, and Marimbu, 1984), and the drug can release prolactin, perhaps by involving the GABA system (Sibilia et al., 1985). Cimetidine-induced seizures in mice were prevented by GABA agonists, but not by phenytoin, which acts on sodium channels. Strychnine, a glycine-site antagonist, had no effect on cimetidine-induced seizures (Amabeoku and Chikuni, 1993). The authors suggest that the NMDA receptor was not involved in this model, perhaps not realizing that the glycine co-agonist site at the NMDA receptor is strychnine-insensitive.

Histaminergic neurons, located in the posterior hypothalamus, suppress interleukin-1 beta (IL-1 beta) levels (Alvarez et al., 1993). I have previously hypothesized that IL-1 beta antagonism might be involved in the pathophysiology of CFS. H_2 blockade could attenuate this IL-1 beta suppression. Increased central IL-1 beta may produce immunosuppression by increasing CRH, thereby decreasing the cytokine excess of acute infectious mononucleosis. Central IL-1 beta also stimulates central histamine release, a process involved in elevating body temperature (Kang et al., 1994).

When a CFS patient responds to an H_2 antagonist (I use ranitidine), the onset of action is similar to that seen in acute infectious mononucleosis, i.e., one or two days at a dose of 150 mg b.i.d.

Usually all symptoms are ameliorated. Some patients are unable to take any dose of ranitidine because it makes them "hyper." Increasing central ACh might produce this effect, particularly acting at the M_4 muscarinic receptor, which enhances glycine secretion and could indirectly increase glutamatergic neurotransmission (Russo et al., 1993). Increasing preganglionic cholinergic transmission could enhance NE production from sympathetic ganglia. Inhibiting GABA certainly could cause stimulation, especially if the patient had a history of panic disorder (Rimon et al., 1995). It is difficult to explain agitation on the basis of dopamine antagonism, although some of the movement disorders attributed to H_2 antagonists could result from dopamine excess in a complex system. A ranitidine analog has enhanced learning and recall in rats. JWS-USC-75-IX blocks the muscarinic M_2 receptor and has anticholinesterase activity. Its effects are antagonized by the anticholinergic drug scopolamine (Terry et al., 1995). Perhaps ranitidine behaves in a similar manner in neurosomatic patients.

Histamine may also induce melatonin secretion by virtue of stimulating pineal cyclic AMP. Vasoactive intestinal peptide is the only other substance known to stimulate pineal cyclic AMP (Nowak and Sek, 1994). Histamine may thus be involved in sleep-wake cycles and other aspects of circadian physiology.

Case Report

A 50-year-old single Caucasian female probation officer was well until she had a surgical repair of an Achilles tendon two years prior to consulting me. Postoperatively she developed typical CFS/FMS symptoms and it was difficult for her to continue to work, even though she stated, "I love my job." She was begun on ranitidine 150 mg b.i.d. and felt much better in two days in all respects. Over the next three years she was prescribed sertraline for depression and did well until she developed cognitive dysfunction which was greatly relieved by the addition of gabapentin. Another physician referred her to a gastroenterologist for evaluation of heartburn. Her ranitidine was discontinued by the gastroenterologist and omeprazole was prescribed with assurances that it would "work even better" than ranitidine for her CFS as well as for her reflux esophagitis. Three days after stopping ranitidine she began sleeping 14 hours a day and experienced severe malaise. After several days of this relapse, she restarted ranitidine and resumed good health in 48 hours.

HYDROCHLOROTHIAZIDE (HYDRODIURIL)

Why include a diuretic in CFS treatment? As is usual with most drugs, hydrochlorothiazide (HCTZ) has more than one pharmacologic effect, and can alter levels of glucose, lipoproteins, and uric acid besides producing diuresis and lowering blood pressure. Benzothiadiazide diuretics, of which HCTZ is one, can inhibit rapid glutamate AMPA (alpha-amino-3-hydroxy-5-methyl-4-isoxazolepropionic acid) receptor desensitization (Yamada and Tang, 1993), a property that may be important in CFS. HCTZ therapy should result in increased secretion of glutamate and nitric oxide. Thus far, this action has been tested only in hippocampal slice preparations (in vitro) and the effects on the intact animal have not been published. HCTZ is not the most potent benzothiadiazide for inhibition of glutamatergic receptor desensitization. Cyclothiazide, a diuretic formerly marketed under the trade name Anhydron by Eli Lilly, is far and away the most potent. When cyclothiazide is given in rats intraperitoneally, however, little crosses the blood-brain barrier, and there is some question about whether systemically administered HCTZ would have a direct central effect (Yamada, personal communication, 1994). Some medications I prescribe for CFS (e.g., naphazoline eyedrops and pyridostigmine) have a peripheral mode of action, but can produce dramatic effects on centrally mediated symptoms and cerebral perfusion. It appears that such agents can alter brain function by stimulating peripheral nerves, autonomic ganglia, or circumventricular organs. Aniracetam, a nootropic agent not available in the United States, also modulates desensitization of responses to glutamate in hippocampal neurons (Tang et al., 1991).

OXYTOCIN

Oxytocin (OXT) has a wide range of behavioral effects besides its classical peripheral endocrine actions. The peripheral effects include milk ejection by contraction of the myoepithelial cells that encircle mammary acini during suckling, its well-known stimulating effect on uterine contractility during labor, and the ability to expedite delivery of the placenta after childbirth. Two areas of the hypothalamus contain OXT-secreting neurons: the magnocellular neurons of the supraoptic nucleus and the paraventricular nucleus. The supraoptic nucleus and the paraventricular nucleus also secrete vasopressin (VP) and corticotropin-releasing hormone (CRH). Both OXT and VP can be found in lateral hypothalamic cells that loosely span several diencephalic nuclei (Sukhov et al., 1993). CRH has been shown to be hyposecreted in chronic fatigue syndrome (CFS) (Demitrack et al., 1991). I have found the CRH secretagogues, including DDAVP, but not fenfluramine, to be ineffective in treating CFS. Vasopressin levels may be normal (Crofford et al., 1994) or low (Bakheit et al., 1993) in CFS. OXT is also a CRH secretagogue, often colocalized with CRH; it is worthy of a trial in treatment-resistant cases of CFS and related neurosomatic disorders.

OXT neurons project to many areas of the limbic system and brainstem, as well as to the frontal cortex. Brain OXT is involved in organization of maternal behavior, female and male sexual behavior, feeding, social behavior, and memory. OXT also has effects on cardiovascular, autonomic, and thermoregulatory processes (de-Wied, Diamant, and Fodor, 1993). OXT, in contrast to VP, has been found to have an amnestic effect on experimental animals and is elevated in the hippocampus and temporal cortex of patients with dementia of the Alzheimer's type. OXT has also been found to inhibit tolerance to morphine and cocaine (Sarnyai and Kovacs, 1994). Other agents with this property, such as nimodipine and nitroglycerin, are effective in treating CFS (Goldstein, 1994a). Cholecystokinin antagonists, which also have this property (Xu et al., 1992), may be useful in CFS therapy. It has been suggested that "OXT acts on adaptive neuronal processes . . . through the modulation of brain monoaminergic transmission" (Sarnyai and Kovacs, 1994). In rats primed with estrogen and progesterone, OXT enhances extracellular NE levels in the VMH (Etgen and Karkanios, 1994).

OXT secretion from the paraventricular nucleus can be stimulated by brainstem catecholaminergic neurons as well as by glutamatergic neurons. It may be influenced by higher centers as well as by brainstem structures, circumventricular organs, autonomic ganglia and cranial nerves (Ericsson, Kovacs, and Sawchenko, 1993). OXT may have particular importance in modulation of hippocampal function, and an oxytocinergic neural network has been demonstrated experimentally (Sawchenko, 1991; Sarnyai and Kovacs, 1994). OXT is also an arterial vasoconstrictor (Altura and Altura, 1984).

Case Report

A 25-year-old married Caucasian health care worker who was previously in good health had a baby three months prior to first consulting me. She did well until she stopped breast-feeding. The next day she developed symptoms of CFS, including exhaustion, memory problems, and myalgias, and was diagnosed by her family physician and a consultant psychiatrist as having postpartum depression. Antidepressants prescribed by the psychiatrist relieved her depression but did not affect her other symptoms. She was unable to work. Her Karnofsky performance scale self-rating was 60 (requires occasional assistance but is able to care for most needs). She did not respond to any medication I prescribed, including a neuroleptic to raise her prolactin levels. I advised her to stop her antidepressants and resume breast-feeding, at which time her symptoms resolved and she was able to return to work part-time. She informed me that a breast pump did not relieve her symptoms; only the suckling of her baby did. She wished to return to work full-time but was unable to because of the need for breast-feeding. "Will I have to breast-feed forever?" she asked.

The next logical step in treatment was to administer OXT, available under the trade name Pitocin. The medical literature does not consider the possible role of OXT withdrawal in postpartum syndromes associated with weaning (Susman and Katz, 1988). Administering ten units intramuscularly relieved her symptoms, which had recurred when I advised her to stop breast-feeding again. She continues to do well on one or two injections daily. Of interest is that the patient's mother has CFS, irritable bowel syndrome, and interstitial cystitis, all neurosomatic disorders, and her symptoms promptly responded to OXT as well.

Approximately one-fifth of my patients have a good response to IM (intramuscular) OXT after failing to respond to numerous oral agents. Cognitive clarity is the most responsive symptom, with fibromyalgia pain being second. Energy is not increased in many responders. One patient with reflex sympathetic dystrophy, another neurosomatic disorder, had all her pain relieved after IM OXT. There may be an inverted U-shaped dose-response curve; some patients do well on 5 units, but become agitated and have some return of symptoms on 10 units. Perhaps this effect should be expected, since OXT is intimately involved in the stress response (Silverman, Hou-Yu, and Kelly, 1989). Overcorrection of OXT hyposecretion could possibly produce symptoms of anxiety.

Oxytocin (OXT) has a marked effect on libido and sexual behavior, both in animals and humans. It stimulates mating behavior in voles (Insel and Shapiro, 1992), and induces penile erection in rats via stimulation of the PVN (Arletti, Benelli, and Bertolini, 1992). OXT increases the excitability of neurons in several brain areas, including the CA1 region of the rat hippocampus (Muhlethaler et al., 1983), where injection also produces penile erection (Argiolas, Melis, and Stancampiano, 1993). Penile erection induced by OXT in rats can be prevented by NO synthase inhibitors acting on a DA-OXT link in the PVN (Melis and Argiolas, 1993). Indeed, OXT neurons may be the main source of NO production in the hypothalamic-pituitary system (Miyagawa, Okamura, and Ibata, 1994). OXT increases sexual arousal in both men and women. Masculine sexual behavior in rats increases Fos expression in PVN OXT neurons (Witt and Insel, 1994). George Flechas, M.D., and I, who both discovered this effect independently, were surprised to hear from several women that they had become multiorgasmic for the first time in their lives. OXT is often colocalized in neurons with met-enkephalin, and thus stimulation of these neurons may produce analgesia (Uvnas-Moberg, Bruzelius, et al., 1992), illustrating the importance of this neuropeptide in human sexual function as well.

Central OXT release can be independent of the release of OXT from the posterior pituitary (Amico, Schallinor, and Cameron, 1990). There are no sex differences in the location and density of human brain OXT receptors, which are most numerous in the nucleus basalis of Meynert, the nucleus of the vertical limb of the diagonal band of Broca, the bed nucleus of the stria terminalis (BNST), the entire hypothalamus, the pars compacta of the substantia nigra (where dopaminergic projections to the basal ganglia originate), and the substantia gelatinosa of the caudal trigeminal nucleus (Loup et al., 1989; Loup et al., 1991).

Systemic administration of OXT does not result in penetration of the blood-brain barrier; as little as 0.003 percent of the dose reaches the brain in some species (Mens et al., 1983). It has a plasma half-life of one to six minutes. Thus OXT must be an extraordinarily effective placebo in neurosomatic patients, or must exert its central effects through peripheral nerves (Uvnas-Moberg, 1994, see below), autonomic ganglia, or circumventricular organs (Bull, Douglas, and Russell, 1994). OXT is present in sympathetic ganglia (Elfvin, Lindh, and Hokfelt, 1993).

In experiments in which OXT has been administered i.c.v. or into specific brain sites, moderate doses can improve memory function (Bohus, Kovacs, and DeWied, 1978). OXT induces grooming behaviors in animals, which may be related to obsessive-compulsive disorder (OCD) in humans, in which CSF OXT levels are elevated (Leckman et al., 1994a; Leckman et al., 1994b). Abnormalities in functional brain imaging in OCD are found in the orbitofrontal cortex, the anterior cingulate area, and the head of the caudate nucleus, all of which are hypermetabolic (Baxter et al., 1992). These are functionally related limbic structures that are part of cortico-striatal-thalamo-cortical (CSTC) circuits. I have previously noted that OCD is extremely uncommon in my neurosomatic patient population (Goldstein, 1993), and decreased CSF OXT in this group could be one reason for this low prevalence rate, as could elevated CFS NE (see below).

OXT, both in my patients and in rats, can be anxiolytic (Uvnas-Moberg, Alster, et al., 1992) and an antidepressant (Arletti and Bertolini, 1987). Oxytocin produced a manic episode in a 58-year-old mildly demented male physician with CFS who was taking sertraline 100 mg QD. Reducing the sertraline dosage prevented further mania, and the combination markedly alleviated his symptoms, including his dementia. No disorders have been characterized by decreased levels of CSF OXT, although fibromyalgia may be (Russell, personal communication, 1994). There are positive correlations between CSF oxytocin levels and CSF 5-HIAA and NE levels (Van de Kar et al., 1995). In another study, medication-free Tourette's syndrome (TS) and OCD patients had various biogenic amines measured in CSF obtained by lumbar puncture. The most significant finding was in CSF NE levels: TS > OCD > normals (Leckman et al., 1994b). CFS/FMS patients have decreased CSF NE levels. Clomipramine treatment of patients with OCD resulted in decreased levels of CRH, VP (vasopressin), 5-HIAA, HVA, and MHPG (3-methoxy-4-hydroxyphenylglycol). The levels of CSF OXT in this group were *increased* with treatment, however (Altemus et al., 1994). This result was somewhat surprising, since stimulation of the 5-HT$_{2C}$ receptor increases oxytocin levels. 5-HT$_{1A}$ stimulation does not, however (Bagdy and Makara, 1994). SRIs used to treat OCD stimulate both receptors.

It is well known that the brain can influence gastrointestinal function, and may do so by the interaction of descending cortical impulses and routine afferent activity of the neurons of the nucleus of the solitary tract. Stimulation of the anterior limbic area depresses responses in the solitary tract that were induced by electrical stimulation of the vagus nerve (Bagaev and Panteleev, 1994). An interesting paper by Kerstin Uvnas-Moberg of the Karolinska Institute in Stockholm (Uvnas-Moberg, 1994) explores the role of central OXT in regulating gastrointestinal function, but also discusses how vagal afferents transfer information from the gut to the brain, a key concept in understanding CNS regulation by peripheral nerves, as well as the food intolerance commonly encountered by patients with neurosomatic disorders. She notes that "90% of the vagal fibres are afferent (from the gut to the brain), allowing an intense impulse traffic in this direction."

Efferent vagal nerves regulate the activity of the gut neuroendocrine system. OXT reaches the vagal motor nucleus, and releases gut hormones that can be measured in plasma. Ingested food causes activation of the "satiety hormone" cholecystokinin (CCK), which binds to vagal receptors and activates vagal afferents to "inform" the brain about how much food is in the gut and whether food-seeking behavior should continue. Both food intake and CCK cause sedation, which may be OXT-mediated. The projections of the solitary tract terminate in the parabrachial nucleus, which in turn projects to the visceral-limbic forebrain. Stimulation of the caudal solitary tract nucleus induces sleep and changes in autonomic regulation (Jones, 1993). Vagotomized rats continue food-seeking exploratory behavior even after they are fed. Vagotomized animals that had been pregnant also stopped suckling, and had lowered OXT levels, suggesting that "a tonic influence from the gut which sustains the activity in the oxytocin neurons has been lost" (Uvnas-Moberg, 1994). The projections of the solitary tract terminate in the parabrachial nucleus, which in turn projects to the visceral-limbic forebrain. Stimulation of the caudal solitary tract nucleus induces sleep and changes in autonomic regulation (Jones, 1993).

OXT also induces maternal behavior in estrogen-primed rats (Argiolas and Gessa, 1991), as does intraperitoneal injection of CCK. Therefore, "afferent vagal mechanisms not only influence gastrointestinal motility and secretion, . . . they also influence behavior and endocrine patterns" (Uvnas-Moberg, 1994). It follows that food intolerance could result from dysregulated PFC gating of vagal afferent sensory input to the solitary tract and the structures with which it synapses. Vagal afferents regulate numerous other CNS functions including fever, *hypothalamic norepinephrine depletion*, elevation in serum corticosteroids, learned taste aversion, suppression of social interaction, pain, and cytokine-to-brain communication (reviewed by Watkins, Maier, and Goehler, 1995b). Other neuropeptides are depleted in the solitary tract after (cervical) vagal stimulation. These include neurotensin, cholecystokinin, substance P, calcitonin gene-related peptide, and somatostatin. Cholecystokinin and somatostatin are selectively released by gastric afferent activation. The others are related to cardiovascular afferent neurons (Saleh and Cechetto, 1995). This phenomenon has recently been described with cytokines (Watkins, Maier, and Goehler, 1995a).

Dihydropyridine calcium channel blockers abolish the secretion of OXT potentiated by dihydropyridine agonists, but have no effect on OXT secretion in rat neurointermediate lobe when administered alone (Jorgensen et al., 1994). Thus, at least in this model, these antagonists could not improve neurosomatic disorders or Tourette's syndrome (Goldstein, 1984), by altering OXT secretion.

Oxytocin levels increase following a CRH challenge, and oxytocin receptor binding in limbic areas is significantly reduced by adrenalectomy. Thus OXT receptors are upregulated by glucocorticoids (Liberzon et al., 1994), as they are by gonadal steroids (Johnson, 1992). A model for stress response override by OXT receptors sensitive to circulating glucocorticoids has been proposed by Liberzon and co-workers. They also suggest a neurobiologic link between hippocampal oxytocin and glucocorticoids (Liberzon et al., 1994).

Giving OXT on an ongoing basis appears to be safe thus far, with one caveat. A 56-year-old male physician with CFS and treatment-resistant depression was refused electroconvulsive therapy because of cognitive dysfunction. He resolved all his symptoms 15 minutes after receiving 10 units IM OXT but became flushed and quite hypertensive, necessitating administration of nifedipine. He did not become hypertensive after a subsequent lower OXT dose, however. Blood pressure should be monitored after OXT administration. The effectiveness of OXT in certain patients reinforces the pluripotential nature of virtually all transmitter substances; patient response depends on which cells are affected, not the nature of the transmitter itself.

PENTAZOCINE (TALWIN)

Pentazocine and other sigma agonists inhibit NMDA-stimulated norepinephrine (NE) release from rat hippocampal slices. They also inhibit the reuptake of NE into rat synaptosomes. Neuropeptide Y may be an endogenous sigma receptor ligand (Gonzalez-Alvear and Werling, 1995). Sigma receptors are dense in the locus ceruleus (McQuiston and Colmers, 1992) and are important in the regulation of NE secretion. Pentazocine is a sigma receptor agonist, as is dextromethorphan. Two sigma receptors have now been defined: sigma-1 and sigma-2. Sigma-1 receptors are tenfold more dense in the hindbrain than in the cortex, but the distribution of subtypes varies between rats and guinea pigs. The sigma-2 site is supposedly prevalent in the human brain (Knight et al., 1991). Sigma receptors are said to play a role in motor function and in the motor effects of the antipsychotic drugs. The highest relative proportion of sigma-2 sites is found in the cerebellum (Leitner et al., 1994).

Sigma ligands have been investigated as antipsychotics and can inhibit dopamine cell firing in the substantia nigra (Chavkin, 1990). The sigma site may be responsible for the antitussive properties of dextromethorphan, and, perhaps significant for neurosomatic medicine, can block potassium conductance, thus increasing neuronal excitability. Sigma ligands have inhibited motor neurons in the red nucleus of the rat and caused dystonia (Chavkin, 1990).

Also relevant to possible neurosomatic effects is the finding that pentazocine, administered prior to the NMDA antagonist MK-801, attenuates a decrement in spatial working memory caused by MK-801. Pentazocine and dextromethorphan are stereoselective for the sigma-1 site (Maurice et al., 1994).

A nonspecific sigma receptor ligand, 1, 1i3-di(2-tolyl)guanidine (DTG), potentiates the activation of CA3 dorsal hippocampal neurons induced by application of NMDA in rats (Monnet, Debonnet, and DeMontigny, 1992). DTG also potentiates the release of NE from hippocampal slices (Roman et al., 1991). Thus, pentazocine and dextromethorphan may act as NMDA co-agonists (like glycine) in the neurosomatic patient.

In the basal ganglia, sigma agonists stimulate mRNA for pro-enkephalin and pro-neurotensin, while inhibiting pro-tachykinin A mRNA expression. The sigma agonist SKF 10047 increases the firing rate of nigral and ventral tegmental area (VTA) dopaminergic neurons, most likely by a nondopaminergic receptor mechanism. Sigma receptor activity may be mediated through the dopaminergic system (Angulo and McEwen, 1994). Sigma agonists activate tyrosine hydroxylase in nigrostriatal dopamine neurons, enhancing the formation of dopa (Weiser et al., 1995).

None of my patients has ever responded positively to dextromethorphan. Occasionally, however, an extremely treatment-resistant individual has felt much better after taking pentazocine plus naloxone (Talwin-Nx). Talwin has been reformulated to minimize its potential for addiction or abuse.

Case Report

A 30-year-old single unemployed Caucasian woman was referred to me by her most recent biological psychiatrist. She had a ten-year history of suicidal depression, severe fatigue, cognitive impairment, marked insomnia, and fibromyalgia. She had failed treatment with every standard psychotropic agent, alone and in combination, and had not responded to multiple courses of ECT. She had severe panic disorder and was taking 10 mg of clonazepam a day as well as 100 mg of sertraline when she consulted me. She was bitter, and hopeless, and spent virtually all her time in a small apartment, immobilized from fatigue and anhedonia.

She did not respond to most of the medications I tried, but felt "10 percent" better on baclofen and gabapentin. I referred her for possible cingulotomy because it seemed she would kill herself at any time. Further psychiatric hospitalization seemed useless, per her psychiatrist.

While she was waiting for her neurosurgical consultation, I administered one tablet of pentazocine with naloxone (Talwin-Nx). She rapidly felt much better: less depressed, much less anxious; she had less pain and more energy. Since pentazocine made her feel somewhat "goofy" she reduced the dose to one-fourth of a tablet. She could sleep much better taking pentazocine h.s. The effect of pentazocine was enhanced by high-dose oral glycine. Captopril further relieved her depression. As of this writing she is working part-time in a boutique and has a boyfriend.

Case Report

A 59-year-old female married Caucasian former political worker was well until 1987 when she received a flu shot. Within hours she became extremely ill and remained so until seeing me in 1994. She endorsed every item on my CFS questionnaire, and gave a history of being intolerant to 15 medications. Prior to developing CFS she had several hospitalizations for depression. She experienced severe exhaustion, diffuse pain, and significant cognitive dysfunction. Past history revealed an abusive family structure with possible depersonalization and dissociation in adolescence. (Patients with somatization disorder sometimes have dissociative experiences as well [Saxe et al., 1994]). She had not responded to any psychotropic medication and of the first 20 treatments tried in the office she improved only with naphazoline, which eliminated a headache. All her symptoms abated with pentazocine/naloxone. She demonstrated the characteristic global reduction in cerebral perfusion on pre- and post-treatment brain SPECT. Neuropsychological testing revealed significant problems with encoding and distractibility. She made 17 errors on the Proactive Inhibition Subtest of the Irvine Memory Battery. One hour after pentazocine, she made three errors, a fairly common response to effective treatment in CFS patients. She is now doing well on one pentazocine/naloxone tablet five times a day.

PINDOLOL

Pindolol, a beta-blocker that is also a $5\text{-}HT_{1A}$ antagonist, would seem to be an ideal drug with which to treat neurosomatic disorders. If we assume that these illnesses are characterized by noradrenergic denervation hypersensitivity, then it would be desirable to enhance LC norepinephrine secretion. The PFC sends glutamatergic projections to brainstem monoaminergic nuclei to regulate the secretion of neurotransmitters, and CSF MHPG, an NE metabolite, was low in CFS/FMS patients in one study (Russell et al., 1992), although it was normal in another (Bearn and Wessely, 1994).

It has been shown that serotonin selectively attenuates glutamate-evoked activation of noradrenergic locus ceruleus neurons (Aston-Jones et al., 1991), and that this effect is mimicked by $5\text{-}HT_{1A}$ agonists such as buspirone. It would thus seem reasonable to treat neurosomatic disorders with a $5\text{-}HT_{1A}$ antagonist, and would explain why almost none of my patients, many of whom are quite anxious, have improved by taking buspirone.

SRIs do not increase serotonin levels in the projection areas of the raphe nuclei after a single dose. This lack of effect is thought to be due to stimulation of a $5\text{-}HT_{1A}$ presynaptic autoreceptor by the excess of 5-HT that follows reuptake blockade. Thus it appears that blocking of the $5\text{-}HT_{1A}$ autoreceptor could augment the antidepressant effect of SRIs by enabling serotonergic nerve terminals to release more serotonin. There is no selective $5\text{-}HT_{1A}$ receptor antagonist available for human use, but pindolol has a similar effect. Stimulating both the $5\text{-}HT_{1A}$ and $GABA_B$ receptors results in an increase in K conductance in the hippocampal CA1 region, causing hyperpolarization and decreased activation. Activation of the hippocampal MR (mineralocorticoid receptor) attenuates this effect (Joels and deKloet, 1992), giving further credence to the suggestion that fludrocortisone (Florinef) could augment the response of SRIs, particularly when combined with pindolol.

The $5\text{-}HT_2$ receptor, when coupled to a G protein, closes potassium channels. When coupled to phosphatidylinositol, it stimulates protein kinase C and opens the K channel (Harrington et al., 1992). Pindolol is not a pure $5\text{-}HT_{1A}$ antagonist, but is actually a partial agonist. It therefore blocks 5-HT-induced prolactin secretion by a

5-HT$_{1A}$ antagonist mechanism, and increases basal cortisol secretion by an agonist mechanism. There is also cooperativity between the 5-HT$_{1A}$ receptor and the 5-HT$_{1C}$ receptor, which is antagonized by ritanserin and risperidone (Meltzer and Maes, 1994).

When my patients respond to pindolol, 5 mg PO, they do so within 30 minutes. When pindolol is used to augment MAOIs or SRIs, the effect takes longer. Pindolol has produced a dramatic reduction in latency of onset of the effect of paroxetine and response of treatment-resistant patients to MAOIs and SRIs. One week was as long as it took pindolol to have an effect in one study (Artigas, Perez, and Alvarez, 1994). Thus pindolol could benefit neurosomatic patients by increasing glutamate-stimulated NE release, and also serotonin release in association with antidepressants. Fluoxetine and meclobemide, but not desipramine, trimipramine, or maprotiline, increase the release of [^{3}H] norepinephrine stimulated by a 5-HT$_3$ agonist (Mongeau, DeMontigry, and Blier, 1994). This property may explain the superiority of SRIs and MAOIs in the treatment of neurosomatic disorders.

Case Report

A 57-year-old married Caucasian female clinical psychologist recalled having severe headaches and diffuse musculoskeletal and abdominal pain since the fourth grade. She was told by her family doctor that "It was all in my head." Her stepfather was abusive and alcoholic. She suffered recurrent depression since adolescence. She was also diagnosed by a neurologist as having migraine headaches. There was a question of a developmental learning disorder. Cognitive dysfunction was limiting her ability to work. She was taking 31 medications for varous symptoms at the time of her consultation. Her physical exam was unremarkable except for the presence of 18 out of 18 of the characteristic fibromyalgia tender points.

She had no response to naphazoline or nitroglycerin, but 30 minutes after taking nimodipine she was symptom-free, and remained so for two months. Then she began to develop symptoms of allergic rhinitis and had a mild relapse. All symptoms were relieved by pyridostigmine and gabapentin and she did very well for the next four months, taking only seven medications. She then developed severe bronchitis and had multiple root canal surgeries, causing her to relapse again. She experienced a three-inch burning dysesthesias over her left elbow, as well as her typical CFS/FMS symptoms. These were all promptly (within 20 to 30 minutes) relieved by 5 mg of pindolol, which she now takes three times a day. She can tell when it is time to take another dose of pindolol because her elbow starts to burn again. It is also useful as an augmenting agent with mood stabilizers and SRIs (Keck et al., 1995), when treating mixed depression, schizoaffective disorder, and OCD (Jacobsen, 1995).

RISPERIDONE (RISPERDAL)

Risperidone is marketed as an antipsychotic. It is closely related to ritanserin, a serotonin ($5\text{-}HT_2$) receptor antagonist that produced impressive results in an open study I performed in my office several years ago. Risperidone is a high-affinity $5\text{-}HT_2$ antagonist and a low-affinity dopamine (D_2) antagonist (Megans et al., 1994). At the low doses used for CFS, the D_2 antagonist effect, useful in schizophrenia, is not very prominent. The antidepressant nefazodone (Serzone) is a $5\text{-}HT_2$ receptor antagonist as well as a serotonin reuptake inhibitor. In the prefrontal cortex, nucleus accumbens, and striatum of the rat, risperidone increases dopamine levels by about 100 percent. It also increases serotonin release in the frontal cortex by 70 percent (Hertel et al., 1995).

The $5\text{-}HT_2$ receptor is implicated in neurosomatic disorders for several reasons:

A. It is located in the cortex, caudate, limbic system, midbrain, and hypothalamus. Antagonism of the $5\text{-}HT_2$ receptor could enhance midbrain dopamine release (Meltzer, 1992).

B. It influences vasoconstriction, migraine, anxiety, depression, and sleep (Dubovsky, 1994), all functions relevant to CFS. The $5\text{-}HT_{1C}$ receptor, perhaps being eliminated in current nomenclature (there are now 15 serotonin receptors), is closely related to the $5\text{-}HT_2$ receptor, and is also involved in appetite, learning, and aversion. $5\text{-}HT_2$ antagonists may also release dopamine from midbrain sites (Megans et al., 1994). Risperidone, like ritanserin, blocks frontal cortex $5\text{-}HT_2$ sites, but is even more potent at doing so (Megans et al., 1994). It increases stage 3 and stage 4 slow-wave sleep, which may be impaired in CFS. A drug profile of risperidone has recently been published in the *Lancet* (Livingston, 1994). Remember, only very low doses are necessary in CFS. Drug effects usually occur in 30 to 45 minutes but peak plasma levels are not reached for two hours.

C. The $5\text{-}HT_2$ receptor is also involved in upregulating limbic (especially hippocampal) glucocorticoid receptor density (Meaney et al., 1993). There is reason to believe that hippocampal glucocorticoid receptor (GR) density, and possibly mineralocorticoid receptor (MR) density are increased in CFS, especially since CFS patients have decreased CRH secretion (Demitrack et al., 1991). Although this topic is too complex to cover extensively in an article on CFS treatment, hippocampal corticosteroid receptors are involved in the inhibitory influence of glucocorticoids over adrenocortical activity. Antidepressants upregulate these receptors and increase MR and GR mRNA (Meaney et al., 1993). Recent evidence indicates that the density of these receptors can be affected for a lifetime by genetic predisposition interacting with early life experiences (at least in rats) (Herman, 1993), thus altering the stress response later in life and possibly deranging other limbic functions. Such an alteration may also occur in extremely premature infants with prolonged hospitalizations in neonatal intensive care units (Grunau et al., 1994). $5\text{-}HT_2$ antagonists decrease limbic glucocorticoid receptor density and should have a beneficial effect in this scenario.

> Mineralocorticoid receptors are involved in the sensitivity of the stress response system: this concerns processes related to the evaluation of situations and the corresponding response selection resulting in the reactivity of an animal to its environment. Glucocorticoid receptors are involved in the termination of the stress response: in processes concerning the consolidation of information, i.e., learning and memory. As corticosteroid receptor changes occur in relation to environmental, developmental, and pharmacological challenges, we have to be aware that the animal's ability to respond to its environment adaptively (behavioral plasticity) will be determined by the balance of mineralocorticoid and glucocorticoid receptors. (deKloet, Oitzl, and Joels, 1993)

A regulatory influence of alpha-1 adrenoreceptors on hippocampal glucocorticoid receptors has been postulated. Thus there is an anatomical substrate for potential regulatory interactions between noradrenergic transmission and glucocorticoid regulation in stress (Petit, Williams, and Morilak, 1995). Administration of a mineralocorticoid receptor antagonist concomitantly with risperidone should have a beneficial effect in this paradigm, since a MR receptor agonist may attenuate serotonin responses if there is an imbalance between MR- and GR-mediated effects (Joels and deKloet, 1992). A recent study showed that if rats are reexposed to a compartment previously associated with a stressor, the MR is implicated in fear-motivated immobility exerted by corticosterone. An MR antagonist reduced this fear-motivated immobility. GR antagonists are ineffective in this paradigm. MR antagonists are anxiolytic only when the rat was previously exposed to the fear-producing situation. The presence of corticosteroids is necessary to produce this reversible anxiety, since it does not occur in adrenalectomized animals. Steroid-serotonin interactions in the raphe-hippocampal system are thought to underlie these MR-mediated behavioral effects (Korte et al., 1995). Since spironolactone is the only MR antagonist clinically available, it would be interesting to prescribe it in conditions such as posttraumatic stress disorder (PTSD). Occasionally, a patient will report exacerbation of symptoms with treatment for downregulated hippocampal corticosteroid receptors. This individual may respond to agents besides antidepressants that could upregulate these receptors. I have used baclofen (Lioresal), a $GABA_B$ agonist, with fludrocortisone (Florinef), a mineralocorticoid agonist. Baclofen modulates slow inhibitory postsynaptic potentials at hippocampal corticosteroid receptors, and fludrocortisone can also increase intravascular volume in the dysautonomic neurosomatic patient with orthostatic hypotension, although I rarely find it to be beneficial in general symptomatic improvement.

SPIRONOLACTONE (ALDACTONE)

Spironolactone (a mineralocorticoid receptor antagonist) has been used for several years to treat premenstrual syndrome (PMS). One double-blind study found it to be effective and another did not (Hellberg, Chesson, and Nilsson, 1991; Burnet et al., 1991). The mode of action for this agent in PMS has not been identified. If we accept that

PMS is a limbic disorder involving altered sensitivity to the neuronal plasticity that usually occurs after ovulation (Goldstein, 1994a), there would be a benefit in trying to regulate this process in CFS, a related disorder. The symptoms of CFS are quite similar to PMS, and women with CFS usually report a premenstrual exacerbation of their symptomatology. My experience with spironolactone is that it helps only occasionally, but the effect is rapid (30 minutes or so), and thus can be assessed while the patient is in the office.

SUMATRIPTAN

It is now generally agreed that migraine headaches are caused by dysfunctional neural transmission through the trigeminovascular system and not by changes in brain vessel diameter (Markowitz, Saito, and Moskowitz, 1987). A "neurogenic inflammatory response" is postulated that causes release of numerous peptide mediators that could be responsible for the pain, nausea, photophobia, auras, and phonophobia of the migraine attack, even though the generator of the migraine phenomenon is still elusive. Headaches may represent a pain modulation disorder such as is seen in fibromyalgia syndrome (FMS) and may be the cranial equivalent of pain from other visceral organs (Mayer and Gebhart, 1994; Moskowitz, 1991; Nicolodi et al., 1994). Conduction of the pain through the trigeminovascular system involves the trigeminal nucleus caudalis and the mesencephalic tract of the trigeminal nerve, the latter of which then projects to both higher and lower structures.

Sumatriptan, an agonist at the $5-HT_{1D}$ receptor, is postulated to prevent the release of peptides by neurogenic inflammation, thus stopping the train of excitation, and also impeding the expression of c fos in the trigeminal nucleus caudalis (Nozaki, Moskowitz, and Boccalini, 1992). It may act at the level of the meninges, since sumatriptan penetrates the blood-brain barrier poorly. The drug may also block trigeminal nerve transmission directly, which would explain its rapidity of effect in patients who respond in two or three minutes. This mechanism of action may be related to that of the topical ophthalmic agent proparacaine, which may be effective in cluster headaches and trigeminal neuralgia, most likely by altering neurotransmission through the gasserian ganglion (Goldstein,

1993). Lidocaine also blocks neurogenic plasma extravasation in the dura mater with a time course similar to that of sumatriptan (Moskowitz, 1992b), perhaps explaining why mexiletine, a lidocaine analog, is often effective in reducing the headaches of some neurosomatic patients, as is intravenous lidocaine itself.

311C90, a 5-HT$_{1D}$ agonist that acts both peripherally and centrally, may be superior to sumatriptan. It attenuates the secretion of calcitonin gene-related peptide (CGRP) and vasoactive intestinal peptide (VIP), but does not alter levels of NPY or beta endorphin. The inhibition of VIP release appears to occur at the synapse of the trigeminal nucleus caudalis (Goadsby and Edvinsson, 1994).

Endothelin-3, acting at the ET$_B$ receptor, can cause neurogenic inflammation by release of SP and related compounds. The ET$_B$ receptor can be blocked by bosentan, which is being investigated as a migraine treatment (Brandli et al., 1996). Bosentan should be useful to ameliorate other neurosomatic disorders. Sumatriptan and ergotamine derivatives decrease headaches of many sorts, including cluster headaches, classic and common migraine headaches, tension-type headaches, and the headaches of drug withdrawal, as well as headaches caused by meningovascular irritations such as meningitis and subarachnoid hemorrhage (Moskowitz, 1992a). Sumatriptan works rapidly when administered subcutaneously, aborting 74 percent of migraine headaches within 15 minutes (Ferrari and Saxena, 1993). Adverse effects can include chest pain, thought to be of esophageal origin, vertigo, fatigue, worsening of the headache, nausea, numbness, and a feeling of dysphoria or "strangeness." The chest pain may also result from dysfunctional thalamic stimulation (Lenz et al., 1994), which may also cause "chest pain of unknown etiology" in neurosomatic disorders. I have had success eliminating these reactions with the nonselective serotonin receptor antagonist cyproheptadine, 4 mg orally. Cyproheptadine usually aborts reactions to fenfluramine as well, especially when the fenfluramine is given with an SRI. Serious adverse events have occurred when sumatriptan has been given to patients with undetected subarachnoid hemorrhage or significant coronary artery disease, or to those who were receiving monoamine oxidase inhibitors (Palmer, 1994). Headaches can recur after sumatriptan administration, and there is controversy about giving a second dose on the same day.

The problem of rebound headache encountered with ergot alkaloids does not seem to occur with sumatriptan (Saper, 1987).

When administered to patients with neurosomatic disorders, the most important neuroendocrine effects of sumatriptan are an increase in growth hormone (Herdman et al., 1994) and a tripling of neuropeptide Y (NPY) levels (Goadsby and Edvinsson, 1993). Many patients with fibromyalgia who may have decreased growth hormone levels (Bennett et al., 1992), respond to sumatriptan. In most patients only pain is decreased. A minority of responders report improvement of all neurosomatic symptoms. Neurosomatic patients require administration of the drug on an almost daily basis to suppress their symptoms. Even though sumatriptan is not a vasoconstrictor in vivo (Kobari et al., 1993a; Ferrari and Saxena, 1993), when effective it produces global hypoperfusion in the CFS/FMS patients we have studied with pre- and post-treatment brain SPECT. All other successful agents tested in this patient group, notably alpha-adrenergic eyedrops, which appear to act through the first division of the trigeminal nerve, produce global cerebral hypoperfusion.

The ventral two-thirds of the main sensory trigeminal nucleus gives rise to the trigeminal lemniscus, which projects to the contralateral nucleus ventralis posteromedialis of the thalamus (Fromm, 1987), which then projects to layer IV of the primary sensory cortex in the face area and to the secondary somatosensory region. Corticothalamic afferents may subsequently alter the function of the reticular nucleus and decrease diffuse pain. The mesencephalic tract of the trigeminal nerve synapses with the locus ceruleus and the reticular formation (LW Swanson, 1993). Depending upon how these structures are modulated by higher centers, sumatriptan might have a diffuse effect on neurosomatic symptoms. The fact that it markedly increases NPY levels provides another mechanism for generalized improvement. It may also bind to the dorsal raphe nucleus in a manner similar to dihydroergotamine (DeKeyser et al., 1993), and focus projections to the trigeminal sensory complex and forebrain structures (Li et al., 1993), by altering signal-to-noise ratio.

Case Report

A 46-year-old married male Caucasian minister was seen for the first time in 1988 for feelings of intermittent fatigue, tingling all over, headaches, panic attacks, cognitive dysfunction, and numbness in both arms and his left leg. All of these symptoms were made worse by stress. He also had a tic disorder of his head. He complained of feeling weak in his calves and in his hands and triceps muscles, which were also painful. Physical examination revealed the typical tender points of fibromyalgia. The patient had received several orthopedic, immunologic, rheumatologic, and neurologic consultations. It had been projected that the patient might develop multiple sclerosis in later years. He continued to have paresthesias and dysesthesias in various parts of his body and diffuse myalgias and arthralgias. He had lost most of his sense of taste and had significant cognitive dysfunction, especially problems with short-term memory. He had also developed fasciculations, which were diffuse, and experienced intermittent flushing of his face. Laboratory results were essentially within normal limits except for elevated cholesterol and an increased cerebrospinal fluid immunoglobulin.

The patient also had intermittent chest pain and paresthesias in his right great toe and left calcaneal pain. Sometimes he was not able to walk because of the pain in his legs and feet. He had a problem with snoring but had no sleep apnea. He had no vocalizations with his tic. An MRI revealed some unidentified bright objects in the right parietal area but these were not distributed in the periventricular manner that would be consistent with multiple sclerosis.

As the years went on, his dysesthesias became more painful. His tics were partially controlled, first with calcium channel blockers and then with pimozide. These medications did not reduce his other symptoms, however. He had intermittent blurred vision that made it difficult for him to read, and sometimes he was unable to remember what he had said two minutes previously. He denied depression. He had nocturnal panic attacks and significant exertional intolerance. He had not responded to serotonin reuptake inhibitors, tricyclic antidepressants, clonazepam, hydralazine, nimodipine, pyridostigmine, clonidine, captopril, baclofen, mexiletine, felbamate, or nicotine patches. He had an excellent response to sublingual nitroglycerin, which unfortunately only lasted for about two months, after which he developed tolerance to the effect.

He had visual evoked responses that were normal. A repeat MRI of the brain was within normal limits in 1993.

Sometimes his feet became completely numb so that he was not able to feel them. There was a positive family history for peptic ulcer disease and the patient had peptic ulcer disease at age 21. He had been started on H-2 receptor antagonists. Once, in the middle of the night, he had a painful rigor at 3:00 a.m. while lying in bed. This lasted for about 30 minutes, after which he had myasthenia in his legs and was unable to walk. During this time he felt nauseated and had dysesthesias in his chest as well as left flank pain. These symptoms gradually resolved over the next 24 hours.

He stated that the amount of stress at his work place was not unusual. He complained of severe fatigue, was not able to function past noon, and required three- or four-hour naps. He was given a trial of risperidone, which did not help him, and naltrexone, which decreased his tic but made him feel "spacey." Nevertheless, he tried naltrexone at home but did not feel that the risk/benefit ratio was worth his taking it. He also tried tacrine, gabapentin, hydrochlorothiazide, ergoloid mesylates, pindolol, and spironolactone. His tic worsened. He reported that his right leg "gave out" frequently. A trial of colchicine for atypical multiple sclerosis was ineffective. He was given a trial of intramuscular oxytocin, which made his symptoms worse. This response has also occurred in some CFS patients with obsessive-compulsive disorder. A brain SPECT showed extensive bilateral frontotemporal hypoperfusion.

He received sumatriptan, which completely relieved all his symptoms except for his tic. He was seen again two months later, complaining that he had severe pain in his hands and feet, as well as his thighs, face, and calves. He he had burning dysesthesias and hot flashes. He could not hold a pen. Because he could not afford sumatriptan, he had discontinued taking it seven weeks before. He was given sumatriptan 6 mg subcutaneously and, again, all his symptoms resolved. Since he also had headaches that could be termed common migraines, he was enrolled in a postmarketing study of sumatriptan that enabled him to receive the medication at no charge. His symptomatic improvement has been maintained on twice-daily injections of the drug.

TETRAHYDROAMINOACRIDINE
OR TACRINE (COGNEX)

This drug has been approved for use in dementia, Alzheimer's type. It is a centrally acting cholinesterase inhibitor, increasing brain levels of acetylcholine, an important neurotransmitter. It works differently in CFS than the peripherally acting cholinesterase inhibitor, pyridostigmine (Mestinon). Tacrine is sometimes effective when pyridostigmine is not, and vice versa. Those who take the drug require bi-weekly monitoring of liver function tests. Tacrine blocks voltage-gated potassium, sodium, and calcium channels, and is structurally similar to 4-aminopyridine, a well-known potassium channel blocker (Vorobjev and Shanarova, 1994). Tacrine also reduces beta adrenoceptor linked adenylate cyclase activity in the aged brain (Vivas et al., 1995). Other agents useful in CFS also block potassium channels. These include gamma globulin (Abrahams and Sutter, 1994), dihydropyridine calcium channel blockers (Ellory et al., 1994), and 5-HT$_2$ agonists (Aghajanian, 1992). Tacrine also seems to block NMDA channels in the *open* state, prolonging NMDA response (Vorobjev and Shanarova, 1994). It is not clear what is the role of potassium channels in CFS, but they help to modulate cellular excitability (Swanson, 1993).

In order for excitable cells to be electrically active, charged ions must be distributed unequally between intracellular and extracellular compartments to produce the "resting membrane potential." A major process in producing this potential is sequestration of potassium (K) ions intracellularly. When K leaves the cell rapidly through K channels, the cell becomes hyperpolarized, or less excitable. When the rate of K efflux is sufficiently decreased the cell will be quite excitable and depolarize. Drugs that can further open or close existing channels can therefore have profound pharmacologic effects. Medications in use now, besides tacrine and gamma globulin, which block K channels, include sulfonylureas and the antiarrhythmic sotalol. Those that open potassium channels, e.g., cromakalim, pinacidil, and nicorandil, are in the pipeline for use as antihypertensive and antiasthma medications (Weston and Edwards, 1992). Research on CNS K channels has lagged behind those in peripheral tissues even though they are "ubiquitous" in the brain (Gehlert and Robertson, 1994).

There are three large families of K channels (Rudy, 1988). One is regulated by electrical transmission, a second by neurotransmitters and hormones linked to G proteins, and a third by ions such as calcium or by nucleotides such as ATP. K channel blockers should be useful in neurosomatic disorders because they produce membrane depolarization and release of neurotransmitters. There may even be an endogenous ligand for CNS K channels (Virsolvy-Vergine et. al., 1988). Conversely, K channel openers could be antiepileptic drugs. Carbamazepine is a possible example. Agonists and antagonists for CNS K channel subtypes are being developed for clinical use.

The K blocker tacrine also normalizes the lipid viscosity of brain synaptosomes and modulates sodium channels (Burov, 1994). Furthermore, tacrine increases hippocampal nitric oxide synthase activity in rats pretreated with lithium chloride, probably by ACh-esterase inhibition. It does not have this effect in the frontoparietal cortex, which has a relatively low concentration of NO synthase (Bagetta et al., 1993). Tacrine also can presynaptically inhibit glutamatergic transmission in the rat amygdala (Wang, Huang, and Gean, 1995).

Case Report

A 30-year-old married Caucasian female was well until five years before seeing me when she developed amoebic dysentery and giardiasis after white-water rafting. Although these parasitic infestations were appropriately treated she subsequently developed CFS and had to drop out of her doctoral program. By the time she saw me she had consulted 19 other health care professionals and was still disabled.

She had a history of endometriosis and interstitial cystitis. She did not benefit from multiple antidepressants, IV ascorbic acid, antifungals, or kutapressin. She had transient improvement after one dose of intravenous immunoglobulin but could not continue it due to the expense. She complained of multiple chemical sensitivities and a disorder of initiating and maintaining sleep (DIMS), for which she took oxazepam. She had a lifelong history of allergic rhinitis. All symptoms worsened after exposure to an "insect bomb" in her home two years prior to seeing me. Her mother had a probable cyclothymic disorder. Family and past medical history was otherwise noncontributory. Physical examination revealed 18 out of 18 of the characteristic fibromyalgia tender points.

She had moderate responses to naphazoline, nitroglycerin, and nimodipine, which increased her energy somewhat. Gabapentin 100 mg made her "much more alert" but she stated she felt too "speedy."

The next day she took 100 mg of gabapentin and then took hydralazine 25 mg, which eliminated her tender points. By this time she was up to 40 percent of her premorbid energy level, from 10 percent (she could barely walk). After tacrine 10 mg she stated, "I feel a lot better," and after 10 mg more reported that she felt the best she had in five years. She continued on this regimen and was planning to return to graduate school. She stated that tacrine, the most beneficial medication she tried, made her more alert, increased her energy, enhanced her "cognitive processing" and assimilation of information, and gave her a general feeling of well-being. I wonder whether the intravenous immunoglobulin, also a potassium channel blocker, helped her in a similar fashion.

VENLAFAXINE (EFFEXOR)

Marketed as the best thing since sliced bread, venlafaxine is approved for use in depression, especially treatment-resistant depression. Its adverse reaction profile is similar to that of the serotonin reuptake inhibitors (SRIs), except that it can raise blood pressure in certain patients and frequently causes nausea. As of this writing, venlafaxine has been only recently available, but I have been using it for over a year and see it only as another alternative treatment, rather than the most effective antidepressant. Since it can raise blood pressure, I prescribe the SRIs and bupropion (Wellbutrin) before venlafaxine. The drug blocks serotonin, norepinephrine, and dopamine reuptake, and is chemically unrelated to any other medication. Patients typically take two or more weeks to respond to venlafaxine. It is sometimes helpful to use risperidone and venlafaxine concomitantly. Initially, venlafaxine should be taken with meals in an 18.75 mg dose. Its most common adverse reaction, nausea, may be ameliorated by low-dose cisapride (Russell, personal communication, 1996). Venlafaxine has been reported to rapidly resolve panic disorder at low doses (Geracioti, 1995), an effect which I have never seen in my patient population, even though FMS is related to panic disorder (Tanum and Malt, 1995). It may also be effective in attention deficit disorder (Findling et al., 1996).

A CLOSING NOTE

Finally, if alpha-adrenergic eyedrops help a patient to feel better, they will also alleviate panic attacks (if the patient has them). Panic disorder is commonly diagnosed in CFS patients. The eyedrops are effective in a few seconds and are not addictive, although tolerance may develop to this effect. Anti-panic eyedrops should be a helpful addition to the therapeutic armamentarium. I believe that many of the new treatments I have described for CFS are effective in treatment-resistant cases of other neurosomatic disorders.

Conclusion

. . . that the comprehensive understanding of the human mind requires an organismic perspective; that not only must the mind move from a nonphysical cogitum to the realm of biological tissue, but it must also be related to a whole organism possessed of integrated body proper and brain fully interactive with a physical and social environment.

–Antonio R. Damasio
Descartes' Error (1994)

What new ideas have I proposed in this book? The most important one is that the broad spectrum of disorders of central information processing that I term "neurosomatic" can be explained on a neurologic basis. Viewing them as limbic dysfunction, which is still correct, is too provincial; they are dysregulations of widely distributed neural networks that use parallel computational strategy.

The large majority of neurosomatic patients do not have structural deficits, but appear to have problems with regulation of receptors, and probably post-receptor messengers. A corollary to this statement is that a full complement of gene products are still expressed, but perhaps in abnormal amounts. The genes affected may be those that influence the capacity for neural plasticity, i.e., alterations in receptor-coupled signal transduction pathways that modulate the adaptive capabilities of neurons and, hence, neuronal networks.

Neurosomatic disorders are usually state-dependent. They commonly wax and wane in severity and thus may be amenable to rapidly acting therapeutic agents, as opposed to drugs such as antidepressants, which probably act by altering gene regulation and manufacture of proteins. Such a mechanism would explain their prolonged latent period of effect. Treating neurosomatic disorders seems to be a matter of pushing the right neurochemical button.

Patients who have been sick for twenty years can feel normal in a few minutes. Patients who have been completely refractory to fifty medications can feel better with the fifty-first. Patients whose symptoms do not wax and wane may have structural lesions and/or genetic dysfunctions that are not amenable to rapid remediation, even if they are not apparent on structured brain imaging or currently available laboratory tests. These patients tend to respond poorly to rapidly acting treatments on my neurosomatic protocol but may improve with antidepressants. Therapy may alter expression of one gene, or compensate for a genetically, developmentally, or environmentally impaired pathway by altering the function of other signal transduction pathways. The most effective medications are nimodipine, baclofen, gabapentin, oxytocin, and intravenous lidocaine; this latter treatment is perhaps the most efficacious of all.

A central noradrenergic deficit appears likely, perhaps accompanied by a neuropeptide Y and an oxytocin deficiency. This deficit is worsened by activities which may exacerbate symptoms, such as exercise, sustained attention, ejaculation, infection, and vaccination. Noradrenergic denervation hypersensitivity is easily demonstrated by instilling a 0.05 percent or less solution of topical tropicamide into the conjunctival sac and performing pupillometry, which differentiates patients from controls although there is some overlap. The noradrenergic deficit is global, since reduction in post-treatment regional cerebral blood flow is diffuse. The role of endothelin in this process remains obscure to me as of this writing, although it is tempting to postulate that endothelin is responsible for symptoms related to baseline decreases in rCBF, as well as those induced by various stressors, which usually further decrease cerebral perfusion. Endothelin stimulates the secretion of substance P, and both peptides are elevated in the CSF of FMS patients. Substance P levels tend to have an inverse relationship with norepinephrine, in part (or entirely) as a result of neuronal competition for nerve growth factor (Davis, Albers et al., 1994). Substance P widens receptive fields, which may be an aspect of neurosomatic pathophysiology, and could neurochemically explain the evolution of fibromyalgia from a regional myofascial pain syndrome. Substance P also decreases the signal-noise ratio of sensory input, perhaps a desirable outcome in certain hypervigilant states, but maladaptive under ordinary conditions. The mechanism of reduction of rCBF after exercise may relate to dysregulation of the vascular response to hyperventilation. The core neurochemical deficit, however, may be that of reduced excitatory amino acid secretion from the prefrontal cortex causing hyposecretion of biogenic amines and possibly acetylcholine. Structural defects on a microscopic level may occur in mesencephalic neurosecretory nuclei as well as in the hippocampus and in corticothalamic projections.

The role of the thalamic reticular nucleus in the pathophysiology of neurosomatic disorders has not been previously considered, as far as I can tell. Its role in coordination of thalamic information has just recently been elucidated, and the function of the dense corticothalamic projections are still not understood. Indeed, the reason why there is a thalamus at all is not apparent to many thalamic researchers.

The importance of cortico-striatal-thalamico-cortical loops in the pathophysiology of neurosomatic disorders cannot be denied. These complex feedforward and feedback systems modulate numerous non-motor functions. The case of the physician with parkinsonian dyskinesia who had marked contralateral relief of his fibromyalgia after pallidotomy is so striking as to be a landmark. The role of the basal ganglia in pain modulation and other sensory gating functions is of extreme importance, a fact little recognized until recently.

The confluence of genetic and developmental influences creating a predisposition for response to diverse environmental triggering agents in the etiology of neurosomatic disorders should be quite apparent. Patients with neurosomatic disorders have an impaired ability to make the appropriate adaptive response to a stimulus situation due to improper sensory gating, which may be related to a defect in the regulation of normal gene products that produce abnormal neural plasticity and adaptability. In this paradigm the distinction between "mental" and "physical" causation is virtually meaningless, and the unprovable nature of most psychoanalytic constructs is highlighted. I am reminded of a two-week period during my medical student psychiatry rotation when I was able to discuss every patient in the context of his/her having an oral impregnation fantasy. It took quite a while for my supervisors to realize that I was parodying the illusory certainty that contemporary psychiatric thinking provided. Scientifically generated hypothesis testing is much more rational and measurable, and more beneficial to patients. Cognitive-behavioral therapy can be a useful aspect of neurosomatic treatment.

It has been of great interest to me that medications that do not cross the blood-brain barrier can still have a marked effect on CNS function. Although this principle has been obvious for years in the literature, many researchers and clinicians still do not appreciate how profoundly the brain can be modulated by molecules acting at the level of peripheral nerves, autonomic ganglia, or circumventricular organs. Acupuncture also has this mode of action.

Most neurosomatic patients can be markedly improved in a short time with medications that have a good risk/benefit ratio and act by increasing central levels of norepinephrine in various ways thus raising signal-to-noise ratio of sensory input, perhaps the primary deficit in neurosomatic disorders. Some drugs, e.g., lidocaine, also decrease substance P. Neural plasticity can be enhanced by increasing secretion of glutamate, with resultant modulation of retrograde messengers such as nitric oxide. In this era of cost containment in health care, when often the bottom line seems more important than clinical outcome, the paradigms and treatment techniques described in this book make financial sense as well as being scientifically and ethically reasonable. It is extremely gratifying for me to apply what I learn to making low-cost "miracles" (as they are often called by patients) occur every day. I look forward to the time when all physicians will do the same.

References

Abrahams Z, Sutter MC. (1994) Effects of K^+ channel openers on the vascular actions of human gamma globulin. *Eur J Pharmacol* 252: 195-203.

Adams ML, Kalick JM, Meyer ER, Ciccro TJ. (1993) Inhibition of the morphine withdrawal syndrome by a nitric oxide synthase inhibitor N^G-nitro-L-arginine methyl ester. *Life Sci* 52: PL 245-249.

Aghajanian GK. (1992) Central 5-HT receptor subtypes: Physiological responses and signal transduction mechanisms. In Marsden CA, Heal DJ (Eds.), *Central Serotonin Receptors and Psychotropic Drugs* (pp. 116-143). London: Blackwell Scientific Publications.

Alborch E, Salom JB, Perales AJ, Torregrosa G, Miranda FJ, Alabadi JA, Jover T. (1992) Comparison of the anticonstrictor action of dihydropyridines (nimodipine and nicardipine) and Mg^{++} in isolated human cerebral arteries. *Eur J Pharmacol* 229(1): 83-89.

Alexander GE, Crutcher MD. (1990) Functional architecture of basal ganglia circuits: Neural substrates of parallel processing. *Trends Neurosci* 13: 266-271.

Alexander RW, Mountz JM, Mountz JD, Triana M, Aaron LA, Alarcon GS, Bradley LA, Martin M, Alberts K, Stewart KE. (1994) SPECT imaging of caudate nucleus (CN) regional cerebral blood flow (rCBF): A sensitive physiological marker of fibromyalgia (FM). *Arth Rheum* 37(9): S346.

Alreja M, Liu W. (1995) Norepinephrine excites septohippocampal GABAergic neurons via alpha-1 adrenoceptors. *Abstracts, Soc for Neurosci* 21: 44.4, p. 94.

Altemus M, Swedo SE, Leonard HL, Richter D, Rubinow DR, Potter WZ, Rapoport JL. (1994) Changes in cerebrospinal fluid neurochemistry during treatment of obsessive-compulsive disorder with clomipramine. *Arch Gen Psychiatry* 51: 794-803.

Altman J. (1995) Deciding what to do next. *Trends Neurosci* 18: 117-118.

Altura BM, Altura BT. (1984) Actions of vasopressin, oxytocin and synthetic analogs on vascular smooth muscle. *Fed Proc* 43: 80-86.

Alvarez XA, Franco A, Fernandez-Novoa L, Cacabelos R. (1993) Effects of neurotoxic lesions in histaminergic neurons on behavior and brain cytokines. *Neuropsychopharmacol* 9(2S): 164S.

Amabeoku GJ, Chikuni O. (1993) Cimetidine-induced seizures in mice: Antagonism by some GABAergic agents. *Biochem Pharmacol* 46(12): 2171-2175.

Amico JA, Schallinor SM, Cameron JL. (1990) Pattern of oxytocin concentrations in the plasma and cerebrospinal fluid of lactating rhesus monkeys (Mascaca mulatta): Evidence for functionally independent oxytocinergic pathways in primates. *J Clin Endocrinol Metab* 71: 1531-1535.

Andreasen NC, Arndt S, Swayze V, Cizadlo T, Flaum M, O'Leary D, Ehrhardt JC, Yuh WTC. (1994) Thalamic abnormalities in schizophrenia visualized through magnetic resonance average imaging. *Science* 266: 294-298.

Angulo JA, McEwen BS. (1994) Molecular aspects of neuropeptide regulation and function in the corpus striatum and nucleus accumbens. *Brain Res Rev* 19: 1-28.

Argiolas A, Gessa GL. (1991) Central functions of oxytocin. *Neurosci Biobehav Rev* 15(2): 217-231.

Argiolas A, Melis MR, Stancampiano R. (1993) Role of central oxytocinergic pathways in the expression of penile erection. *Regul Pep* 45: 139-142.

Arletti R, Bertolini A. (1987) Oxytocin acts as an antidepressant in two animal models of depression. *Life Sci* 41: 1725-1730.

Arletti R, Benelli A, Bertolini A. (1992) Oxytocin involvement in male and female sexual behaviors. In Pedersen CA, Caldwell JD, Jirkouoski GF, Fasel TR (Eds.), *Oxytocin in Maternal, Sexual and Social Behaviors–Annals of the New York Academy of Science* (pp. 180-193). New York: The New York Academy of Sciences.

Arnsten AFT, Cai JX, Goldman-Rakic PS. (1988) The alpha-2 adrenergic agonist guanfacine improves memory in aged monkeys without sedative or hypotensive side effects. *J Neurosci* 8: 4287-4298.

Artigas F, Perez V, Alvarez E. (1994) Pindolol induces a rapid improvement of depressed patients treated with serotonin reuptake inhibitors. *Arch Gen Psychiatry* 51: 248-251.

Arvat E, Cappa M, Casanueva FF, Dieguez C, Ghigo E, Nicolosi M, Valcavi R, Zini M. (1993) Pyridostigmine potentiates growth hormone (GH)-releasing hormone-induced GH release in both men and women. *J Clin Endocrinol Metab* 76(2): 374-377.

Aston-Jones GA, Akaoka H, Charlety P, Chowet G. (1991) Serotonin selectively attenuates glutamate-evoked activation of noradrenergic locus coeruleus neurons. *J Neurosci* 11(3): 760-769.

Autret E, Mercier C, Marimbu J. (1984) Convulsion and cimetidine. *Arch Fr Paediatr* 41: 729.

Azmitia EC, Whitaker-Azmitia PM. (1991) Awakening the sleeping giant: Anatomy and plasticity of the brain serotonergic system. *J Clin Psychiatry* 52(12/suppl.): 4-16.

Azmitia EC, Kramer HK, Kim-Pak WK. (1993) Nimodipine blocks the efflux of $^{45}Ca^{2+}$ and enhances the depolarization-induced release of $[^{3}H]$5-HT from CNS synaptosomes. In Scriabine A, Janis RA, Triggle DJ (Eds.), *Drugs in Development* (vol. 2: Ca^{2+} Antagonists in the CNS, pp. 407-415). Brandford, Connecticut: Neva Press.

Babey A-M, Kolesnikov Y, Cheng J, Intorrisi CE, Trifilletti RR, Pasterna KGW. (1994) Nitric oxide and opioid tolerance. *Neuropharmacol* 35: 1463-1470.

Bach-y-Rita P. (1993a) Neurotransmission in the brain by diffusion through the extracellular fluid: A review. *NeuroReport* 4: 343-350.

Bach-y-Rita P. (1993b) Nonsynaptic diffusion neurotransmission (NDN) in the brain. *Neurochem Int* 23(4): 297-318.

Backonja M, Miletic V. (1991) Responses of neurons in the rat ventrolateral orbital cortex to phasic and tonic nociceptive stimulation. *Brain Res* 557: 353-355.

Bacon NM, Bacon SF, Atkinson JW, Slater MA, Patterson TL, Grant I, Garfin SR. (1994) Somatization symptoms in chronic low back pain patients. *Psychosom Med* 56(22): 118-127.

Bacon SJ, Smith AD. (1993) A monosynaptic pathway from an identified vasomotor centre in the medial prefrontal cortex to an autonomic area in the thoracic spinal cord. *Neurosci* 54(3): 719-728.

Bagaev VA, Panteleev SS. (1994) Limbic cortical influences to the vagal input neurones of the solitary tract nucleus. *NeuroReport* 5(148): 1705-1708.

Bagdy G, Makara GB. (1994) Hypothalamic paraventricular nucleus lesions differentially affect serotonin-1A (5-HT$_{1A}$) and 5-HT$_2$ receptor agonist-induced oxytocin, prolactin, and corticosterone responses. *Endocrinol* 134: 1127- 1131.

Bagetta G, Massoud R, Rodino P, Federici G, Nistico G. (1993) Systemic administration of lithium chloride and tacrine increases nitric oxide synthase activity in the hippocampus of rats. *Eur J Pharmacol* 237: 61-64.

Bakheit AMO, Behan PO, Watson WS, Morton JJ. (1993) Abnormal arginine-vasopressin secretion and water metabolism in patients with postviral fatigue syndrome. *Acta Neurol Scand* 87: 234-238.

Bakhle YS, Bell C. (1994) Increased number of substance P-containing sensory neurons in a rat strain with a genetic neurotrophic defect. *Neuropep* 27: 169-174.

Balster RL. (1994) Behavioral effects of glycine-site NMDA antagonists. *Neuropsychopharmacol* 10(3S/Pt.1): 100S.

Barinaga M. (1992) Playing "telephone" with the body's message of pain. *Science* 258: 1085.

Barinaga M. (1994) To sleep, perchance to . . . learn? New studies say yes. *Science* 265: 603-604.

Barinaga M. (1996) The cerebellum: Movement coordinator or much more? *Science* 272: 482-483.

Barsky AJ, Barnett MC, Cleary PD. (1994) Hypochondriasis and panic disorder: Boundary and overlap. *Arch Gen Psychiatry* 51: 918-925.

Bartus RT, Levere TE. (1977) Functional decortication in rhesus monkeys: A test of the interference hypothesis. *Brain Res* 119: 233-249.

Bauman WA, Spungen AM, Zhong Y-G, Tsitouras PD. (1994) Chronic baclofen therapy improves the blunted growth hormone response to intravenous arginine in subjects with spinal cord injury. *J Clin Endocrinol Metab* 78: 1135-1138.

Baumeister AA. (1991) The effects of bilateral intranigral microinjection of selective opioid agonists on behavioral responses to noxious thermal stimuli. *Brain Res* 557: 136-145.

Baumeister AA, Anticich TG, Hawkins MF, Liter JC, Thibodeaux HF, Guillory EC. (1988) Evidence that the substantia nigra is a component of the endogenous pain suppression system in the rat. *Brain Res* 447: 116-121.

Baumeister AA, Hawkins MF, Anderson-Moore LL, Anticich TG, Higgins TD, Griffin P. (1988) Effects of bilateral injection of GABA into the substantia nigra on spontaneous behavior and measures of analgesia. *Neuropharmacol* 27: 817-821.

Baxter LR, Schwartz JM, Bergman KS, Szuba MP, Guze BH, Mazziotta JC, Alazraki A, Selin CE, Ferng H-K, Munford P, Phelps ME. (1992) Caudate glucose metabolic rate changes with drug and behavior therapy for obsessive-compulsive disorder. *Arch Gen Psychiatry* 49: 681-689.

Beal JE, Olson R, Laubenstein L, Morales JO, Bellman P, Yangco B, Lefkowitz L, Plasse TF, Shepard KV. (1995) Dronabinol as a treatment for anorexia associated with weight loss in patients with AIDS. *J Pain Symptom Manage* 10(2): 89-97.

Bear MF, Kirkwood A. (1993) Neocortical long-term potentiation. *Curr Opin Neurobiol* 3: 197-202.

Bearn J, Wessely S. (1994) Neurobiological aspects of the chronic fatigue syndrome. *Eur J Clin Invest* 24: 79-90.

Beauclair L, Vinogradov S, Riney SJ, Czernansky JG, Hollister LE. (1987) An adjunctive role for ascorbic acid in the treatment of schizophrenia? *J Clin Psychopharmacol* 7: 282-283.

Beck AT. (1978) *Depression*. Philadelphia: University of Pennsylvania Press.

Beck AT. (1979) *Cognitive Therapy of Depression*. New York: Guilford Press.

Bekkers JM. (1993) Enhancement by histamine of NMDA-mediated synaptic transmission in the hippocampus. *Science* 261: 104-107.

Bell KM, Widmark C, DeMet E, Milne N. (1994) SPECT Diamox response augmented in cocaine dependent patients. *Biol Psychiatry* 35: 683.

Benington JH, Heller HC. (1995) Restoration of brain energy metabolism as the function of sleep. *Prog Neurobiol* 45(4): 347-360.

Benjamin J, Levine J, Fux M, Aviv A, Levy D, Belmaker RH. (1995) Double-blind, placebo-controlled, crossover trial of inositol treatment for panic disorder. *Am J Psychiatry* 152: 1084-1086.

Bennett GJ, Kajander KC, Schera Y, Iadaroza MJ, Sugimoto T. (1989) Neurochemical and anatomical changes in the dorsal horn of rats with an experimental painful peripheral neuropathy. In Cervaro F, Bennett GJ, Headley DM (Eds.), *Processing of Sensory Information in the Superficial Dorsal Horn of the Spinal Cord* (pp. 463-471). New York: Plenum.

Bennett RM, Clark SR, Campbell SM, Burckhardt CS. (1992) Low levels of somatomedin C in patients with the fibromyalgia syndrome: A possible link between sleep and muscle pain. *Arth Rheum* 35: 1113-1116.

Benson DF. (1993) Prefrontal abilities. *Behav Neurol* 6: 75-81.

Benton D, Owens DA. (1993) Blood glucose and human memory. *Psychopharmacol* 113: 83-88.

Bergen DC, Ristanovic RK, Waicosky K, Kanner A, Hoeppner TJ. (1995) Weight loss in patients taking felbamate. *Clin Neuropharmacol* 18(1): 23-27.

Berridge CW, Arnsten AFT, Foote SL. (1993) Noradrenergic modulation of cognitive function: Clinical implications of anatomical, electrophysiological, and behavioural studies in animal models. *Psychol Med* 23: 557-564.

Bickford PC, Luntz-Leybman V, Freedman F. (1993) Auditory sensory gating in the rat hippocampus: Modulation by brainstem activity. *Brain Res* 607: 33-38.

Biello SM, Janik D, Mrosovsky N. (1994) Neuropeptide Y and behaviorally induced phase shifts. *Neurosci* 62(1): 273-279.

Billiard M, Besset A, Montplaisir J, Laffont F, Goldenberg F, Weill JS, Lubin S. (1994) Modafinil: A double-blind multicentric study. *Sleep* 17: S107-S112.

Bittiger H, Froestl W, Mickel SJ, Olpe H-R. (1993) GABA$_B$ receptor antagonists: From synthesis to therapeutic applications. *Trends Pharmacol Sci* 14: 391-393.

Blandini F, Greenamyre JT. (1995) Effect of subthalamic nucleus lesion on mitochondrial enzyme activity in the rat basal ganglia. *Brain Res* 669: 59-66.

Bloedel JR. (1993) "Involvement in" versus "storage of." *Trends Neurosci* 16(11): 451-452.

Bohus B, Kovacs G, de Wied D. (1978) Oxytocin, vasopressin, and memory: Opposite effects on consolidation and retrieval processes. *Brain Res* 157: 414-417.

Bolwig TG. (1994) ECS induces synaptic remodeling and increases synthesis of neuropeptide Y in rat limbic system. *Neuropsychopharmacol* 10(3S/Pt.1): 566S.

Bonneau RH, Sheridan JF, Feng N, Glaser R. (1993) Stress-induced modulation of the primary cellular immune response to herpes simplex virus infection is mediated by both adrenal-dependent and independent mechanisms. *J Neuroimmunol* 42: 167-176.

Bonnin A, Ramos JA, deFonseca FR, Ceveira M, Fernandez-Ruiz JJ. (1993) Acute effects of Δ^9-tetrahydrocannabinol on tuberoinfundibular dopamine activity, anterior pituitary sensitivity to dopamine and prolactin release vary as a function of estrous cycle. *Neuroendocrinol* 58: 280-286.

Bouzamondo E, Ladogana A, Tsiang H. (1993) Alteration of potassium-evoked 5-HT release from virus-infected rat cortical synaptosomes. *NeuroReport* 4: 555-558.

Bowery N. (1990) GABA$_B$ receptors and their significance in mammalian pharmacology. *Trends Pharmacol Sci* 10: 401-407.

Bowman ES. (1993) Etiology and clinical course of pseudoseizures: Relationship to trauma, depression, and dissociation. *Psychosom Med* 34(4): 333-340.

Bradette M, Delvaus M, Staumont G, Fioramonti J, Bueno L, Frexinos J. (1994) Octreotide increases thresholds of colonic visceral perception in IBS patients without modifying muscle tone. *Dig Dis Sci* 39(6): 1171-1178.

Brady LS. (1994) Stress, antidepressant drugs, and the locus coeruleus. *Brain Res Bull* 35: 545-556.

Brandli P, Loffler B-M, Breu V, Osterwalder R, Maire J-P, Clozel M. (1996) Role of endothelin in mediating neurogenic plasma extravasation in rat dura matter. *Pain* 64: 315-322.

Breiter HC, Seidman LJ, Goodman JM, Goldstein JM, O'Craven KM, Weisskoff RM, Woodruff PRW, Savoy R, Jiang A, Kennedy D, Kennedy W, Tsuang MT, Rosen BR. (1995) Functional MRI of auditory effortful attention in humans. *Abstracts, Soc for Neurosci* 21: 229.9, p. 1988.

Bremner JD, Randall P, Scott TM, Bronen RA, Seibyl JP, Southwick SM, Delaney RC, McCarthy G, Charney DS, Innis RB.

(1995) MRI-based measurements of hippocampal volume in patients with combat-related post-traumatic stress disorder. *Am J Psychiatry* 152: 973-981.

Breneman SM, Moynihan JA, Grota LJ, Felten DL, Felten SY. (1993) Splenic norepinephrine is decreased in MRL-1pr/1pr mice. *Brain Behav Immun* 7(2): 135-143.

Brenneman DE, Schultzberg M, Bartgai T, Gozes I. (1992) Cytokine regulation of neuronal survival. *J Neurochem* 58: 454-460.

Breslow MF, Fankhauser MP, Potter RL, Meredith KE, Misiaszek J, Hope DG. (1989) Role of gamma-aminobutyric acid in antipanic drug efficacy. *Am J Psychiatry* 146: 353-356.

Brown HD, Kosslyn SM. (1993) Cerebral lateralization. *Curr Opin Neurobiol* 3:183-186.

Bubser M, Koch M. (1994) Prepulse inhibition of the acoustic startle response of rats is reduced by 6-hydroxydopamine lesions of the medial prefrontal cortex. *Psychopharmacol* 113: 487-492.

Bull PM, Douglas AJ, Russell JA. (1994) Opioids and the coupling of the anterior peri-third ventricular input to oxytocin neurons in anaesthetized pregnant rats. *J Neuroendocrinol* 6: 267-274.

Burnet RB, Radden HS, Easterbrook EG, McKinnon RA. (1991) Premenstrual syndrome and spironolactone. *Aust NZ J Obstet Gynaecol* 31(4): 366-368.

Burov Y. (1994) New generation of drugs to treat dementia on the basis of tacrine and amiridine. *Neuropsychopharmacol* 10(3S/Pt.1): 669S.

Burstein R, Borsook D, Strassman A. (1993) The trigeminohypothalamic tract (THT): Properties of nociceptive trigeminal neurons that project directly to the hypothalamus. *Abstracts, 7th World Congress on Pain* (p. 258). Seattle: IASP Publications.

Buzy J, Brenneman DE, Pert CB, Martin A, Salazar A, Ruff MR. (1992) Potent gp120-like neurotoxic activity in the cerebrospinal fluid of HIV-infected individuals is blocked by peptide T. *Brain Res* 598(1-2): 10-18.

Calignano A, Persico P, Mancuso F, Sorrentino L. (1993) Endogenous nitric oxide modulates morphine-induced changes in locomotion and food intake in mice. *Eur J Pharmacol* 231: 415-419.

Calogero AE, Gallucci WT, Chrousos GP, Gold PW. (1988) Interaction between GABAergic neurotransmission and rat hypothalamic corticotropin-releasing hormone in vitro. *Brain Res* 463(1): 28-36.

Calogero AE, Kling MA, Gallucci WT, Bernardini R, Chrousos GP, Gold PW. (1990) Procaine and lidocaine stimulate corticotropin-releasing hormone secretion by explanted rat hypothalami through a sodium conductance-independent mechanism. *Horm Metab Res* 22(1): 25-28.

Cantello R, Aguaggia M, Gilli M, Deseldine M, Cutin I, Riccio A. (1989) Major depression in Parkinson's disease and the mood response to intravenous methylphenidate: Possible role of the "hedonic" dopamine synapse. *J Neurol Neurosurg Psychiatry* 52: 724-731.

Cardinal DP, Esquifino AI, Arce A, Vara E, Ariznavaretta C, Tresguerres JAF. (1994) Changes in serum growth hormone and prolactin levels, and in hypothalamic growth hormone-releasing hormone, thyrotropin-releasing hormone and somatostatin content, after superior cervical sympathectomy in rats. *Neuroendocrinol* 59: 42-48.

Carelli RM, West MO. (1991) Representation of the body by single neurons in the dorsolateral striatum of the awake, unrestrained rat. *J Comp Neurol* 309: 231-249.

Carlson SL, Albers KM, Beiting DJ, Parish M, Conner JM, Davis BD. (1995) NGF modulates sympathetic innervation of lymphoid tissues. *Abstracts, Soc for Neurosci* 21: 814.7, p. 2072.

Carpenter DO, Hubbard JH, Humphrey DR, Thompson HK, Marshall WH. (1972) Carbon dioxide effects on nerve cell function. In Nahag G, Schafer KE (Eds.), *Carbon Dioxide and Metabolic Regulation.* Heidelberg: Springer.

Cascella NG, Macciardi F, Cavallini C, Smeraldi E. (1994) D-Cycloserine adjuvant therapy to conventional neuroleptic treatment in schizophrenia: An open-label study. *J Neural Transm* 95: 105-111.

Castellano C, McGaugh JL. (1991) Oxotremorine attenuates retrograde amnesia induced by post-training administration of the GABAergic agonists muscimol and baclofen. *Behav Neural Biol* 56(1): 25-31.

Cesaro P, Nguyen-Legros J, Berger B, Alvarez C, Albe-Fessard D. (1979) Double labelling of branched neurons in the central nervous system of the rat by retrograde axonal transport of horseradish peroxidase and iron dextran complex. *Neurosci Lett* 15: 1-7.

Chan JYH, Tsuo M-Y, Len W-B, Lee T-Y, Chan SHH. (1995) Participation of noradrenergic neurotransmission in the enhancement of baroreceptor reflex response by substance P at the nucleus tractus solitarii of the rat: A reverse microdialysis study. *J Neurochem* 64: 2644-2652.

Chao CC, Jannoff EN, Hu S, Thomas K, Gallagher M, Tsong M, Peterson PK. (1991) Altered cytokine release in peripheral blood mononuclear cell cultures from patients with the chronic fatigue syndrome. *Cytokine* 3(4): 292-298.

Chao LL, Knight RT. (1995) Human prefrontal cortex gates distracting sensory input. *Abstracts, Soc for Neurosci* 21: 476.1, p. 1212.

Chave S, Kushikata T, Ohkawa H, Ishiara H, Grimand D, Matsuki A. (1996) Effects of two volatile anesthetics (sepoflurane and halothane) on the hypothalamic noradrenaline release in rat brain. *Brain Res* 706: 293-296.

Chavkin C. (1990) The sigma enigma: Biochemical and functional correlates emerge for the haloperidol-sensitive sigma binding site. *Trends Pharmacol Sci* 11: 213-215.

Chen N-H, Reith MEA. (1994) Effects of locally applied cocaine, lidocaine, and various uptake blockers on monoamine transmission in the ventral tegmental area of freely moving rats: A microdialysis study on monoamine interrelationships. *J Neurochem* 63(5): 1701-1713.

Chen X, Pozo MA, Gallar J, Belmonte C. (1993) Response of corneal nociceptors to CO_2: Blockade by calcium antagonists. *Abstracts, 7th World Congress on Pain* (p. 47). Seattle: IASP Publications.

Chibasaki T, Imaki T, Hotta M, Ling N, Demura H. (1993) Psychological stress increases arousal through brain corticotropin-releasing hormone without significant increase in adrenocorticotropin and catecholamine secretion. *Brain Res* 618: 71-75.

Chudler EH, Dong WK. (1995) The role of the basal ganglia in nociception and pain. *Pain* 60: 3-38.

Clapham J, Kilpatrick GJ. (1994) Thioperamide, the selective H_3 receptor antagonist, attenuates stimulant-induced locomotor activity in the mouse. *Eur J Pharmacol* 259: 107-114.

Clarke AS, Kammerer CM, George KP, Kupfer DJ, McKinney WT, Spence MA, Kraemer GW. (1995) Evidence for heritability of biogenic amine levels in the cerebrospinal fluid of rhesus monkeys. *Biol Psychiatry* 38: 572-577.

Clauw DJ, Schmidt M, Sabot M, Gaumund E, Radulovic D, Katz P, Barbniuk JC. (1994) The role of neuropeptides in fibromyalgia. *Proc Amer Assoc Chr Fatigue*, Fort Lauderdale, Florida, October 7-9.

Cleare AJ, Bearn J, Allain T, McGregor A, Wessely S, Murray RM, O'Keane V. (1995) Contrasting neuroendocrine responses in depression and chronic fatigue syndrome. *J Aff Dis* 35: 283-289.

Clouse RE. (1994) Antidepressants for functional gastrointestinal symptoms. *Dig Dis Sci* 39(11): 2352-2363.

Clouse RE, Lusthan PJ, Geisman RA, Alpers DH. (1994) Antidepressant therapy in 138 patients with irritable bowel syndrome: A five-year clinical experience. *Aliment Pharmacol Ther* 8(4): 409-416.

Coderre TJ, Katz J, Vaccarino AL, Melzack R. (1993) Contribution of central neuroplasticity to pathological pain: Review of clinical and experimental evidence. *Pain* 52(3): 259-286.

Cook EH, Metz J, Leventhal BL, Lebovitz M, Nathan M, Semerdjian SA, Brown T, Cooper MD. (1994) Fluoxetine effects on cerebral glucose metabolism. *NeuroReport* 5: 1745-1748.

Cooper JR, Bloom PE, Roth RH. (1982) *The Biochemical Basis of Neuropharmacology.* New York: Oxford University Press.

Cope H, David A, Mann A. (1994) "Maybe it's a virus": Beliefs about viruses, symptom attributional style and psychological health. *J Psychosom Res* 38(2): 89-98.

Coplan J, Pine D, Goetz R, Rosenblum L, Papp L, Klein D, Gorman J. (1994) Monoamine and HPA function in panic: Clinical and preclinical approaches. *Neuropsychopharmacol* 10(3S/Pt.1): 218S.

Coplan JD, Pine D, Papp L, Martinez J, Cooper T, Rosenblum LA, Gorman JM. (1995) Uncoupling of the noradrenergic-hypothalamic-pituitary-adrenal axis in panic disorder patients. *Neuropsychopharmacol* 13: 65-73.

Coplan JD, Sharma T, Rosenblum LA, Friedman S, Bassoff TB, Barbour RL, Gorman JM. (1992) Effects of sodium lactate infusion on cisternal lactate and carbon dioxide levels in nonhuman primates. *Am J Psychiatry* 149(10): 1369-1373.

Covenas R, DeLeon M, Chadi G, Cintra A, Gustafsson J-A, Marvaez JA, Fuxe K. (1994) Adrenalectomy increases the number of substance P and somatostatin immunoreactive nerve cells in the rat lumbar dorsal root ganglia. *Brain Res* 680: 325-356.

Crabtree JW, Killackey HP. (1989) The topographic organization and axis of projection within the visual sector of the rabbit thalamic reticular nucleus. *Eur J Neurosci* 1: 94-109.

Cramer H, Just S, Reuner C, Milios E, Geiger J, Mundinger F. (1991) Ventricular fluid neuropeptides in Parkinson's disease. II. Levels of substance P-like immunoreactivity. *Neuropep* 18: 69-73.

Crick F. (1984) Function of the thalamic reticular complex: The searchlight. *Proc Natl Acad Sci USA* 81: 4586-4590.

Crofford LJ, Pillemer SR, Kalogeras KT, Cash JM, Michelson D, Kling MA, Sternberg EM, Gold PW, Chrousos GP, Wilder RL. (1994) Hypothalamic-pituitary-adrenal axis perturbations in patients with fibromyalgia. *Arth Rheum* 37: 1583-1592.

Cuesta MC, Suarez-Roca J, Arcavo JL, Gomez G, Cano G, Enriquez R, Bonilla E, Maixner W. (1995) Glutamate inhibits substance P release from trigeminal nucleus caudalis capsaicin-sensitive primary afferents. *Abstracts, Soc for Neurosci* 21: 554.9, p. 1413.

Cummings JL. (1994) Frontal-subcortical dysfunction and neuropsychiatric illness. *J Neuropsychiatry Clin Neurosci* 6: 299.

Curtis AL, Valentino RJ. (1994) Corticotropin-releasing factor neurotransmission in locus coeruleus: A possible site of antidepressant action. *Brain Res Bull* 35: 581-587.

Dall'olio R, Rimondini R, Gandolfi O. (1994) The NMDA positive modulator D-Cycloserine inhibits dopamine-mediated behaviors in the rat. *Neuropharmacol* 33(1): 55-59.

Dalterio SL, Michael SK, MacMillan BT, Bartke A. (1981) Differential effects of cannabinoid exposure and stress on plasma prolactin, growth hormone and corticosterone levels in male mice. *Life Sci* 28: 761-765.

Damasio AR. (1994) *Descartes' Error: Emotion, Reason, and the Human Brain.* New York: GP Putnam.

Damasio H, Grabowski T, Frank R, Galaburda AM, Damasio AR. (1994) The return of Phineas Gage: Clues about the brain from the skull of a famous patient. *Science* 264: 1102-1105.

Daum I, Ackerman. (1995) Cerebellar contributions to cognition. *Behav Brain Res* 67(2): 201-210.

Davis BJ, Aul EA, Granner MA, Rodnitzky RL. (1994) Ranitidine-induced cranial dystonia. *Clin Neuropharmacol* 17(5): 489-491.

Davis BM, Albers KM, Seroogy KB, Katz DM. (1994) Overexpression of nerve growth factor in transgenic mice induces novel sympathetic projections to primary sensory neurons. *J Comp Neurol* 349: 464-474.

Davis KD, Tasker RR, Kiss ZHT, Hutchinson WD, Dostrovsky JO. (1995) Visceral pain evoked by thalamic microstimulation in humans. *NeuroReport* 6: 369-374.

Davis KI, Powchik P. (1995) Tacrine. *Lancet* 345: 625-630.

Davis R, Bloedel JR. (1984) *Cerebellar Stimulation for Spasticity and Seizures*. Boca Raton, Florida: CRC Press.

Deale A, David AC. (1994) Chronic fatigue syndrome: Evaluation and management. *J Neuropsychiatry Clin Neurosci* 6(2): 189-194.

deAngelis L. (1995) Ascorbic acid and atypical antipsychotic drugs: Modulation of amineptine-induced behavior in mice. *Brain Res* 670: 303-307.

De Bellis MD, Chrousos GP, Dorn LD, Burke L, Helmers K, Kling MA, Trickett PK, Putnam FW. (1994) Hypothalamic-pituitary-adrenal axis dysregulation in sexually abused girls. *J Clin Endocrinol Metab* 78(2): 249-255.

de Campos-Lima P-O, Gavioli R, Zhang Q-J, Wallace LE, Dolcetti R, Rowe M, Rickinson AB, Masucci MG. (1993) HLA-A11 epitope loss isolates Epstein-Barr virus from a highly A11[+] population. *Science* 260: 98-100.

DeGroat WC. (1989) Neuropeptides in pelvic afferent pathways. In Polak JM (Ed.), *Regulatory Peptides* (pp. 334-361). Basel: Birkhauser Verlag.

de Jonge M, Griedl A, De Vry J. (1993) CNS pharmacology of nimodipine: Antidepressant effects, drug discrimination, and Ca^{2+} imaging. In Scriabine A, Janis RA, Triggle DJ (Eds.), *Drugs in Development* (vol. 2: Ca^{2+} Antagonists in the CNS, pp. 165-174). Brandford, Connecticut: Neva Press.

DeKeyser J, Vauquelin G, De Backer J-P, De Vos H, Wilczaky N. (1993) What intracranial tissues in humans contain sumatriptan-sensitive 5-HT$_1$-type neurons? *Neurosci Lett* 164: 63-66.

deKloet ER, Oitzl MS, Joels M. (1993) Functional implications of brain corticosteroid receptor diversity. *Cell Mol Neurobiol* 13(4): 433-459.

Delgado PL, Miller HL, Salomon RM, Licinio J, Heninger GR, Gelenberg AJ, Charney DS. (1994) Monoamines and the mechanism of antidepressant action: Effects of catecholamine depletion on mood of patients treated with antidepressants. *Psychopharmacol Bull* 29(3): 389-395.

Demitrack MA, Greden JF. (1991) Chronic fatigue syndrome: The need for an integrative approach. *Biol Psychiatry* 30: 714-752.

Demitrack MA, Dale JK, Straus SE, Laue L, Listwak SJ, Kruesi MJ, Chrousos GP, Gold PW. (1991) Evidence for impaired activation of the hypothalamic-pituitary-adrenal axis in patients with chronic fatigue syndrome. *J Clin Endocrinol Metab* 73(6): 1224-1234.

Desole MS, Kim W-K, Rabin RA, Laychock SG. (1994) Nitric oxide reduces depolarization-induced calcium influx in PC12 cells by a cyclic GMP-mediated mechanism. *Neuropharmacol* 33: 193-198.

DeSouza E. (1993) Personal communication.

Deutsch SI, Rosse RB, Kendrick KA, Fay-McCarthy M, Collins JP, Wyatt RJ. (1993) Famotidine adjunctive pharmacotherapy for schizophrenia: Preliminary data. *Clin Neuropharmacol* 16(6): 518-524.

Devane WA, Axelrod J. (1994) Characterization of the enzymatic synthesis of anandamide: Properties and distribution in the brain. *Neuropsychopharmacol* 10(3S/Pt.1): 145S.

Devane WA, Hanus L, Breuer A, Pertwee RG, Stevenson LA, Griffin G, Gibson D, Mandelbaum A, Etinger A, Mechoulam R. (1992) Isolation and structure of a brain constituent that binds to the cannabinoid receptor. *Science* 258: 1946-1949.

Dewey WL. (1986) Cannabinoid pharmacology. *Pharmacol Rev* 38: 151-178.

deWied D, Diamant M, Fodor M. (1993) Central nervous system effects of the neurohypophyseal hormones and related peptides. *Front Neuroendocrinol* 14(4): 251-302.

Dey P, Wu W, Yarmush J, Zbuzek VK. (1993) The analgesic effect of epidural injection of nifedipine in rats. *Abstracts, 7th World Congress on Pain* (p. 47). Seattle: IASP Publications.

Dicpinigaitis PV, Spungen AM, Bauman WA, Absgarten A, Almenoff PL. (1994) Inhibition of bronchial hyperresponsiveness by the GABA-agonist baclofen. *Chest* 106(3): 758-761.

Diehl DL, Fullerton S, Mayer EA. (1995) Functional bowel disease symptoms in patients with chronic fatigue syndrome (CFS): Prevalence and quality of life. Presented at the American Gastroenterologic Association Digestive Disease Week, San Diego, May 14-17.

Dimitrova SS, Felten SY, Felten DL. (1995) Sympathetic noradrenergic innervation of spleen, thymus and mesenteric lymph nodes: A comparison between Sprague-Dawley, Lewis and Fischer 344 rats. *Abstracts, Soc for Neurosci* 21: 814.6, p. 207.

Disterhoft JF, Moyer JR, Thompson LT, Kowalska M. (1993) Functional aspects of calcium channel modulation. *Clin Neuropharmacol* 16(suppl. 1): 512-524.

Dolan RJ, Bench CJ, Liddle PF, Friston KJ, Frith CD, Grasby PM, Frackowiak RSJ. (1993) Dorsolateral prefrontal cortex dysfunction in the major psychoses: Symptom or disease specificity? *J Neurol Neurosurg Psychiatry* 56: 1290- 1294.

Domeney AM. (1994) Angiotensin converting enzyme inhibitors as potential cognitivie enhancing agents. *J Psychiatry Neurosci* 19: 46-50.

Donati F, Fagioli L, Komaroff AL, Duffy FH. (1994) Quantified EEG findings in patients with chronic fatigue syndrome. Proc AACFS Research Conf, p. 37.

Drake ME. (1993) Conversion hysteria and dominant hemisphere lesions. *Psychosom* 34(6): 524-529.

Drevets WC, Raichle ME. (1992) Neuroanatomical circuits in depression: Implications for treatment mechanisms. *Psychopharmacol Bull* 28(3): 261-274.

Dubner R. (1992) Hyperalgesia and expanded receptive fields. *Pain* 48: 3-4.

Dubovsky SL. (1994) Beyond the serotonin reuptake inhibitors: Rationales for development of new serotonergic agents. *J Clin Psychiatry* 55(2/suppl.): 33-44.

Duffy JD, Campbell JJ. (1994) The regional prefrontal syndromes: A theoretical and clinical overview. *J Neuropsychiatry Clin Neurosci* 6: 379-387.

Duggan AW, Hopo PJ, Lang CW, Williams CA. (1991) Sustained isometric contraction of skeletal muscle results in release of immunoreactive neurokinins in the spinal cord of the anesthetized cat. *Neurosci Lett* 122: 191-194.

Duman RS, Heninger GR, Nestler EJ. (1994) Adaptations of receptor-coupled signal transduction pathways underlying stress- and drug-induced neural plasticity. *J Nerv Ment Dis* 182: 692-700.

Dun NJ, Dun SL, Forstermann U. (1994) Nitric oxide synthase immunoreactivity in rat pontine medulla neurons. *Neurosci* 59: 429-445.

Dunn AJ. (1993) Role of cytokines in infection-induced stress. *Ann NY Acad Sci* 697: 189-202.

Dunn AJ, Vickers SL. (1994) Neurochemical and neuroendocrine responses to Newcastle disease virus administration in mice. *Brain Res* 645: 103-112.

Dunn AJ, Swiergel AH, Stone EA. (1995) The role of cerebral norepinephrine in the Fos response to interleukin-1. *Abstracts, Soc for Neurosci* 21: 45.2, p. 97.

Dutar P, Nicoll RA. (1988) A physiological role for $GABA_B$ receptors in the central nervous system. *Nature* 332(6160): 156-158.

Edeline JM, Manunta Y. (1995) Norepinephrine (NE) increases selectivity in frequency receptive fields (FRF) of auditory cortex neurons. *Abstracts, Soc for Neurosci* 21: 257.18, p. 636.

Edvinsson L, MacKenzie ET, McCulloch J. (1993) *Cerebral Blood Flow and Metabolism*. New York: Raven Press.

Ehnis M, Aston-Jones G. (1988) Activation of locus coerulus from paragigantocellularis: A new excitatory amino acid pathway in the brain. *J Neurosci* 8: 3644-3657.

Eisendrath SJ, Valan MN. (1994) Psychiatric predictors of pseudoepileptic seizures in patients with refractory seizures. *J Neuropsychiatry Clin Neurosci* 6: 257-260.

Elfvin L-G, Lindh B, Hokfelt T. (1993) The chemical neuroanatomy of sympathetic ganglia. *Ann Rev Neurosci* 16: 471-507.

Ellis WV. (1990) Octreotide, a small peptide, alleviates burning pain and hyperesthesia: A preliminary report. *Pain Clin* 3: 239-242.

Ellory JC, Culliford SJ, Smith PA, Wolowy KMW, Knaus EE. (1994) Specific inhibition of Ca-activated K channels in red cells by selected dihydropyridine derivatives. *Br J Pharmacol* 111: 903-905.

Ericsson A, Kovacs KJ, Sawchenko PE. (1993) A functional anatomical analysis of central pathways subserving the effects of interleukin-1 on stress-related neuroendocrine neurons. *J Neurosci* 14(2): 897-913.

Etgen AM, Karkanios GB. (1994) Estrogen regulation of noradrenergic signalling in the hypothalamus. *Psychoneuroendocrinol* 19 (5-7): 603-610.

Evans J, Wilson B, Wraight EP, Hodges JR. (1993) Neuropsychological and SPECT scan findings during and after transient global amnesia: Evidence for the differential impairment of remote episodic memory. *J Neurol Neurosurg Psychiatry* 56: 1227-1230.

Fanelli RJ, McMonagle-Strucko K, Johnson DE, Janis RA. (1993) Behavioral and neurochemical effects of sustained-release pellets of nimodipine. In Scriabine A, Janis RA, Triggle DJ (Eds.), *Drugs in Development* (vol. 2: Ca^{2+} Antagonists in the CNS, pp. 407-415). Brandford, Connecticut: Neva Press.

Faria M, Navarra P, Tsagarakis S, Basser GM, Grossman AB. (1991) Inhibition of CRH-41 release by substance P, but not substance K, from the rat hypothalamus in vitro. *Brain Res* 538: 76-78.

Farkkila M, Palo J, Saijonmaa O, Fyhrquist F. (1992) Raised plasma endothelin during acute migraine attack. *Cephalalgia* 12: 383-384.

Felten DL, Felten SY, Bellinger DL, Lorton D. (1992) Noradrenergic and peptidergic innervation of secondary lymphoid organs: Role in experimental rheumatoid arthritis. *Eur J Clin Invest* 22 (suppl. 1): 37-43.

Fernandez-Ruiz JJ, Navarro M, Hernandez ML, Vaticon D, Ramos JA. (1992) Neuroendocrine effects of an acute dose of Δ^9-tetrahydrocannabinol: Changes in hypothalamic biogenic amines and anterior pituitary hormone secretion. *Neuroendocrinol Lett* 14: 349-355.

Ferrari MD, Saxena PR. (1993) Clinical and experimental effects of sumatriptan in humans. *Trends Pharmacol Sci* 14: 129-133.

Ferreira SH, Duarte IDG, Lorenzetti BB. (1991) The molecular mechanism of action of peripheral morphine analgesia: Stimulation of the cGMP system via nitric oxide release. *Eur J Pharmacol* 201: 121-122.

Fickling SA, Williams D, Vallance P, Mussey SS, Whitley GS. (1993) Plasma concentrations of endogenous inhibitor of nitric oxide synthesis in normal pregnancy and pre-eclampsia. *Lancet* 342 (8865): 242-243.

Findling RL, Schwartz MA, Flannery DJ, Manos MJ. (1996) Venlafaxine in adults with attention-deficit/hyperactivity disorder: An open clinical trial. *J Clin Psychiatry* 57(5): 184-189.

Fisher LA. (1989) Corticotropin-releasing factor: Endocrine and autonomic integration of responses to stress. *Trends Pharmacol Sci* 10: 189-193.

Fleckenstein AE, Lookingland KJ, Moore KE. (1994a) Differential role of histamine in mediating stress-induced changes in central dopaminergic neuronal activity in the rat. *Brain Res* 653: 267-272.

Fleckenstein AE, Lookingland KJ, Moore KE. (1994b) Histaminergic neurons mediate restraint stress-induced increases in the activity of noradrenergic neurons projecting to the hypothalamus. *Brain Res* 653: 273-277.

Fleishmann J. (1994) Calcium channel antagonists in the treatment of interstitial cystitis. *Urol Clin N Am* 21(2): 107-111.

Fleshner M, Goehler LE, Hermann J, Relton JK, Maier SF, Watkins LR. (1995) Interleukin-1 beta induced corticosterone elevation and hypothalamic NE depletion is vagally mediated. *Brain Res Bull* 17(6): 605-610.

Fort P, Luppi P-H, Jouvet M. (1993) Glycine-immunoreactive neurones in the cat brain stem reticular formation. *NeuroReport* 4: 1123-1126.

Freeman U. (1993) Meclobemide. *Lancet* 342: 1528-1532.

Freeman T, Karson C, Garcia RHE. (1993) Locus ceruleus neuropathology in anxiety disorders. *Biol Psychiatry* 33: 148A.

Frith CD, Friston K, Liddle PF, Frackowiak RS. (1991) Willed action and the prefrontal cortex in man: A study with PET. *Pro R Soc Lond B Biol Sci* 224(1311): 241-246.

Fromm C. DeLeo JA, Coombs DW, Colburn RW, Twitchell BB. (1993) The ganglioside GM1 decreases autotomy but not substance P depletion in a peripheral mononeuropathy rat model. *Anesth Analg* 77(3): 501-506.

Fromm GH. (1987) Anatomy and physiology of the trigeminal system. In Fromm GH (Ed.), *Medical and Surgical Management of Trigeminal Neuralgia* (pp. 46-72). Mount Kisco, New York: Futura.

Fromm GH. (1991) Pathophysiology of trigeminal neuralgia. In Fromm GH, Sessle BJ (Eds.), *Trigeminal Neuralgia: Current Concepts Regarding Pathogenesis and Treatment* (pp. 105-130). Boston: Butterworth-Heinemann.

Fromm GH. (1994) Gabapentin: Discussion. *Epilepsia* 35 (suppl. 5): 77-80.

Fry R. (1993) Adult physical illness and childhood sexual abuse. *J Psychosom Res* 37(2): 89-103.

Fuster J. (1989) *The Prefrontal Cortex: Anatomy, Physiology and Neuropsychology of the Frontal Lobe.* New York: Raven.

Fuster J. (1993) Frontal lobes. *Curr Opin Neurobiol* 3: 160-165.

Fuxe K, Kurosawa N, Cintra A, Hallstrom A, Goiny M, Rosen L, Agnati LF, Ungerstedt U. (1992) Involvement of local ischemia in endothelin-1 induced lesions of the neostriatum of the anesthetized rat. *Exp Brain Res* 88(1): 131-139.

Gard PR, Mandy A, Whiting JM, Nickels DPD, Meakin AJLS. (1994) Reduction of responses to angiotensin II by antidepressant drugs. *Eur J Pharmacol* 264: 295-300.

Gardier AM, Kachaner S, Shaghaghi EK, Biot C, Bohuon C, Jacquot C, Pallardy MJ. (1994) Effects of a primary immune response to T-cell dependent antigen on serotonin metabolism in the frontal cortex: In vivo microdialysis study in freely moving rat. *Brain Res* 645: 150-156.

Gedye A. (1992) Serotonin-GABA treatment is hypothesized for self-injury in Lesch-Nyhan syndrome. *Med Hypotheses* 38(4): 325-328.

Gehlert DR, Robertson DW. (1994) ATP sensitive potassium channels: Potential drug targets in neuropsychopharmacology. *Prog Neuropsychopharmacol Biol Psychiatry* 18: 1093-1102.

Gehlert DR, Schober DA, Hipskind PA, Nixon J, Gitter BD, Houbert JJ. (1995) Characterization of the guinea pig NK-1 receptors using the potent antagonist ligand [^{3}H]-LY303870. *Abstracts, Soc for Neurosci* 21: 532.16, p. 135.

George MS, Ketter TA, Parekh PI, Gill DS, Huggins T, Marangell L, Pazzaglia PJ, Post RM. (1994) Spatial ability in affective illness. *Neuropsychiatry Neuropsychol Behav Neurol* 7(3): 143-153.

George MS, Ketter TA, Parekh PI, Horwitz B, Hersovich P, Post RM. (1995) Brain activity during transient sadness and happiness in healthy women. *Am J Psychiatry* 152: 341-351.

Geracioti TD. (1995) Venlafaxine treatment of panic disorder: A case series. *J Clin Psychiatry* 56: 408-410.

Gerfen CR, Staines WA, Arbuthnot GW, Fibiger HC. (1982) Crossed connections in the substantia nigra in the cat. *J Comp Neurol* 207: 283-303.

Gerra G, Caccavari R, Reali N, Bonvicini P, Marcato A, Fertonani G, Delsignore R, Passeri M, Brambilla F. (1993) Noradrenergic and hormonal responses to physical exercise in adolescents. *Neuropsychobiol* 27(2): 65-71.

Giannini AJ, Loiselle RH, DiMarzio LR, Giannini MC. (1987) Augmentation of haloperidol by ascorbic acid in phencyclidine intoxication. *Am J Psychiatry* 144: 1207-1209.

Gibbs DM. (1992) Hyperventilation-induced cerebral ischemia in panic disorder and the effect of nimodipine. *Am J Psychiatry* 149: 1589-1591.

Gioiditta A (Ed.). (1995) *The Function of Sleep*. Special issue of *Behav Brain Res* 69(1-2).

Gispen WH. (1993) Neuronal plasticity and function. *Clin Neuropharmacol* 16(suppl.1): S5-551.

Giuliani S, Evangelista S, Borsini F, Meli A. (1988) Intracerebroventricular phaclofen antagonizes baclofen antinociceptive activity in hot plate test with mice. *Eur J Pharmacol* 154(2): 225-226.

Glick SD, Ross DA, Hugh LB. (1982) Lateral asymmetry of neurotransmitters in the human brain. *Brain Res* 234: 53-63.

Glickstein M. (1993) Motor skills but not cognitive tasks. *Trends Neurosci* 16(11): 450-451.

Goadsby P, Edvinsson L. (1993) The trigeminovascular system and migraine: Studies characterizing cerebrovascular and neuropeptide changes seen in humans and cats. *Ann Neurol* 33(1): 48-56.

Goadsby P, Edvinsson L. (1994) Peripheral and central trigeminovascular activation in cat is blocked by the serotonin (5HT$_{1D}$) receptor agonist 311C90. *Headache* 34: 394-399.

Goland RS, Conwell IM, Warren WB, Wardlaw SL. (1992) Placental corticotropin-releasing hormone and pituitary-adrenal function during pregnancy. *Neuroendocrinol* 56: 742-749.

Goldberg E, Podell K, Lovell M. (1994) Lateralization of frontal lobe functions and cognitive novelty. *J Neuropsychiatry Clin Neurosci* 6: 371-378.

Goldenberg DL. (1993) Fibromyalgia, chronic fatigue syndrome, and myofascial pain syndrome. *Curr Opin Rheumatol* 5: 199-208.

Goldman-Rakic PS. (1987) Circuitry of the primate prefrontal cortex and the regulation of behavior by representational memory. In F. Plum (Ed.), *Handbook of Physiology, The Nervous System, Higher Functions in the Brain,* (sect. 1, vol. V, pt. 1, pp. 373-417). Bethesda, Maryland: American Physiological Society.

Goldstein, JA. (1983) Cimetidine and mononucleosis. *Ann Int Med* 99(3): 410-411.

Goldstein JA. (1984) Nifedipine treatment of Tourette's syndrome. *J Clin Psychiatry* 45: 360.

Goldstein JA. (1985) Calcium channel blockers in the treatment of panic disorder. *J Clin Psychiatry* 4(12): 546.

Goldstein, JA. (1986a) Cimetidine, ranitidine, and Epstein-Barr virus infection. *Ann Int Med* 105(1): 139.

Goldstein, JA. (1986b) Treatment of chronic Epstein-Barr disease with H-2 blockers. *J Clin Psychiatry* 47(11): 572.

Goldstein JA. (1990) *Chronic Fatigue Syndrome: The Struggle for Health.* Los Angeles: Chronic Fatigue Syndrome Institute.

Goldstein JA. (1992) CFS: Limbic encephalopathy in a dysfunctional neuroimmune network. In Hyde BW (Ed.), *The Clinical and Scientific Basis of Myalgic Encephalomyelitis/Chronic Fatigue Syndrome* (pp. 247-252). Ottawa: Nightingale Research Foundation.

Goldstein JA. (1993) *Chronic Fatigue Syndromes: The Limbic Hypothesis.* Binghamton, New York: The Haworth Medical Press.

Goldstein JA. (1994a) Fibromyalgia syndrome: A pain modulation disorder related to altered limbic function? In Masi A (Ed.), *Fibromyalgia and Myofascial Pain Syndromes* (pp. 777-800). London: Balliere.

Goldstein JA. (1994b) New treatments for CFS. *CFIDS Chron* Summer: 2-6.

Goldstein JA, Daly J. (1993) Neuroimmunoendocrine findings in chronic fatigue syndrome before and after exercise. Cited in *Chronic Fatigue Syndromes: The Limbic Hypothesis.* Binghamton, New York: The Haworth Medical Press.

Goldstein JA, Mena I. (1994) Pre- and post-nimodipine brain SPECT in patients with chronic fatigue syndrome. Presented at American Association for Chronic Fatigue Syndrome Research Conference, Fort Lauderdale, Florida, October 8.

Goldstein JA, Mena I. (1995) unpublished.

Goldstein JA, Sandman CA. (1990) Encoding deficits in fibromyalgia patients with no subjective cognitive deficits. Unpublished.

Goldstein JA, Terasaki P. (1990) HLA typing in chronic fatigue syndrome. Cited in *Chronic Fatigue Syndrome: The Struggle for Health.* Los Angeles: Chronic Fatigue Syndrome Institute.

Goldstein JA, Mena I, Yunus MB. (1993) Regional cerebral blood flow by SPECT in chronic fatigue syndrome with and without fibromyalgia syndrome. *Arth Rheum* 39(9/suppl.): 205.

Goldstein JA, Russell IJ, Gilbert V. (1995) Could low levels of cerebrospinal fluid endothelin explain the vasoconstriction response to nimodipine seen in pre- and post-treatment brain SPECT of CFS/FMS patients? *J Musculoskel Pain* 3(suppl. 1): 14.

Goldstein JA, Sandman C, Hetrick W, van de Wal E. (1994) Decreased event-related potential N-100: A possible neurologic marker for CFS impairment. *Proc AACFS Research Conf,* (p. 40).

Goldstein JA, Mena I, Jouanne E, Lesser I. (1995) The assessment of vascular abnormalities in late life chronic fatigue syndrome by brain SPECT; comparison with late life major depressive disorder. *J Chron Fatigue Syn* 1: 55-80.

Gonzalez-Alvear GM, Werling LL. (1995) Sigma receptor regulation of norepinephrine release from rat hippocampal slices. *Brain Res* 673(1): 61-69.

Goodwin GM, Austin M-P, Dougall N, Ross M, Murray C, O'Carroll RE, Moffoot A, Prentice N, Ebmeier KP. (1993) State changes in brain activity shown by the uptake of ^{99m}Tc-exametazime with single photon emission tomography in major depression before and after treatment. *J Aff Dis* 29: 243-253.

Gorard DA, Farthing MJ. (1994) Intestinal motor function in irritable bowel syndrome. *Dig Dis Sci* 12: 72-84.

Gotz E, Feverstein TJ, Lais A, Meyer DK. (1993) Effects of gabapentin on release of gamma-aminobutyric acid from slices of rat neostriatum. *Arzneimittelforschung* 43: 636-638.

Grady CL, VanMeter JW, Maisog JM, Pietrini P, Krasuki J, Rauschecker JP. (1995) Changes in auditory cortex activation during selective attention. *Abstracts, Soc for Neurosci* 21: 779.5, p. 1988.

Grasby PM, Friston KJ, Bench CJ, Cowen PJ, Frith CD, Liddle PF, Frackowiak RS, Dolan RJ. (1993) The effect of the dopamine agonist, apomorphine, on regional cerebral blood flow in normal volunteers. *Psychol Med* 23(3): 605-612.

Grassetto M, Varotto A. (1994) Primary fibromyalgia is responsive to S-adenosyl-L-methionine. *Curr Ther Res* 55(7): 797-806.

Greenbaum DS, Mayle JE, Vanergeren LE, Jerome JA, Mayor JW, Greenbaum RB, Matson RW, Stein GE, Dean HA, Haworsen NA, Rosen LW. (1987) Effects of desipramine on irritable bowel syndrome compared with atropine and placebo. *Dig Dis Sci* 32: 257-266.

Greene P. (1992) Baclofen in the treatment of dystonia. *Clin Neuropharmacol* 15(4): 276-288.

Green-Johnson JM, Zalcman S, Vriend CY, Dolina S, Nance DM, Greenberg AH. (1995) Role of norepinephrine in antibody production: Suppressed IgG production in epilepsy-prone mice. *Abstracts, Soc for Neurosci* 21: 814.10, p. 2072.

Greenough WT, Bailey CH. (1988) The anatomy of a memory: Convergence of results across a diversity of tests. *Trends Neurosci* 11: 142-147.

Gresch PJ, Sved AF, Zigmond MJ, Finlay JM. (1995) Local influence of endogenous norepinephrine on extracellular dopamine in the rat prefrontal cortex. *J Neurochem* 63: 111-116.

Grider JR, Jin J-G. (1993) Induced nitric oxide (NO) production and relaxation in isolated muscle cells of the gut in human and other mammalian species. *Gastroenterol* 104(4): A515.

Griep EN, Boersma JW, de Kloet ER. (1993) Altered reactivity of the hypothalamic-pituitary-adrenal axis in the primary fibromyalgia syndrome. *J Rheumatol* 20: 469-474.

Groenewegen HJ, Berendse HW. (1994) The specificity of the "nonspecific" midline and intralaminar thalamic nuclei. *Trends Neurosci* 17(2): 52-57.

Groenewegen HJ, Berendse HW, Wolters JG, Lohman AHM. (1990) In Uylings HMB, van Eden CG, DeBruin JPC, Corner MA, Feenstra MGD (Eds.), *The Prefrontal Cortex: Its Structure, Function, and Pathology* (Prog Brain Res, vol. 85, pp. 95-118). New York: Elsevier.

Gross PM, Zochodine DW, Wainmain DS, Ho LT, Espinosa FJ, Weaver DF. (1992) Intraventricular endothelin-1 uncouples the blood flow: Metabolism relationship in periventricular structures of the rat brain: Involvement of L-type calcium channels. *Neuropep* 22: 155-165.

Grunau RVE, Whitfield MF, Petrie JH, Fryer EL. (1994) Early pain experience, child and family factors as precursors of somatization: A prospective study of extremely premature and full-term infants. *Pain* 56: 353-359.

Grundemar L, Hakanson R. (1994) Neuropeptide Y effector systems: Perspectives for drug development. *Trends Pharmacol Sci* 15: 153-159.

Grunewald RA, Fillenz M. (1984) Release of ascorbate from a synaptosomal fraction of rat brain. *Neurochem Int* 6: 491-500.

Grunewald RA, Thompson PJ, Corcoran R, Corden Z, Jackson GD, Duncan JS. (1994) Effects of vigabatrin on partial seizures and cognitive function. *J Neurol Neurosurg Psychiatry* 57: 1057-1063.

Guberman A, Stuss D. (1983) The syndrome of bilateral paramedian thalamic infarction. *Neurol* 33: 540-546.

Guze BH, Gitlin M. (1994) The neuropathologic basis of major affective disorder: Neuroanatomical insights. *J Neuropsychiatry Clin Neurosci* 6(2): 114-121.

Hadcock JR, Wang HY, Malbon CC. (1989) Attenuation of glucocorticoid-induced up-regulation of beta-adrenergic receptors. *J Biol Chem* 264: 19928-19933.

Hampel H, Korschenhauser D, Becker I, Hegraty A, Muller N, Ackenheil M. (1994) Evidence of cytomegalovirus in postmortem frontal lobe brain tissue of schizophrenic patients by two-dimensional gel electrophoresis. *Neuropsychopharmacol* 10(3S/Pt.1): 231S.

Hanbauer I, Wink D, Osawa Y, Edelman GM, Gally JA. (1992) Role of nitric oxide in NMDA-evoked release of [^{3}H]dopamine from striatal slices. *NeuroReport* 3(5): 409-412.

Harlow JM. (1868) *Recovery after Severe Injury to the Head.* Publication of the Massachusetts Medical Society 2: 327-346.

Harrington MA, Zhong P, Garlow SJ, Ciaranello RD. (1992) Molecular biology of serotonin receptors. *J Clin Psychiatry* 53(10/suppl.): 8-27.

Hasler WL, Soudah HC, Owyang C. (1993) A somatostatin analog inhibits afferent pathways mediating perception of rectal distension. *Gastroenterol* 104: 1390-1397.

Hasselmo ME. (1995) Neuromodulation and cortical function: Modeling the physiological basis of behavior. *Behav Brain Res* 67(1): 1-27.

Hata F, Kuo C-H, Matsuda T, Yoshida H. (1976) Factors required for co-sensitive acetylcholine release from crude synaptic vesicles. *J Neurochem* 27: 139-144.

Hausdorff WP, Pitcher JA, Luttrell DK, Linder ME, Kurose H, Parsons SJ, Caron MG, Lefkowitz RJ. (1992) Tyrosinic phosphorylation of G protein alpha subunits by PP60C-5rc. *Proc Natl Acad Sci USA* 89: 5720-5724.

Hayes S. (1993) Acetazolamide neuropharmacology in primary psychiatric disorder. *Neuropsychopharmacol* 9(25): 131.

Haynes WG, Davenport AP, Webb DJ. (1993) Endothelin: Progress in pharmacology and physiology. *Trends Pharmacol Sci* 14: 225-228.

Heefner JD, Russell MW, Wilson ID. (1978) Irritable colon and depression. *Psychosom* 19: 540-547.

Heider LM, Vorce DE, Pettibon WH, Klimas NG, Keller RH, Reiter WM. (1994) Psychological correlates of physical symptoms in patients with chronic fatigue syndrome (CFS). *Proc Amer Assoc CFS*: 61.

Heilig M, Widerlov E. (1990) Neuropeptide Y: An overview of central distribution, functional aspects, and possible involvement in neuropsychiatric illnesses. *Acta Psychiatr Scand* 82(2): 95-114.

Heilig M, McLeod S, Brot M, Heinrichs SC, Menzaghi F, Koob GF, Britton KT. (1993) Anxiolytic-like action of neuropeptide Y: Mediation by Y_1 receptors in amygdala and dissociation from food intake effects. *Neuropsychopharmacol* 8: 357-363.

Heinrichs SC, Menzaghi F, Pich EM, Tilders ST, Koob GF. (1993) Corticotropin-releasing factor in the paraventricular nucleus modulates feeding induced by neuropeptide Y. *Brain Res* 611: 18-24.

Hellberg D, Chesson B, Nilsson S. (1991) Premenstrual tension: A placebo-controlled efficacy study with spironolactone and medroxyprogesterone acetate. *Int J Gynaecol Obstet* 34(3): 243-248.

Herdman JRE, Delva NJ, Hockney RE, Campling GM, Cowen PJ. (1994) Neuroendocrine effects of sumatriptan. *Psychopharmacol* 113: 561-564.

Herkenham M, Lynn AB, Johnson MR, Melvin LS, de Costa CR, Rice KC. (1991) Characterization and localization of cannabinoid receptors in rat brain: A quantitative in vitro autoradiographic study. *J Neurosci* 11: 563-583.

Herman JP. (1993) Regulation of adrenocorticosteroid receptor mRNA expression in the central nervous system. *Cell Mol Neurobiol* 13(4): 349-370.

Hertel P, Nomikas GG, Andersson JL, Iurlo M, Svensson TH. (1995) Preferential activation by risperidone of serotonin but not dopamine metabolism in the rat medial prefrontal cortex. *Abstracts, Soc for Neurosci* 21: 191.14, p. 469.

Hey JA, Mingo G, Bosler DC, Kreutner W, Krobatson D, Chapman RW. (1995) Respiratory effects of baclofen and 3-aminopropylphosphinic acid in guinea-pigs. *Br J Pharmacol* 114: 735-738.

Hickie I, Wilson A. (1994) A catecholamine model of fatigue. *Br J Psychiatry* 165: 275-276.

Hill RR, Stagno SJ, Tesar GE. (1995) Secondary mania associated with the use of felbamate. *Psychosom* 36: 404-407.

Hirai M, Miyabo S, Ooya E, Miyanaga K, Aoyagi N, Kimura K, Kishida S, Nakai P. (1991) Endothelin-3 stimulates the hypothalamic-pituitary-adrenal axis. *Life Sci* 48(24): 2359-2363.

Hoffman A, Keiser HR, Grossman E, Goldstein DS, Gold PW, Kling M. (1989) Endothelin concentrations in cerebrospinal fluid in depressives. *Lancet* 2(8678-8679): 1519.

Hoheisel U, Mense S, Simons DG, Yu X-M. (1993) Appearance of new receptive fields in rat dorsal horn neurons following noxious stimulation of skeletal muscle: A model for referral of muscle pain? *Neurosci Lett* 153: 9-12.

Hohenfellner M, Nunes L, Schmidt RA, Lampel A, Thuroff JW, Tanagho EA. (1992) Interstitial cystitis: Increased sympathetic innervation and related neuropeptide synthesis. *J Urol* 147(3): 587-591.

Hokanson CL, Mohankumar SMJ, Quadri SL. (1995) Effects of chronic administration of interleukin-1 beta. *Abstracts, Soc for Neurosci* 21: 45.6, p. 98.

Hollander E, Wong CM. (1995a) Introduction to obsessive-compulsive spectrum disorders. *J Clin Psychiatry* 56(suppl. 3).

Hollander E, Wong CM. (1995b) Developments in the treatment of obsessive-compulsive disorder. *Prim Psychiatry* 2(2): 28-33.

Horton RW, Lowther S, Chivers J, Jenner P, Marsden CD, Testa SO. (1988) The interaction of substituted benzamides with brain benzodiazepine binding sites in vitro. *Br J Pharmacol* 94(4): 1234-1240.

Howlett AC, Bidaut-Russell M, Devane MA, Melvin LS, Johnson MR, Herkenham M. (1990) The cannabinoid receptor: Biochemical, anatomical and behavioral characterization. *Trends Neurosci* 13: 420-423.

Huang S-K, Pan J-T. (1993) Potentiating effects of serotonin and vasoactive intestinal peptide on the action of glutamate on suprachiasmatic neurons in brain slices. *Neurosci Lett* 159: 1-4.

Huang SK, Simonson MS, Dunn MJ. (1993) Manidipine inhibits endothelin-1-induced $[Ca^{2+}]$ signalling but potentiates endothelin's effect on c-fos and c-jun induction in vascular smooth muscle and glomerular mesangial cells. *Am Heart J* 125: 589-597.

Hudson JI, Goldenberg DL, Pope HG, Keck PE, Schlesinger L. (1992) Comorbidity of fibromyalgia with medical and psychiatric disorders. *Am J Med* 92(4): 363-367.

Huggins JP, Pelton JT, Miler RC. (1993) The structure and specificity of endothelin receptors: Their importance in physiology and medicine. *Pharmacol and Therapeutics* 59: 55-123.

Hughes PJ, Michell RH. (1993) Novel inositol-containing phospholipids and phosphates: Their synthesis and possible new roles in cellular signalling. *Curr Opin Neurobiol* 3: 383-400.

Huie RE, Padmaja S. (1993) The reaction of NO with superoxide. *Free Rad Res Comm* 18(4): 195-199.

Iacono, R. (1995) Personal communication.

Iadarola MJ, Max MB, Berman KF, Byas-Smith MG, Coghill RC, Gracely RH, Bennett GJ. (1995) Unilateral decrease in thalamic activity observed with positron emission tomography in patients with neuropathic pain. *Pain* 63: 55-64.

Iadecola C, Faris PL, Hartman BX, Xu X. (1993) Localization of NADPH diaphorase in neurons of the rostral ventral medulla: Possible role of nitric oxide in central autonomic regulations and chemoreception. *Brain Res* 603: 173-179.

Ichise M, Salit IE, Abbey SE, Chung DG, Gray B, Kirsh JC, Freedman M. (1992) Assessment of regional cerebral perfusion in ^{99m}Tc-HMPAO SPECT in chronic fatigue syndrome. *Nuc Med Comm* 13: 767-772.

Ignatowski TA, Spengler RN. (1994) Tumor necrosis factor-alpha: Presynaptic sensitivity is modified after antidepressant drug administration. *Brain Res* 665: 293-299.

Imaki J, Nahon J-L, Rivier C, Sawchenko PE, Vale W. (1991) Differential regulation of corticotropin releasing factor mRNA in rat brain cell types by glucocorticoid and stress. *J Neurosci* 11: 585-599.

Imperato A. (1994) Cocaine and D-amphetamine enhance acetylcholine release in the hippocampus through action of dopamine on both D_1 and D_2 receptors. *Neuropsychopharmacol* 10(3S/Pt.1): 69S.

Imperato A, Gessa GL. (1994) Evidence for dopamine-gaba-acetylcholine interaction in regulation of cognition. *Neuropsychopharmacol* 10(3S/Pt.1): 671S.

Insel TR, Shapiro LE. (1992) Central oxytocin administration reflects social organization in monogamous and polygamous voles. *Proc Natl Acad Sci USA* 89: 5981-5985.

Irwin PP, Galloway NTM. (1994) Surgical management of interstitial cystitis. *Urol Clin N Am* 21(1): 153-162.

Ito Y, Teicher MH, Glod CA, Harper D, Magnus E, Gelbard HA. (1993) Increased prevalence of electrophysiological abnormalities in children with psychological, physical, and sexual abuse. *J Neuropsychiatry Clin Neurosci* 5(4): 401-408.

Iverson S. (1994) Modulation of dopamine function by glycine site antagonists: Atypical neuroleptic profile? *Neuropsychopharmacol* 19(3S/Pt.1): 98S.

Jacobs BL. (1995) Personal communication ("Would you like to work in my lab on this for a year as a post-doc?").

Jacobsen FM. (1995) Risperidone in the treatment of affective illness and obsessive-compulsive disorder. *J Clin Psychiatry* 56: 423-429.

Jaffe JH. (1990) Drug addiction and drug abuse. In Gilman AG, Rall TW, Nies AS, Taylor P (Eds.), *Goodman and Gilman's the Pharmacological Basis of Therapeutics* (8th ed.). New York: Pergamon Press.

Jankovic J, Gilden JL, Hiner BC, Kaufmann H, Brown DC, Coughlan CH, Rubin M, Fouad-Tarazi FM. (1993) Neurogenic orthostatic hypotension: A double-blind placebo-controlled study with midodrine. *Am J Med* 95: 38-48.

Janowsky DS, Davis JM, El-Youssef J, Sekerke HJ. (1972) A cholinergic-adrenergic hypothesis of mania and depression. *Lancet* ii: 632-635.

Javitt DC, Zylberman I, Zukin SR, Heresco-Levy U, Lindemayer J-P. (1994) Amelioration of negative symptoms in schizophrenia by glycine. *Am J Psychiatry* 151: 1234-1236.

Jeanmonod D, Magnin M, Morel A. (1993) Thalamus and neurogenic pain: Physiological, anatomical, and clinical data. *NeuroReport* 4(5): 475-478.

Jensen I, Llewellyn-Smith IJ, Pilowsky P, Minson JB, Chalmers J. (1995) Serotonin inputs to rabbit sympathetic preganglionic neurons projecting to the superior cervical ganglion or adrenal medulla. *J Comp Neurol* 353: 427-438.

Jerusalinsky D, Quillfeldt JA, Walz R, DaSilva RC, Medina JH, Izquierdo I. (1994) Post-training intrahippocampal infusion of protein kinase C inhibitors causes amnesia in rats. *Behav Neurol Biol* 61: 107-109.

Joels M, deKloet ER. (1992) Coordinative mineralocorticoid and glucocorticoid receptor-mediated control of responses to serotonin in the rat hippocampus. *Neuroendocrinol* 55: 344-350.

Johnson AE. (1992) The regulation of oxytocin receptor binding in the ventromedial hypothalamic nucleus by gonadal steroids. *Ann NY Acad Sci* 652: 357-373.

Johnson PA, Chahl LA. (1992) Chronic treatment with ascorbic acid inhibits the morphine withdrawal response in guinea-pigs. *Neurosci Lett* 135: 23-27.

Joly E, Mucke L, Oldstone MBA. (1991) Viral persistence in neurons explained by lack of major histocompatibility class I expression. *Science* 253: 1283-1285.

Jones BE. (1993) Basic mechanisms of sleep-wake states. In Kryger ME, Roth T, Dement WC (Eds.), *Principles and Practice of Sleep Medicine* (pp. 145-162). Philadelphia: Saunders.

Jones NM, Loiacono RE, Moller M, Beart PM. (1994) Diverse roles for nitric oxide in synaptic signalling after activation of NMDA release-regulating receptors. *Neuropharmacol* 33: 1351-1356.

Jorgensen A, Fjalland B, Christensen JD, Threiman M. (1994) Dihydropyridine ligands influence the evoked release of oxytocin and vasopressin dependent on stimulation conditions. *Eur J Pharmacol* 259: 151-163.

Kalivas PW, Duffy P. (1989) Similar effects of daily cocaine and stress on mesocorticolimbic dopamine neurotransmission in the rat. *Biol Psychiatry* 25: 913-928.

Kamei C, Okumura Y, Tasaka K. (1993) Influence of histamine depletion on learning and memory recollection in rats. *Psychopharmacol* 111: 376-382.

Kamei J, Hitosugi H, Kawashima N, Aoki T, Ohhashi Y, Kasuya Y. (1992) Antinociceptive effects of mexiletine in diabetic mice. *Res Comm Chem Path Pharmacol* 77: 245-248.

Kandel ER. (1994) The long and short of short-term memory. *Neuropsychopharmacol* 10 (3S/Pt.1): 2S-4S.

Kandel ER, Hawkins RD. (1992) The biochemical basis of learning and individuality. *Sci Am* 267(3): 79- 86.

Kang M, Yoshimatso H, Ogawa R, Kurokawa M, Oohara A, Tamari Y, Sakata T. (1994) Thermoregulation and hypothalamic histamine turnover modulated by interleukin-1 beta in rats. *Brain Res Bull* 35(4): 299-301.

Kapas L, Fang J, Kruger JM. (1994) Inhibition of nitric oxide synthase inhibits rat sleep. *Brain Res* 664: 189-196.

Kapp BS, Whalan PJ, Supple WF, Pascoe JP. (1992) Amygdaloid contributions to conditional arousal and sensory information processing. In Aggleton JP (Ed.), *The Amygdala: Neurobiological Aspects of Emotion, Memory, and Mental Dysfunction* (pp. 229-254). New York: Wiley-Liss.

Kapur S, Meyer J, Wilson AA, Houle S, Brown GM. (1994) Modulation of cortical neuronal activity by a serotonergic agent: A PET study in humans. *Brain Res* 646: 292-294.

Karler R, Calder LD, Thai LH, Bedingfield JB. (1995) The dopaminergic, glutamatergic, GABAergic bases for the action of amphetamine and cocaine. *Brain Res* 671: 100-104.

Karni A, Tanne D, Rubenstein BS, Askenasy JJ, Sagi D. (1994) Dependence on REM sleep of overnight improvement of a perceptual skill. *Science* 265 (5172): 679-682.

Katafuchi T, Okada E, Take S, Hori T. (1994) The biphasic changes in splenic natural killer cell activity following ventromedial hypothalamic lesions in rats. *Brain Res* 652: 164-168.

Kataoka A, Imai H, Inayoshi S, Tsuda T. (1993) Intermittent high-dose vitamin C therapy in patients with HTLV-I associated myelopathy. *J Neurol Neurosurg Psychiatry* 56: 1213-1216.

Kataoka Y, Koizumi S, Kohzuma M, Shibaguchi H, Shigematsu K, Niwa M, Taniyama K. (1995) NMDA receptor involvement in endothelin neurotoxicity in rat striatal slices. *Eur J Pharmacol* 273: 285-289.

Kavanau JL. (1994) Sleep and dynamic stabilization of neural circuitry: A review and synthesis. *Behav Brain Res* 63: 111-126.

Kay DSG, Naylor GJ, Smith AHW, Greenwood C. (1984) The therapeutic effect of ascorbic acid and EDTA in manic-depressive psychosis: Double-blind comparisons with standard treatments. *Psychol Med* 14: 533-539.

Keck PE, Wilson DR, Strakowski SM, McElroy SL, Kizer DL, Balistreti TM, Holtman HM, DePriest M. (1995) Clinical predictors of acute risperidone response in schizophrenia, schizoaffective disorder, and psychotic mood disorders. *J Clin Psychiatry* 56: 466-470.

Kehne JH, Baron BM, Harrison BL, McDonald IA, Palfreyman MG, Salituro FG, McCloskey TC, White HS. (1993) Glycine antagonists as potential anxiolytic agents. *J Neurochem* 61(suppl.): 551.

Keller RH, Lane JL, Klimas N, Reiter WM, Fletcher MA, van Riel F, Morgan R. (1994) Association between HLA class II antigens and the chronic fatigue immune dysfunction syndrome. *Clin Infect Dis* 18: (suppl. 1): S154-S156.

Kennedy MB. (1992) Second messengers and neuronal function. In Hall ZW (Ed.), *An Introduction to Molecular Neurobiology* (pp. 207-246). Sunderland, Massachusetts: Sinauer.

Kennedy MB, Marder E. (1992) Cellular and molecular mechanisms of neuronal plasticity. In Hall ZW (Ed.), *An Introduction to Molecular Neurobiology* (pp. 463-495). Sunderland, Massachusetts: Sinauer.

Kent-Braun JA, Sharma KR, Weiner MW, Massie B, Miller RG. (1993) Central basis of muscle fatigue in chronic fatigue syndrome. *Neurol* 43(1): 125-131.

Kessler JA, Black IB. (1982) Regulation of substance P in the adult rat sympathetic ganglia. *Brain Res* 234(1): 182- 187.

Kim S-G, Ugurbil K, Strick PL. (1994) Activation of a cerebellar output nucleus during cognitive processing. *Science* 265: 949-951.

King JH, Nuss S. (1993) Reflex sympathetic dystrophy treated by electroconvulsive therapy: Intractable pain, depression, and bilateral electrode ECT. *Pain* 55(3): 393-396.

Kitayama I, Makamura S, Yaga T, Murase S, Nomura J, Kayahara T, Nakano K. (1994) Degeneration of locus coeruleus axons in stress-induced depression model. *Brain Res Bull* 35: 573-580.

Klein E, Uhde TW. (1988) Controlled study of verapamil for treatment of panic disorder. *Am J Psychiatry* 145: 431-434.

Klimas N. (1993) Immune correlates and mechanisms in chronic fatigue syndrome. Presented at Medical Neurobiology of Chronic Fatigue Syndrome and Fibromyalgia: The Fourth Annual Conference, Bel Air, California, May. (1993) *CFIDS Chron* Summer: 1-11.

Knight AR, Gillard J, Wong EH, Middlemiss DN. (1991) The human sigma site, which resembles that in NCB 20 cells, may correspond to a low affinity site in guinea pig brain. *Neurosci Lett* 131: 233.

Knight RT, Hillyard SA, Woods DL, Neville HJ. (1981) The effects of frontal cortex lesions on event-related potentials during auditory selective attention. *Electroencephalogr Clin Neurophysiol* 52: 571-582.

Kobari M, Fukuuchi Y, Tomita M, Tanahashi N, Konno S, Takeda H. (1993a) Effects of sumatriptan on the cerebral intraparenchymal microcirculation in the cat. *Eur J Pharmacol* 110: 1445-1448.

Kobari M, Fukuuchi Y, Tomita M, Tanahashi N, Yamawaki T, Takeda H, Matsuoka S. (1993b) Transient cerebral vasodilatory effect of neuropeptide Y by nitric oxide. *Brain Res Bull* 31: 443-448.

Kocsis JD, Honmou D. (1994) Gabapentin increases GABA-induced depolarization in rat neonatal optic nerve. *Neurosci Lett* 169(1-2): 181-184.

Koller WC. (1984) Sensory symptoms in Parkinson's disease. *Neurol* 34: 957-959.

Komai M, Bryant BP. (1993) Acetazolamide specifically inhibits lingual trigeminal nerve responses to carbon dioxide. *Brain Res* 612: 122-129.

Koob GF, Heinrichs SC, Menzaghi F, Pich EM, Britton KT. (1994) Corticotropin releasing factor, stress and behavior. *Sem Neurosci* 6: 221-229.

Kopelman MD, Panayiotopoulous CP, Lewis P. (1994) Transient epileptic amnesia differentiated from psychogenic "fugue": Neuropsychological, EEG, and PET findings. *J Neurol Neurosurg Psychiatry* 57: 1002-1004.

Korbut R, Gryglewski RJ. (1992) Nitric oxide from polymorphonuclear leukocytes modulates red blood cell deformability in vitro. *Eur J Pharmacol* 234: 17-22.

Korte SM, deBoer SF, deKloet ER, Bohus B. (1995) Anxiolytic-like effects of selective mineralocorticoid and glucocorticoid antagonists on fear-enhanced behavior in the elevated plus-maze. *Psychoneuroendocrin* 20: 385-394.

Kostic VS, Dijoric BM, Covickovic-Stemic N, Bumbasirevic L, Nikolic M, Mrsulja BB. (1987) Depression and Parkinson's disease: Possible role of serotonergic mechanisms. *J Neurol* 234: 94-96.

Koyana K, Mito T, Takashima S, Suzuki S. (1990) Effects of phenylephrine and dopamine on cerebral blood flow, blood volume, and oxygenation in young rabbits. *Ped Neurol* 6(2): 87-90.

Kudrow L, Kudrow DB, Sandweiss JH. (1995) Rapid and sustained relief of migraine attacks with intranasal lidocaine: Preliminary findings. *Headache* 35: 79-82.

Kuo CH, Hata F, Yoshida H, Yamatodani A, Wada H. (1979) Effect of ascorbic acid on release of acetylcholine from synaptic vesicles prepared from different species of animals and release of noradrenaline from synaptic vesicles of rat brain. *Life Sci* 24 (10): 911-915.

Kurosawa M, Fuxe K, Hallstrom A, Goiny M, Cintra A, Ungerstedt U. (1991) Responses of blood flow, extracellular lactate, and dopamine in the striatum to intrastriatal injection of endothelin-1 in anesthetized rats. *J Cardiovasc Pharmacol* 17(suppl. 7): S340-S342.

Kyrakis JM, Hausman RE, Peterson SW. (1987) Insulin stimulates choline acetyltransferase activity in cultured embryonic chicken retina neurons. *Proc Natl Acad Sci USA* 84(21): 7463-7467.

Laitinen LV, Bergenheim T, Hariz MI. (1992) Leksell's posteroventral pallidotomy in the treatment of Parkinson's disease. *J Neurosurg* 76: 53-61.

Lapp CW, Cheney PR, Ouyang G. (1994) Specialist evaluation in chronic fatigue syndrome: A cost/benefit analysis. Poster: International Meeting on Chronic Fatigue Syndrome, Dublin, May 18-20.

Larsen PJ, Jessop D, Patel H, Lightman SL, Chowdrey HS. (1993) Substance P inhibits the release of anterior pituitary adrenocorticotrophin via a central mechanism involving corticotrophin-releasing factor-containing neurons in the hypothalamic paraventricular nucleus. *J Neuroendocrinol* 5(1): 99-105.

Lauterback EC, Price ST, Wilson AN, Jackson G. (1994) Pallidothalamocortical circuits in subcortical poststroke mood disorders. *J Neuropsychiatry Clin Neurosci* 6: 317.

Lavi E, Fisman PS, Highkin MH. (1988) Limbic encephalitis after inhalation of murine coronavirus. *Lab Invest* 58(1): 31-36.

Leckman JF, Goodman WK, North WG, Chappell PB, Price LH, Pauls DL, Anderson GM, Riddle MA, McSwiggan-Hardin M, McDougle CJ, Barr LC, Cohen DJ. (1994a) Elevated cerebrospinal fluid levels of oxytocin in obsessive-compulsive disorder. *Arch Gen Psychiatry* 51: 782-792.

Leckman JF, Goodman WK, North WG, Chappell PB, Price LH, Pauls DL, Anderson GM, Riddle MA, McDougle CJ, Barr LC, Cohen DJ. (1994b) The role of central oxytocin in obsessive compulsive disorder and related normal behavior. *Psychoneuroimmunol* 19(8): 723-749.

LeDoux JE. (1993) Emotional memory systems in the brain. *Behav Brain Res* 58: 69-79.

LeDoux JE. (1994) The amygdala: Contributions to fear and stress. *Sem Neurosci* 6: 231-237.

LeDoux JE, Ruggiero DA, Forest R, Stornetta R, Reis DJ. (1987) Topographic organization of convergent projections to the thalamus from the inferior colliculus and spinal cord in the rat. *J Comp Neurol* 246(1): 123-146.

Lee J-H, Price RAH, Williams FG, Mayer B, Beitz AJ. (1993) Nitric oxide synthase is found in some spinothalamic neurons and in neuronal processes that appose spinal neurons that express Fos induced by noxious stimulation. *Brain Res* 608: 324-333.

Lee MK, Graham SN, Gold PE. (1988) Memory enhancement with posttraining intraventricular glucose injections in rats. *Behav Neurosci* 102(4): 591-595.

Lee S, Rivier C, Torres G. (1994) Induction of c-fos and CRF mRNA by MK-801 in the parvocellular paraventricular nucleus of the rat hypothalamus. *Mol Brain Res* 24: 192-198.

Lees AJ. (1987) A sustained-released formulation of L-dopa (Madopar HBS) in the treatment of nocturnal and early-morning disabilities in Parkinson's disease. *Eur Neurol* 27: 5126-5134.

Lefkowitz RJ, Hoffman BB, Taylor P. (1990) Drugs acting at synaptic and neuroeffector junctional sites: Neurohumoral transmission: The autonomic and somatic motor nervous systems. In Gilman AG, Rall TW, Nies AJ, Taylor P (Eds.), *Goodman and Gilman's the Pharmacological Basis of Therapeutics* (pp. 84-121). New York: Pergamon Press.

Leiner HC, Leiner AL, Dow RS. (1993) Cognitive and language functions of the human cerebellum. *Trends Neurosci* 16(11): 444-447.

Leitner ML, Hohmann AG, Patrick SL, Walker JM. (1994) Regional variation in the ratio of sigma-1 to sigma-2 binding in rat brain. *Eur J Pharmacol* 259: 65-69.

Len WB, Tsuo M-Y, Chan SHH, Chan JYH. (1994) Substance P suppresses the activity of alpha-2 adrenoceptors of the nucleus reticularis gigantocellularis involved in cardiovascular regulation in the rat. *Brain Res* 638: 227-234.

Lenz FA, Gracely RH, Hope EJ, Baker FH, Rowland LH, Dougherty PM, Richardson RT. (1994) The sensation of angina can be evoked by stimulation of the human thalamus. *Pain* 59(1): 119-126.

Leonard BE. (1992) Sub-types of serotonin receptors: Biochemical changes and pharmacological consequences. *Int Clin Psychopharmacol* 7: 13-21.

Levine J, Borak Y, Gonsalves M, Szor H, Elizur A, Kofman O, Belmaker RH. (1995) Double-blind, controlled trial of inositol treatment of depression. *Am J Psychiatry* 152(5): 792-794.

Levine J, Gonsalves M, Babur I, Stier S, Elizur A, Kofman O, Belmaker RH. (1993) Inositol 6 g daily may be effective in depression but not in schizophrenia. *Human Psychopharmacol* 8: 49-53.

Levy A, Cachir S, Kadar T, et al. (1993) Nimodipine, stress and central cholinergic function. In Scriabine A, Janis RA, Triggle DJ (Eds.), *Drugs in Development* (vol. 2: Ca^{2+} Antagonists in the CNS, pp. 223-229). Brandford, Connecticut: Neva Press.

Lewis S, Cooper CL, Bennett D. (1994) Psychosocial factors and chronic fatigue syndrome. *Psychol Med* 24: 661-671.

Lewis SJ, Davisson RL, Bates JN, Johnson AK. (1993) Functional evidence that nitric oxide factors are released from post-ganglionic sympathetic nerves in rats. *FASEB Journal* 7(1): A432.

Li Y-Q, Takada M, Matsuzaki S, Shinonoga Y, Mizuno N. (1993) Identification of periaqueductal gray and dorsal raphe nucleus neurons projecting to both the trigeminal sensory complex and forebrain structures: A fluorescent retrograde double-labeling study in the rat. *Brain Res* 623: 267-277.

Liberzon I, Chalmers DT, Mansour A, Lopez JF, Watson SJ, Young EA. (1994) Glucocorticoid regulation of hippocampal oxytocin receptor binding. *Brain Res* 650: 317-322.

Linde A, Andersson B, Svenson SB, Ahrne H, Carlsson M, Forsberg P, Hugo H, Korstorp A, Lenkel R, Lindwall A, Luflenius A, Sall C, Anderson J. (1992) Serum levels of lymphokines and soluble cellular receptors in primary Epstein-Barr virus infection and in patients with chronic fatigue syndrome. *J Infect Dis* 165: 994-1000.

Lipton SA. (1993) Prospects for clinically tolerated NMDA antagonists: Open-channel blockers and alternative redox states of nitric oxide. *Trends Neurosci* 16(12): 527-532.

Lipton SA, Gendelman HE. (1995) Seminars in medicine of the Beth Israel Hospital, Boston. Dementia associated with the acquired immunodeficiency syndrome. *N Engl J Med* 332(14): 934-940.

Lipton SA, Rosenberg PA. (1994) Excitatory amino acids as a final common pathway for neurologic disorders. *N Engl J Med* 330(9): 613-622.

Livingston MG. (1994) Risperidone. *Lancet* 343: 457-459.

Lloyd A, Hickie I, Brockman A, Dwyer J, Wakefield D. (1991) Cytokine levels in serum and cerebrospinal fluid in patients with chronic fatigue syndrome and control subjects. *J Infect Dis* 164(5): 1023-1024.

Lohse MJ. (1993) Molecular mechanisms of beta-adrenergic membrane receptor desensitization. *Biochim Biophys Acta* 1179: 171-188.

Lohse MJ, Andexinger S, Pitcher J, Trukawinski S, Codina J, Faure J-P, Caron MG, Lefkowitz RJ. (1992) Molecular mechanisms of beta-adrenergic receptor desensitization. *J Biol Chem* 267: 8558-8564.

Lomasney J, Allen L. (1993) Mechanisms of receptor desensitization. *Trends Pharmacol Sci* 14: suppl. 1.

Lorenc-Koci E, Ossowska K, Wardos J, Konieczky J, Wolfarth S. (1994) Involvement of the nucleus accumbens in the myorelaxant effect of baclofen in rats. *Neurosci Lett* 170: 125-128.

Lorrain DS, Hull EN. (1993) Nitric oxide increases dopamine and serotonin release in the medial preoptic area. *NeuroReport* 5(1): 87-89.

Loscher W, Honack D, Taylor CP. (1994) Gabapentin increases aminooxyacetic acid-induced GABA accumulation in several regions of the rat brain. *Neurosci Lett* 128: 150-154.

Lottenberg S. (1993) PET in CFS: Possible hypometabolism in a neural network. Presented at Medical Neurobiology of Chronic Fatigue Syndrome and Fibromyalgia: The Fourth Annual Conference, Bel Air, California, May. *CFIDS Chron* Summer: 1-11.

Loup T, Tribollet E, Dubois-Dauphin M, Dreifuss JJ. (1991) Localization of high-affinity binding sites for oxytocin and vasopressin in the human brain: An autoradiographic study. *Brain Res* 563: 220-232.

Loup T, Tribollet E, Dubois-Dauphin M, Pizzolato G, Dreifuss JJ. (1989) Localization of oxytocin binding sites in the human brainstem and upper spinal cord: An autoradiographic study. *Brain Res* 500: 223-230.

Lukas RJ, Bencherif M. (1993) Channels, channels everywhere: Local anesthetic-mediated blockade of high-affinity neurotransmitter uptake and of Na^+-K^+ exchange. *J Neurochem* 61(suppl.): S214A.

Madsen PL, Sperling BK, Warming T, Schmidt JF, Secher NH, Wildschiodtz G, Holm S, Lassen NA. (1993) Middle cerebral artery blood velocity and cerebral blood flow and O_2 uptake during dynamic exercise. *J Appl Physiol* 74: 245-250.

Mains RE. (1993) Amidation of neuropeptides: A site for regulation by hormones, ascorbic acid, and copper. *Neuropsychopharmacol* 9(25): 465.

Malcongio M, Bowery NG. (1995) Possible therapeutic application of $GABA_B$ receptor agonists and antagonists. *Clin Neuropharm* 18(4): 285-305.

Malick A, Burnstein R. (1995) Direct projection of trigeminal brainstem neurons to the hypothalamus of the rat. *Abstracts, Soc for Neurosci* 21: 456.7, p. 1165.

Markowitz S, Saito K, Moskowitz MA. (1987) Neurogenically mediated leakage of plasma protein occurs from blood vessels in dura mater but not brain. *J Neurosci* 7(12): 4129-4136.

Marrocco RT, Witte EA, Davidson MC. (1994) Arousal systems. *Curr Opin Neurobiol* 4: 166-170.

Martin FC, Anton PA, Gornbein JA, Shanahan F, Merrill JE. (1993) Production of interleukin-1 by microglia in response to substance P: Role for a non-classical NK-1 receptor. *J Neuroimmunol* 42(1): 53-60.

Martin WJ. (1995) Personal communication.

Martin WJ, Glass RT. (1995) Acute encephalopathy induced in cats with a stealth virus isolated from a pateint with chronic fatigue syndrome. *Pathobiol* 63: 115-118.

Martin WJ, Zeng LC, Ahmed K, Roy M. (1994) Cytomegalovirus-related sequence in an atypical cytopathic virus repeatedly isolated from a patient with chronic fatigue syndrome. *Am J Pathol* 145(2): 440-451.

Martin WJ, Ahmed KN, Zeng LC, Olsen JC, Seward JG, Sechrai JS. (1995) African green monkey origin of the atypical cytopathic stealth virus isolated from a patient with chronic fatigue syndrome. *Clin Diag Virol* (4):93-103.

Mathe AA, Agren H, Srinivasan GR, Theodorsson E, Van Kamman DP. (1994) Calcitonin gene-related peptide (CGRP), endothelin (ET) and neuropeptide Y (NPY) in cerebrospinal fluid (CSF) of patients with schizophrenia and major depression. *Acta Psychiatr Scand*: B3.

Mathew RJ. (1995) Sympathetic control of cerebral circulation: Relevance to psychiatry. *Biol Psychiatry* 37(5) 283-285.

Mathias JR, Clench MH, Roberts PH, Reeves-Darby VG. (1994) Effect of leuprolide acetate in patients with functional bowel disease: Long-term follow-up after double-blind, placebo-controlled study. *Dig Dis Sci* 39(6): 1163-1170.

Mathias JR, Clench MH, Reeves-Darby VG, Fox LM, Hsu PH, Roberts PH, Smith LL, Stiglich NJ. (1994) Effect of leuprolide acetate in patients with moderate to severe functional bowel disease: Double-blind, placebo-controlled study. *Dig Dis Sci* 39(6): 1155-1162.

Mathis C, Lehmann J, Ungerer A. (1992) The selective protein kinase C inhibitor, NCP 15437, induces specific deficits in memory retention in mice. *Eur J Pharmacol* 220: 107.

Matsui TA, Takuwa Y, Johshita H, Yamashita K, Asano T. (1991) Possible role of protein kinase C-dependent smooth muscle contraction in the pathogenesis of chronic cerebral vasospasm. *J Cereb Blood Flow Metab* 11: 143-149.

Matsumoto H, Suzuki N, Shiota K, Inoue K, Tsuda M, Fujino M. (1990) Insulin-like growth factor-1 stimulates endothelin-3 secretion from rat anterior pituitary cells in primary culture. *Biochem Biophys Res Comm* 172(2): 661-668.

Maurice T, Hiramatsu M, Itoh J, Kameyama T, Hasegawa T, Nabeshinin T. (1994) Low dose of 1, 3-di (2-tolyl) guanidine (DTG) attenuates MK-801-induced spatial working memory in mice. *Psychopharmacol* 114: 520-522.

Maxton DG, Morris J, Whorwell PJ. (1991) More accurate diagnosis of irritable bowel syndrome by the use of "non-colonic" symptomatology. *Gut* 32: 784-786.

Mayberg HS. (1994) Frontal lobe dysfunction in secondary depression. *J Neuropsychiatry Clin Neurosci* 6(4): 428- 442.

Mayberg HS, Sarkstein SE, Sadzot B, Preziosi T, Andrezejewski PL, Dannals RF, Wagner HN, Robinson RG. (1990) Selective hypometabolism in the inferior frontal lobe in depressed patients with Parkinson's disease. *Ann Neurol* 28: 57-64.

Mayer EA, Gebhart GF. (1993) Functional bowel disorders and the visceral hyperalgesia hypothesis. In Mayer EA, Raybould HE, (Eds.), *Basic and Clinical Aspects of Chronic Abdominal Pain.* New York: Elsevier.

Mayer EA, Raybould H (Eds.). (1993) *Basic and clinical aspects of chronic abdominal pain.* New York: Elsevier.

Mayer ML. (1994) Modulation of NMDA-subtype glutamate receptor ion channels by Mg. *Neuropsychopharmacol* 10(3S/Pt.1): 486S.

Mayeux R, Stern Y, Sano M, Williams JB, Cote LJ. (1988) The relationship of serotonin to depression in Parkinson's disease. *Mov Disord* 3(3): 237-244.

McAllister H. (1994) D-cycloserine enhances social behavior in individually-housed mice in the resident-intruder test. *Psychopharmacol* 116: 317-325.

McBride WJ, Murphy JM, Lumeng L, Li TK. (1986) Effects of ethanol on monoamine and amino acid release from cerebral cortical slices of the alcohol-preferring P line of rats. *Alcohol, Clin Exp Res* 10: 205-208.

McCarty R. (1994) Regulation of plasma catecholamine responses to stress. *Sem Neurosci* 6: 197-204.

McEwen BS. (1994) The plasticity of the hippocampus is the reason for its vulnerability. *Sem Neurosci* 6: 239-246.

McGaugh JL, Intromi-Collison IB, Cahill LF, Costellano C, Dalmaz C, Parent MB, Williams CL. (1993) Neuromodulatory systems and memory storage: Role of the amygdala. *Brain Res* 58: 81-90.

McIntyre MB, Pemberton JH. (1994) Pathophysiology of colonic motor disorders. *Surg Clin North Am* 73(6): 1225- 1243.

McQuiston AR, Colmers WF. (1992) Neuropeptide Y does not alter NMDA conductances in CA3 pyramidal neurons: A slice-patch study. *Neurosci Lett* 138(2): 261-264.

Meaney MJ, Tannenbaum B, Francis D, Bhatnagar S, Shanks N, Viav V, O'Donnell D, Plotsky PM. (1994) Early environmental programming of hypothalamic-pituitary-adrenal responses to stress. *Sem Neurosci* 6: 247-259.

Meaney MJ, Bhatnagar S, Diorio J, Sarocque S, Francis D, O'Donnell D, Shatiks S, Sharma S, Smythe J, Viau V. (1993) Molecular basis for the development of individual differences in the hypothalamic-pituitary-adrenal stress response. *Cell Mol Neurobiol* 13(4): 321-348.

Mega MS, Cummings JL. (1994) Frontal-subcortical circuits and neuropsychiatric disorders. *J Neuropsychiatry Clin Neurosci* 6(4): 358-370.

Megans AAHP, Awauters FHL, Meert TF, Dugovic C, Niemegeers CJE, Leysen JE. (1994) Survey on the pharmacodynamics of the new antipsychotic risperidone. *Psychopharmacol* 114: 9-23.

Mehta S, Parsons LM, Webb HE. (1993) Effect of amitriptyline on neurotransmitter levels in adult mice following infection with the avirulent strain of Semliki Forest virus. *J Neurol Sci* 116: 110-116.

Melis MR, Argiolas A. (1993) Nitric oxide synthase inhibitors prevent apomorphine- and oxytocin-induced penile erection and yawning in male rats. *Brain Res Bull* 32: 71-74.

Meller ST, Gebhart GF. (1993) Nitric oxide (NO) and nociceptive processing in the spinal cord. *Pain* 52: 127-136.

Meltzer HY. (1992) The importance of serotonin-dopamine interactions in the action of clozapine. *Br J Psychiatry* 60(suppl. 17): 22-29.

Meltzer HY, Maes M. (1994) Effect of pindolol on the L-5-HTP-induced increase in plasma prolactin and cortisol concentrations in man. *Psychopharmacol* 114: 635-643.

Melzack R. (1992) Phantom limbs. *Sci Am* 266(4): 120-127.

Mena I. (1993) Cerebral hypoperfusion in late life chronic fatigue syndrome (CFS) and late life depression (D). Presented at Medical Neurobiology of Chronic Fatigue Syndrome and Fibromyalgia: The Fourth Annual Conference, Bel Air, California, May. (1993) *CFIDS Chron* Summer: 1-11.

Mens WBJ, Witter A, Van Wimersma B, Greidanus TB. (1983) Penetration of neurohypophyseal hormones from plasma into cerebrospinal fluid (CSF): Half-times of disappearances of three neuropeptides from CSF. *Brain Res* 262: 143-149.

Messenheimer JA. (1994) Lamotrigine. *Clin Neuropharmacol* 17: 548-559.

Messier C, Destrade C. (1994) Insulin attenuates scopolamine-induced memory deficits. *Psychobiol* 22: 16-21.

Mesulam M-M. (1985) *Principles of Behavioral Neurology*. Philadelphia: FA Davis.

Mesulam M-M. (1990) Large-scale neurocognitive networks and distributed processing for attention, language, and memory. *Ann Neurol* 28(5): 597-612.

Mesulam M-M, Mufson EJ. (1984) Thalamic connections of the insula in the rhesus monkey and comments on the paralimbic connectivity of the medial pulvinar nucleus. *J Comp Nerol* 227 (1): 109-120.

Meunier M, Bachevalier J, Mishkin M, Murray EA. (1993) Effects on visual recognition of combined and separate ablations of the entorhinal and perirhinal cortex of rhesus monkeys. *J Neurosci* 13: 5418-5432.

Middleton D, Savage DA, Smith DG. (1991) No association of HLA class II antigen in chronic fatigue syndrome. *Dis Mark* 9: 47-49.

Middleton FA, Strick PF. (1994) Anatomical evidence for cerebellar and basal ganglia involvement in higher cognitive function. *Science* 266: 458-461.

Mielle M, Boutelle MG, Fillenz M. (1994) The physiologically induced release of ascorbate in rat brain is dependent on impulse traffic, calcium influx, and glutamate uptake. *Neurosci* 42(1): 87-91.

Mikuni M, Muneoka K, Kitera K, Saitoh K, Ogawa T, Takahashi K. (1994) Neonatal and prenatal stresses alter hypothalamic-pituitary-adrenal responses to stressful stimuli in adulthood. *Neuropsychopharmacol* 10(3S/Pt.1): 750S.

Minami M, Kimura M, Iwamoto N, Arai H. (1995) Endothelin-1-like immunoreactivity in cerebral cortex of Alzheimer-type dementia. *Prog Neuropsychopharmacol Biol Psyciatry* 19: 509-513.

Minciacchi D et al. (Eds.). (1993) Thalamic networks for relay and modulation. New York: Pergamon Press.

Minokoshki Y, Okano Y, Shimazu T. (1994) Regulatory mechanism of the ventromedial hypothalamus in enhancing glucose uptake from skeletal muscles. *Brain Res* 649: 343-347.

Mishkin M, Murray EA. (1994) Stimulus recognition. *Curr Opin Neurobiol* 4: 200-206.

Mishkin M, Phillips RR. (1990) A corticolimbic memory path revealed through its disconnection. In Trevarthen C (Ed.), *Brain Circuits and Functions of the Mind: Essays in Honor of Roger W. Sperry* (pp. 197-210). Cambridge: Cambridge University Press.

Mitchell JH, Kaufman MP, Iwamoto GA. (1983) The exercise pressor reflex: Its cardiovascular effects, afferent mechanisms, and central pathways. *Ann Rev Physiol* 43: 229-242.

Mitler MM, Hadjukovic R, Erman MK. (1993) Treatment of narcolepsy with methamphetamine. *Sleep* 16(4): 306-317.

Mitrofanis J. (1992) Patterns of antigenic expression in the thalamic reticular nucleus of developing rats. *J Comp Neurol* 320: 161-181.

Mitrofanis J. (1994) Development of the pathway from the reticular and perireticular nuclei to the thalamus in ferrets: A Dil study. *Eur J Neurosci* 6: 1864-1882.

Mitrofanis J, Guillery RW. (1993) New views of the thalamic reticular nucleus in the adult and developing brain. *Trends Neurosci* 16(6): 240-245.

Miyagawa A, Okamura H, Ibata Y. (1994) Coexistence of oxytocin and NADPH-diaphorase in magnocellular neurons of the paraventricular and supraoptic nuclei of the rat hypothalamus. *Neurosci Lett* 171: 13-16.

Miyamoto A, Nishio A. (1993) Characterization of histamine receptors in isolated pig basilar artery by functional and radioligand studies. *Life Sci* 53: 1259-1266.

Mochizuki T, Okakura-Mochizuki K, Horii A, Yamamoto Y, Yamatodani A. (1994) Histaminergic modulation of hippocampal acetylcholine release in vivo. *J Neurochem* 62: 2275-2282.

Moffoot A, O'Carroll RE, Murray C, Dougall N, Ebmeier KP, Goodwin GM. (1993) Effects of clonidine on cognition and rCBF in Korsakoff's psychosis. *Psychol Med* 23: 341-347.

Mohr E, Knott V, Sampson M, Wesnes K, Herting R, Mendis T. (1995) Cognitive and quantified electroencephalographic correlates of cycloserine treatment in Alzheimer's disease. *Clin Neuropharmacol* 18(1): 28-38.

Molchan SE, Atack JR, Sunderland T. (1994) Decreased CSF inositol monophosphatase activity after lithium treatment. *Psychiatry Res* 53: 103-105.

Moldofsky H. (1989) Non-restorative sleep and symptoms after afebrile illness in patients with fibrositis and chronic fatigue syndrome. *J Rheumatol* 19(suppl.): 150-153.

Mongeau R, DeMontigry C, Blier P. (1994) Effect of long-term administration of antidepressant drugs on the 5-HT$_3$ receptors that enhance the electrically evoked release of [^{3}H] noradrenaline in the rat hippocampus. *Eur J Pharmacol* 271: 121-129.

Monnet FP, Debonnet G, DeMontigny C. (1992) In vivo electrophysiological evidence for a selective modulation of N-methyl-D-aspartate-induced neuronal activation in rat CA$_3$ dorsal hippocampus by sigma ligands. *J Pharmacol Exp Ther* 261: 123-130.

Montero VM, Singer W. (1985) Ultrastructural identification of somatic and neural processes immunoreactive to antibodies against glutamic acid decarboxylase (GAD) in the dorsal lateral geniculate nucleus of the cat. *Exp Brain Res* 59: 151-165.

Moskowitz MA. (1991) The visceral organ brain: Implications for the pathophysiology of vascular head pain. *Neurol* 41(2)(pt.1): 182-186.

Moskowitz MA. (1992a) Interpreting vessel diameter changes in vascular headaches. *Cephalalgia* 12(1): 5-7.

Moskowitz MA. (1992b) Neurogenic versus vascular mechanisms of sumatriptan and ergot alkaloids in migraine. *Trends Pharmacol Sci* 13(8): 307-312.

Mountz JM, Bradley L, Modell JG, Triana M, Alexander R, Mountz JD. (1993) Limbic system dysregulation in fibromyalgia measured by regional cerebral blood flow. *Arth Rheum* 36 (suppl. 57):5P.

Mountz JM, Bradley LA, Modell JG, Alexander RW, Triana M, Aaron LA, Stewart KE, Alarcon G, Mountz JD. (1995) Fibromyalgia in women: Abnormalities of regional cerebral blood flow in the thalamus and caudate nucleus are associated with low pain threshold levels. *Arth Rheum* 7: 926-928.

Muhlethaler M, Swayer WH, Manning MM, Dreifuss JJ. (1983) Characterization of uterine-type oxytocin receptor in the rat hippocampus. *Proc Natl Acad Sci USA* 80: 6713-6717.

Munschauer FE, Mador MJ, Ahuja A, Jacobs L. (1991) Selective paralysis of voluntary but not limbically influenced automatic respirations. *Arch Neurol* 48: 1190-1192.

Murphy LL, Newton SC, Dhali J, Chavez D. (1991) Evidence for a direct anterior pituitary site of Δ^9-tetrahydrocannabinol action. *Pharmacol Biochem Behav* 40: 603-608.

Myhrer T, Johannesen TS. (1994) Cognitive and mnemonic dysfunctions in rats with hippocampal-entorhinal lesions: Attenuating effects of glycine injections. *Psychobiol* 11(1): 61-67.

Myslobodsky MS. (1993) Pro- and anticonvulsant effects of stress: the role of neuroactive steroids. *Neurosci Biobehav Rev* 17: 129-139.

Nadler V, Mechoulan R, Sokolovsky M. (1993) Blockade of $^{45}Ca^{2+}$ influx through the N-methyl-D-aspartate receptor ion channel by non-psychoactive cannabinoid HU-211. *Brain Res* 622: 79-85.

Naftolin F, Leranth C, Perez J, Garcia-Segura LM. (1993) Estrogen induces synaptic plasticity in adult primate neurons. *Neuroendocrinol* 57: 935-939.

Nair MPN, Cilik JM, Schwartz SA. (1986) Histamine-induced suppressor factor inhibition of NK cells: reversal with interferon and interleukin 2. *J Immunol* 136(7): 2456-2462.

Narita K, Nishihara M, Takahashi M. (1993) Concomitant regulation of running activity and metabolic change by the ventromedial nucleus of the hypothalamus. *Brain Res* 642: 290-296.

Narita K, Yokawa T, Nishihara M, Takahashi. (1993) Interaction between excitatory and inhibitory amino acids in the ventromedical nucleus of the hypothalamus in inducing hyper-running. *Brain Res* 603(2): 243-247.

Narkowicz CK, Vial JH, McCartney PW. (1993) Hyperbaric oxygen therapy increases free radical levels in the blood of humans. *Free Rad Res Comm* 19(2): 71-80.

Nasstrom J, Karlsson U, Berge O-G. (1993) Systemic or intracerebroventricular injection of NMDA receptor antagonists attenuates the antinociceptive activity of intrathecally administered NMDA receptor antagonists. *Abstracts, 7th World Congress on Pain* (p. 45). Seattle: IASP Publications.

Nathanson JA. (1992) Nitrovasodilators as a new class of ocular hypotensive agents. *J Pharmacol Exp Ther* 260(3): 956-965.

Nauta WJ. (1971) The problem of the frontal lobe: A reinterpretation. *J Psychiatr Res* 8(3): 167-187.

Nemeroff CB, Owens MJ, Weiss JM. (1994) Stress, CRF and monoamine activity in lower animals and man. *Neuropsychopharmacol* 10(3S/Pt.1): 220S.

Netti C, Sibilia V, Gluidobono F, Villani P, Pecile A, Braga PC. (1994) Evidence for an inhibitory role of central histamine in carrageenin-induced hyperalgesia. *Neuropharmacol* 33(2): 205-210.

Neubauer JA. (1991) Carbonic anhydrase and sensory function in the central nervous system. In Dudgson SJ, Tashian RE, Gros G, Carter ND (Eds.), *The Carbonic Anyhdrases: Cellular Physiology and Molecular Genetics* (pp. 333-346). New York: Plenum Press.

Newberry NR, Gilbert MJ. (1989) 5-Hydroxytryptamine evokes three distinct responses on the rat superior cervical ganglion in vitro. *Eur J Pharmacol* 162(2): 197-205.

Nguyen PV, Abel T, Kandel ER. (1994) Requirement of a critical period of transcription for induction of a late phase of LTP. *Science* 265: 1104-1107.

Nicolodi M, Sicuteri R, Coppola G, Greco G, Pietrini U, Sicuteri F. (1994) Visceral pain threshold is deeply lowered far from the head in migraine. *Headache* 34: 12-19.

Nikolov R, Maslarova J, Semkova I, Moyanova S. (1992) Intracerebroventricular endothelin-1 (ET-1) produces Ca^{2+} mediated antinociception in mice. *Meth Find Exp Clin Pharmacol* 14: 229-233.

Nishimura Y, Muramatsu M, Asahara T, Tanaka T, Yamamoto T. (1995) Electrophysiological properties and their modulation by norepinephrine in the ambiguus neurons of the guinea pig. *Brain Res* 702: 213-222.

Nobler MS, Sackheim HA, Prohovnik I, Moeller JR, Roose SP. (1995) Divergent effects of antidepressants and ECT on cerebral perfusion in major depression. *Psychopharmacol Bull* 30(4): 699.

Nobler MS, Sackheim H, Prohovnik I, Moeller JR, Mukherjel S, Schnur DB, Prudic J, Devanand DP. (1994) Regional cerebral blood flow in mood disorders, III: Treatment and clinical response. *Arch Gen Psychiatry* 51: 884-897.

Nonogaki K, Mizuno K, Sakamoto N, Iguchi A. (1994) Effects of central GABA receptor activation on catecholamine secretion in rats. *Life Sci* 55(12): PL 239-243.

Nordholm AF, Thompson JK, Dersarkissian C, Thompson RF. (1993) Lidocaine infusion in a critical region of cerebellum completely prevents learning of the conditioned eyeblink response. *Behav Neurosci* 107(5): 882-886.

Nowak G, Paul I, Popik P, Young A, Skolnick P. (1993) Ca^{++} antagonists exert an antidepressant-like adaptation of NMDA receptor complex. *Eur J Pharmacol-Mol Pharmacol Section* 247: 101-102.

Nowak JZ, Sek B. (1994) Stimulating effect of histamine on cyclic AMP formation in chick pineal gland. *J Neurochem* 63: 1338-1345.

Nozaki K, Moskowitz MA, Boccalini P. (1992) CP-93,129, sumatriptan, dihydroergotamine block c-fos expression within rat trigeminal nucleus caudalis caused by chemical stimulation of the meninges. *Br J Pharmacol* 106(2): 409-415.

Nozaki K, Moskowitz MA, Maynard KI, Koketsu N, Dawson TM, Bredt DS, Snyder SH. (1993) Possible origins and distribution of immunoreactive nitric oxide synthase-containing nerve fibers in cerebral arteries. *J Cereb Blood Flow Metab* 13(1): 70-79.

Nyhlin H, Ford MJ, Eastwood J, Smith JN, Nicol EF, Elton RA, Eastwood MA. (1993) Non-alimentary aspects of the irritable bowel syndrome. *J Psychosom Res* 37(2): 155-162.

O'Dell TJ, Huang PL, Dawson TM, Dinerman JL, Snyder SH, Kandell ER, Fishman MC. (1994) Endothelial NOS and the blockade of LTP by NOS inhibitors in mice lacking neuronal NOS. *Science* 265(5171): 542-546.

Oh K-S, Lee C-J, Gibbs JW, Coulter DA. (1995) Postnatal development of $GABA_A$ receptor function in somatosensory thalamus and cortex: Whole-cell voltage-clamp recordings in acutely isolated rat neurons. *J Neurosci* 15(2): 1341-1351.

Ohno M, Yamamoto T, Watanabe S. (1994) Intrahippocampal administration of glycine site antagonist impairs working memory performance of rats. *Eur J Pharmacol* 253: 183-187.

Ohta K, Gotoh F, Shimazu K, Amano T, Komatsumoto S, Hamada J, Takahashi S. (1991) Locus coeruleus stimulation exerts different influences on the changes of cerebral pial and intraparenchymal vessels. *Neurol Res* 13(3): 164-167.

O'Keane V, Dinan TG. (1994) Cholinergic and adrenergic function in depressed and healthy subjects: A neuroendocrine test battery using the growth hormone axis. *Human Psychopharmacol* 9: 171-179.

Oldstone MBA. (1989) Viral alterations of cell function. *Sci Am* 261(2): 42-49

Ong J, Kerr DIB, Lacey G, Curtis DR, Hughes R, Prager RH. (1994) Differing actions of nitropropane analogs of GABA and baclofen in central and peripheral preparations. *Eur J Pharmacol* 264: 49-54.

Ooboshi H, Sadoshima S, Ibayashi S, Yao H, Uchimura H, Fujishima M. (1993) Isradipine attenuates the ischemia-induced release of dopamine in the striatum of the rat. *Eur J Pharmacol* 233(1): 165-168.

O'Sullivan RL, Greenberg DB. (1993) H_2 antagonists, restless leg syndrome, and movement disorders. *Psychosom* 34(6): 530-532.

Page ME, Valentino RJ. (1994) Locus coeruleus activation by physiological challenges. *Brain Res Bull* 35: 557-560.

Palfreyman MG, Baron BM, Harrison BL, Kehne JH. (1994) Design and therapeutic potential of selective NMDA-glycine antagonists. *Neuropsychopharmacol* 10(3S/Pt.1): 99S.

Palmer JBD. (1994) Labeling changes for sumatriptan. Letter to physicians from Cerenex Pharmaceuticals.

Papadopolous GC, Parnavelas JG. (1991) Monoamine systems in the cerebral cortex: Evidence for anatomical specificity. *Prog Neurobiol* 36: 195-200.

Papp M, Moryl E. (1994) Antidepressant activity of non-competitive and competitive NMDA receptor antagonists in a chronic mild stress model of depression. *Eur J Pharmacol* 263: 1-7.

Parent A, Hazrati L-N. (1995) Functional anatomy of the basal ganglia. I: The cortico-basal ganglia-thalamo-cortical loop. *Brain Res Rev* 20: 91-127.

Parkes D, Kasckow J, Vale W. (1994) Carbon monoxide modulates secretion of corticotropin-releasing factor from rat hypothalamic cell cultures. *Brain Res* 646: 315-318.

Parsadaniantz SM, Gaillet S, Malaval F, Lenoir V, Batsche E, Barbanel G, Gardier A, Terlain B, Jaquot C, Szafarczyk A, Assenmacher I, Kerdelhue B. (1995) Lesions of the afferent catecholaminergic pathways inhibit the temporal activation of the CRH and POMC gene expression and ACTH release induced by human interleukin-1 beta in the male rat. *Neuroendocrin* 62: 586-595.

Parsons CG, Quack G. (1993) Effects of N-methyl-D aspartate antagonists in dementia. *J Neurochem* 61(suppl.): 551.

Pascale A, Milano S, Corsico N, Lucchi L, Battaini F, Martelli EA, Trabucchi M, Govoni S. (1994) Protein kinase C activation and anti-amnestic effect of acetyl-L-carnitine: In vitro and in vivo studies. *Eur J Pharmacol* 265: 1-7.

Passingham RE. (1975) Changes in the size and organization of the brain in man and his ancestors. *Brain Behav Evol* 11: 73-90.

Patterson PH. (1992) Process outgrowth and the specificity of connections. In Hall ZW (Ed.), *An Introduction to Molecular Neurobiology* (p. 422). Sunderland, Massachusetts: Sinauer.

Pavcovich LA, Cancella LA, Volosin M, Molina V, Ramirez O. (1990) Chronic stress-induced changes in locus coeruleus neuronal activity. *Brain Res Bull* 24: 293-296.

Pazzagalia PJ, George MS, Post RM, Rubinow DR, Davis CL. (1995) Nimodipine increases CSF somatostatin in affectively ill patients. *Neuropsychopharmacol* 13: 75-83.

Peck C, Coleman G. (1991) Implications of placebo theory for clinical research and practice in pain management. *Theoret Med* 12(3): 247-270.

Penalza-Rojas JH, Elterman M, Olmos N. (1964) Sleep induced by cortical stimulation. *Exp Neurol* 10: 140.

Penn RD, Goetz CG, Tanner CM, Klawans HL, Shannon KM, Comella CL, Witt TR. (1988) Adrenal medullary transplant operation for Parkinson's disease: Clinical observations in five patients. *Neurosurg* 22: 999-1004.

Pereira IT, Prado WA, Dos Reis MP. (1993) Enhancement of the epidural morphine-induced analgesia by systemic nifedipine. *Pain* 53(3): 341-346.

Peterson SE, Fiez JA. (1993) The processing of single words studied with positron emission tomography. *Ann Rev Neurosci* 16: 509-530.

Peticlerc E, Abel S, deBlois D, Poubelle PE, Marceau F. (1992) Effects of interleukin-1 receptor antagonist on three types of responses to interleukin-1 rabbit isolated blood vessels. *J Cardiovasc Pharmacol* 19(5): 821- 829.

Petit RL, Williams AM, Morilak DA. (1995) Colocalization of alpha-1$_{A/D}$ adrenoceptor mRNA with Type I and Type II glucocorticoid receptor mRNA in rat hippocampus using double in situ hybridization. *Abstracts, Soc for Neurosci* 21: 632.19, p. 1614.

Pierard C, Satabin P, Lagarde D, Barrere B, Guezennec CY, Menu JP, Pener M. (1995) Effects of a vigilance-enhancing drug, modafinil, on rat brain metabolism: A 2D COSY[1]H-NMR study. *Brain Res* 693: 251-256.

Pierce RC, Rebec GV. (1993) Intraneostriatal administration of glutamate antagonists increases behavioral activation and decreases neostriatal ascorbate via nondopaminergic mechanisms. *J Neurosci* 13(10): 4272-4280.

Pierce RC, Clemens AJ, Shapiro LA, Rebec GV. (1994) Repeated treatment with ascorbate or haloperidol, but not clozapine, elevates extracellular ascorbate in the neostriatum of freely moving rats. *Psychopharmacol* 116: 103-109.

Plotsky PM, Meaney MJ. (1993) Early postnatal experience alters hypothalamic corticotropin-releasing factor (CRF) mRNA, median eminence CRF content and stress-induced release in adult rats. *Mol Brain Res* 18: 195-200.

Pogun S, Baumann MH, Kuhar MJ. (1994) Nitric oxide inhibits [^{3}H] dopamine uptake. *Brain Res* 641: 83-91.

Posner IA. (1994) Treatment of fibromyalgia syndrome with intravenous lidocaine: A prospective, randomized pilot study. *J Musculoskel Pain* 2(4): 55-65.

Post RM. (1992) Transduction of psychosocial stress into the neurobiology of recurrent affective disorder. *Am J Psychiatry* 149: 999-1010.

Post RM. (1995) Anatomy and biochemistry of affective illness— Part I. *Audio-Digest Psychiatry* 24:8.

Powell R, Dolan R, Wessely S. (1990) Attributions and self-esteem in depression and chronic fatigue syndromes. *J Psychom Res* 14(6): 665-671.

Prieto J, Camps-Bansell J, Castilla A. (1992) Opioid-mediated monocyte dysfunction in the chronic fatigue syndrome. In Hyde BM (Ed.), *The Clinical and Scientific Basis of Myalgic Encephalomyelitis/Chronic Fatigue Syndrome* (pp. 575-584). Ottawa: Nightingale Research Foundation.

Prisco S, Pagonnone S, Esposito E. (1994) Serotonin-dopamine interaction in the rat ventral tegmental area: An electrophysiological study in vivo. *J Pharmacol Exp Ther* 271(1): 83-90.

Puder M, Weidenfeld J, Chowers I, Nir I, Conforti N, Seigel RA. (1982) Corticotrophin and corticosterone secretion following Δ^9-tetrahydrocannabinol in intact and hypothalamic deafferentiated male rats. *Exp Brain Res* 46:85.

Putnam FW, Trickett PK, Helmers K, Dorn L, Everett B. (1991) Cortisol abnormalities in sexually abused girls. *Proc of the 144th Annual Meeting of the American Psychiatric Association*, p. 107.

Pyner S, Coote JH. (1994) Evidence that sympathetic preganglionic neurones are arranged in target-specific columns in the thoracic spinal cord of the rat. *J Comp Neurol* 342(1): 15-22.

Quock RM, Nguyen E. (1992) Possible involvement of nitric oxide in chloridiazepoxide-induced anxiolysis in mice. *Life Sci* 51: PL255-260.

Ramassamy C, Girbe F, Christen Y, Costentin J. (1993) Gingkobiloaba extract EGB761 or trolox C prevent the ascorbic acid/Fe^{2+} induced decrease in synaptosomal membrane fluidity. *Free Rad Res Comm* 19(5): 341-350.

Raos V, Bentivoglio M. (1993) Crosstalk between the two sides of the thalamus through the reticular nucleus: A retrograde and anterograde tracing study in the rat. *J Comp Neurol* 332: 145-154.

Ratliff TL, Klutke CG, McDougall EM. (1994) The etiology of interstitial cystitis. *Urol Clin N Am* 21(2): 21-30.

Rebec GV. (1994) Amphetamine-induced ascorbate release in the neostriatum: Behavioral and neurophysiological implications. *Neuropsychopharmacol* 10(3S/Pt.1): 72S.

Reilly M, deSoria VG, Shemer A, Quartemain D. (1995) Efficacy of chronic administration of calcium channel blocker amlodipine on learning and retention in mice. *Abstracts, Soc for Neurosci*, 21: 377.6, p. 948.

Reul JMHM. (1994) Neuroendocrine and neuropharmacological correlates of immunological and psychological stress in animal models with an aberrant hypothalamic-pituitary-adrenocortical system. *Neuropsychopharmacol* 10(3S/Pt.1): 513S.

Rezvani AH, Grady D, Pucilowski O, Janowsky DS. (1993) Suppression of alcohol intake in alcohol-preferring rats by the Ca^{2+} channel antagonist nimodipine. In Scriabine A, Janis RA, Triggle DJ (Eds.), *Drugs in Development* (vol. 2: Ca^{2+} Antagonists in the CNS, pp. 143-151). Brandford, Connecticut: Neva Press.

Rho JH, Donevan SD, Rogowski MA. (1994) Mechanism of action of the anticonvulsant felbamate: Opposing effects on N-methyl-D-aspartate and gamma-aminobutyric acid$_A$ receptor. *Ann Neurol* 35(2): 229-234.

Rice ME, Perez-Pinzon MA, Lee EJK. (1994) Ascorbic acid, but not glutathione, is taken up by brain in slices and preserves cell morphology. *J Neurophysiol* 71(4): 1591-1596.

Richter JE, Baldi F, Clouse RE, Diamant NE, Janssens J, Staiano A. (1992) Functional oesophageal disorders. *Gastroenterol Int* 5: 3-17.

Riddle WJR, Scott AIF. (1995) Relapse after successful electroconvulsive therapy: The use and impact of continuation antidepressant drug therapy. *Human Psychopharmacol* 10: 201-205.

Rimon R, Lepola U, Jolkkonen J, Halonen T, Riekkinen P. (1995) Cerebrospinal fluid gamma-aminobutyric acid in patients with panic disorder. *Biol Psychiatry* 38: 737-741.

Rimpel J, Olbrich HM, Pach J, Scheer A, Louemann E, Grastpar M. (1995) Auditory event-related potentials in the course of antidepressant treatment: Amplitudes. *Prog Neuropsychopharmacol Biol Psychiatry* 19: 243-254.

Rivier C. (1993) Effects of interleukins or immune activation on neuroendocrine functions in the rat. Presented at Medical Neurobiology of Chronic Fatigue Syndrome and Fibromyalgia: The Fourth Annual Conference, Bel Air, California, May. *CFIDS Chron* Summer: 1-11.

Robbins TW, Everett BJ. (1993) Arousal systems and attention. In Gazzaniga MS (Ed.), *Handbook of Cognitive Neuroscience.* Cambridge, Massachusetts: MIT Press.

Robertson D. (1993) Autonomic neuropharmacology. *Curr Opin Neurol Neurosurg* 6: 527-530.

Rodriguez-Manzo G, Fernandez-Guasti A. (1995) Participation of the central noradrenergic system in the reestablishment of copulatory behavior of sexually exhausted rats by yohimbine, naloxone, and 8-OH-DPAT. *Brain Res Bull* 38: 399-404.

Roman FJ, Pascau X, Duffy G, Junien JL. (1991) Modulation by neuropeptide Y and peptide YY of NMDA effects in hippocampal slices: Role of sigma receptors. In Kameyama T, Nameshima T, Domino EF (Eds.), *NMDA Receptor Related Agonists: Biochemistry, Pharmacology, and Behavior* (pp. 211-218). Ann Arbor, Michigan: NPP Books.

Romanski LM, Bates JF, Goldman-Rakic PS. (1995) Selective connections of the superior temporal auditory region with the prefrontal cortex in the macaque monkey. *Abstracts, Soc for Neurosci* 21: 371.5, p. 932.

Roozendaal B, Cools AR. (1994) Influence of the noradrenergic state of the nucleus accumbens in basolateral amygdala mediated changes in neophobia of rats. *Behav Neurosci* 108: 1107-1118.

Rose RC. (1993) Cerebral metabolism of oxidized ascorbate. *Brain Res* 628: 49-55.

Rothwell NJ. (1991) Functions and mechanisms of interleukin-1 in the brain. *Trends Pharmacol Sci* 12(11): 430-436.

Rowe PC, Bou-Holaigah I, Kan JS, Calkins H. (1995) Is neurally mediated hypotension an unrecognised cause of chronic fatigue? *Lancet* 345: 623-624.

Rowsey PJ, Kluger MJ. (1994) Corticotropin releasing hormone is involved in exercise-induced elevation in core temperature. *Psychoneuroendocrinol* 19(2): 179-187.

Rudy B. (1988) Diversity and ubiquity of K channels. *Neurosci* 25: 729-749.

Ruggieri MR, Chelsky MJ, Rosen SJ, Shickley TJ, Hanno PM. (1994) Current findings and future research avenues in the study of interstitial cystitis. *Urol Clin N Am* 21(1): 163-176.

Russell IJ. (1994) Personal communication.

Russell IJ. (1995) Personal communication.

Russell IJ. (1996) Personal communication.

Russell IJ, Vaeroy H, Javors N, Nyberg F. (1992) Cerebrospinal fluid biogenic amine metabolites in fibromyalgia/fibrositis syndrome and rheumatoid arthritis. *Arth Rheum* 35: 550-556.

Russell IJ, Orr MD, Littman B, Vipraio GA, Aboukrek D, Michalek JE, Lopez Y, MacKillip F. (1994). Elevated cerebrospinal fluid levels of substance P in patients with the fibromyalgia syndrome. *Arth Rheum* 37: 1593-1601.

Russo C, Marchi M, Andrioli GC, Cavazzani P, Raiteri M. (1993) Enhancement of glycine release from human brain cortex synaptosomes by acetylcholine acting at M_4 muscarinic receptors. *J Pharmacol Exp Ther* 266(1): 142-146.

Ryding E, Decety J, Sjoholm H, Stenberg G, Ingvar DH. (1993) Motor imagery activates the cerebellum regionally. A SPECT rCBF study with 99mTc-HMPAO. *Brain Res Cogn Brain Res* 1: 94-99.

Ryo JH, Yanai K, Watanabe T. (1994) Marked increase in histamine H_3 receptors in the striatum and substantia nigra after 6-hydroxy-dopamine-induced denervation of dopaminergic neurons: An autoradiographic study. *Neurosci Lett* 128: 19-22.

Sackheim HA, Nobler MS, Provhonik I, Moeller JR, Devenand DP, Prodic J. (1994) Acute and short-term effects of ECT on regional cerebral blood flow—a marker of treatment adequacy? *Neuropsychopharmacol* 10(3S/Pt.1): 569S.

Sadun A. (1995) Personal communication.

Saito M, Minokoshi Y, Shimazu T. (1989) Accelerated norepine-phrine turnover in peripheral tissues after ventromedial hypotha-lamic stimulation in rats. *Brain Res* 481(2): 298-303.

Saito K, Saito H, Katsuki H. (1993) Synergism of tocopherol and ascorbate on the survival of cultured brain neurones. *NeuroReport* 4: 1179-1182.

Saleh TM, Cechetto DF. (1995) Neuropeptide changes in the nucleus of the solitary tract following cervical vagal stimulation. *Abstracts, Soc for Neurosci* 21: 259.9, p. 641.

Saletu B, Brandstatter N, Anderer P, Semlitsch HV, Binder G, Decker K, Metka M, Huber J, Knugler W. (1993) Neurophysio-logical investigations in menopausal syndrome with and without depression and normal controls: EEG and EP mapping. *Neuropsychopharmacol* 9(25): 615.

Salloway S, Cummings J. (1994) Subcortical disease and neuropsy-chiatric illness. *J Neuropsychiatry Clin Neurosci* 6(2): 93-99.

Sanchez-Moreno RM, Condes-Lara M, Alvarez-Leefmans FJ. (1995) Electrical stimulation effects of the locus ceruleus (LC) upon the spontaneous and evoked activity in the medial prefron-tal cortex and central lateral thalamic cells. *Abstracts, Soc for Neurosci* 21: 261.3., p. 646.

Sandi C, Guaza C. (1995) Evidence for a role of nitric oxide in the corticotropin-releasing factor release induced by interleukin-1 beta. *Eur J Pharmacol* 274: 17-23.

Sandman CA, Barron JL, Nackoul K, Goldstein J, Fidler F. (1993) Memory deficits associated with chronic fatigue immune dys-function syndrome (CFIDS). *Biol Psychiatry* 33: 618-623.

Saper JR. (1987) Ergotamine dependency–a review. *Headache* 27(8): 435-438.

Saperstein A, Brand H, Audhya T, Nabriski D, Hutchinson B, Ro-senzweig S, Hollander CS. (1992) Interleukin-1 beta mediates stress-induced immunosuppression via corticotropin-releasing factor. *Endocrinol* 130(1): 152-158.

Sapolsky RM. (1994a) Individual differences and the stress re-sponse. *Sem Neurosci* 6: 261-269.

Sapolsky RM. (1994b). *Why Zebras Don't Get Ulcers: A Guide to Stress, Stress-Related Diseases, and Coping.* New York: W. H. Greeman.

Sapolsky RM, Uno H, Rebert CS, Finch CE. (1990) Hippocampal damage associated with prolonged glucocorticoid exposure in primates. *J Neurosci* 10: 2897-2902.

Sara G, Gordon E, Kraiuhin C, Coyle S, Hauson A, Meares R. (1994) The P300 ERP component: An index of cognitive dysfunction in depression? *J Aff Dis* 31: 29-38.

Sara SJ, Vankov A, Herve A. (1994) Locus coeruleus-evoked responses in behaving rats: a clue to the role of noradrenaline in memory. *Brain Res Bull* 35: 457-465.

Sarnyai Z, Kovacs GL. (1994) Role of oxytocin in the neuroadaptation to drugs of abuse. *Psychoneuroendocrinol* 19(1): 85-117.

Sawchenko, PE. (1991) A tale of three peptides: Corticotropin-releasing factor-, oxytocin-, and vasopressin-containing pathways mediating integrated hypothalamic responses to stress. In McCubbin JA, Kaufmann PG, Nemeroff CB (Eds.), *Stress, Neuropeptides, and Systemic Disease.* San Diego: Academic Press.

Saxe GN, Chinman G, Berkowitz R, Hall K, Lieberg G, Schwartz J, van der Kolk BA. (1994) Somatization in patients with dissociative disorders. *Am J Psychiatry* 151: 1329-1334.

Scheibel AB. (1994) The thalamus in neuropsychiatric illness. *J Neuropsychiatry Clin Neurosci* 6(3): 300.

Schmidt CJ, Fadayel GM. (1995) The selective 5-HT$_{2A}$ receptor antagonist, MDL 100,907, increases dopamine efflux in the prefrontal cortex of the rat. *Eur J Pharmacol* 273: 273-279.

Schneider RJ, Friedman DP, Mishkin M. (1993) A modality-specific somatosensory area within the insula of the rhesus monkey. *Brain Res* 621: 116-120.

Schnider A, Regard M, Landis T. (1994) Anterograde and retrograde amnesia following bitemporal infarction. *Behav Neurol* 7: 87-92.

Schulkin J, McEwen BS, Gold PW. (1994) Allostasis, amygdala, and anticipatory angst. *Neurosci Biobehav Rev* 18(3): 385-396.

Schultz W, Romo R. (1987) Responses of nigrostriatal dopamine neurons to high-intensity somatosensory stimulation in the anesthetized monkey. *J Neurophysiol* 57: 407-411.

Schwartzman RJ. (1993) Reflex sympathetic dystrophy. *Curr Opin Neurol Neurosurg* 6: 531-536.

Scott AIF, Dougall N, Ross M, O'Carroll RE, Riddle W, Ebmeier KP, Goodwin GM. (1994) Short effects of electroconvulsive treatment on the uptake of ^{99m}Tc-exametazime into brain in major depression shown with single photon emission tomography. *J Aff Dis* 30: 27-34.

Seasack SR, Pickel VM. (1992) Prefrontal cortical efferents in the rat synapse on unlabeled neuronal targets of catecholamine terminals in the nucleus accumbens septi and on dopamine neurons in the ventral tegmental area. *J Comp Neurol* 320: 145-160.

Serra M, Ghiani CA, Spano S, Biggio G. (1994) Felbamate antagonizes isoniazid- and FG7142-induced reduction of GABA$_A$ receptor function in mouse brain. *Eur J Pharmacol* 265: 185-188.

Seutin V, Johnson SW, North RA. (1994) Effects of dopamine and baclofen on N-methyl-D-aspartate-induced burst firing in rat ventral tegmental neurons. *Neurosci* 58: 201-206.

Sharma RP, Bissette G, Janicak PG, Davis JM, Nemeroff CB. (1995) Elevation of CSF somatostatin concentrations in mania. *Am J Psychiatry* 152: 1807-1809.

Sheehan DV, Sheehan KH. (1982) The classification of anxiety and hysterical states. *J Clin Psychopharmacol* 2(6): 386-393.

Sheline Y, Black K, Bardgett M, Czernansky J. (1995) Platelet binding characteristics distinguish placebo responders from nonresponders in depression. *Psychopharmacol Bull* 30(4): 714.

Shelley WB, Shelley ED. (1994) Portrait of a practice. *Cutis* 54: 307.

Sherif F, Oreland L. (1994) Effects of chronic treatment with the GABA-transaminase inhibitor vigabatrin on exploratory behavior in rats. *Behav Brain Res* 63: 11-15.

Shibasaki T, Imaki T, Hotta M, Ling N, Demura H. (1993) Psychological stress increases arousal through brain corticotropin-releasing hormone without significant increase in adrenocorticotropin and catecholamine secretion. *Brain Res* 618: 71-75.

Shinomura T, Nakao S, Mori K. (1994) Reduction of depolarization-induced glutamate release by heme oxygenase inhibitor: Possible role of carbon monoxide in synaptic transmission. *Neurosci Lett* 166: 131-134.

Shintani F, Kanba S, Nakaki T, Nibuya M, Kinoshita N, Suzuki E, Yagi G, Kato R, Asai M. (1993) Interleukin-1 beta augments release of norepinephrine, dopamine, and serotonin in the rat anterior hypothalamus. *J Neurosci* 13(8): 3574-3581.

Shirakawa T, Moore RY. (1994) Glutamate shifts the phase of the circadian neuronal firing rhythm in the rat suprachiasmatic nucleus in vitro. *Neurosci Lett* 178: 47-50.

Shorter E. (1992) *From Paralysis to Fatigue.* New York: Free Press.

Shorter E. (1995) Sucker-punched again! Physicians meet the disease-of-the-month syndrome. *J Psychosom Res* 39(2): 115-118.

Shukla VK, Lemaire S. (1994) Non-opioid effects of dynorphins: Possible role of the NMDA receptor. *Trends Pharmacol Sci* 15: 420-424.

Sibilia V, Netti C, Guidobono F, Pagani F, Pecile A. (1985) Cimetidine-induced prolactin release—possible involvement of gabaergic system. *Neuroendocrinol* 40: 189-192.

Sibley DR, Daniel K, Strader CD, Lefkowitz RJ. (1987) Phosphorylation of the beta-adrenergic receptor in intact cells: Mechanisms of adenylate cyclase. *Arch Biochem Biophys* 278: 24-32.

Silverman A-J, Hou-Yu A, Kelly DD. (1989) Modification of hypothalamic neurons by behavioral stress. In Cantin M, Szabo S, Tache Y (Eds.), *Neuropeptides and Stress.* New York: Springer-Verlag.

Silverman D, Munakata JA, Ennes H, Mandelkern M, Hoh C, Mayer E. (1996) Regional cerebral activity in normal and pathologic perception of visceral pain. Submitted for publication.

Simpson LO. (1989) Nondiscocytic erythrocytes in myalgic encephalomyelitis. *N Z Med J* 102: 126-127.

Sissons JGP. (1993) Superantigens and infectious disease. *Lancet* 341: 1627-1628.

Skutella T, Criswell H, Moy S, Probst JC, Breese GR, Jirikowski GF, Holsboer F. (1994) Corticotropin-releasing hormone (CRH) antisense oligodeoxynucleotide induces anxiolytic effects in rat. *NeuroReport* 5: 2181-2185.

Smagin GN, Swiergel AH, Dunn AJ. (1995) Corticotropin-releasing factor administered into the locus coeruleus, but not the parabrachial nucleus, stimulates norepinephrine release in the prefrontal cortex. *Brain Res Bull* 36(1): 71-76.

Smith GD, Harrison SM, Birch PJ, Elliott PJ, Malcangio M, Bowery NG. (1994) Increased sensitivity to the antinociceptive activity of (±)-baclofen in animal model of chronic neuropathic, but not chronic inflammatory, hyperalgesia. *Neuropharmacol* 33(9): 1103-1108.

Snyder SH. (1994) Gases as neural messengers in the brain. *Neuropsychopharmacol* 10(3S/Pt.1): 34S-36S.

Snyder SL, Rosenbaum DH, Rowan AJ, Strain JJ. (1994) SCID diagnosis of panic disorder in psychogenic seizure patients. *J Neuropsychiatry Clin Neurosci* 6: 261-266.

Soltesz I, Haby M, Leresche N, Cronelli V. (1988) The $GABA_B$ antagonist phaclofen inhibits the late K^+-dependent IPSP in cat and rat thalamic and hippocampal neurons. *Brain Res* 448: 351-354.

Soltis RP, Anderson LA, Walters JR, Kelland MD. (1994) A role for non-NMDA excitatory amino acid receptors in regulating the basal activity of rat globus pallidus neurons and their activation by the subthalamic nucleus. *Brain Res* 666: 21-30.

Sotomayor EM, DiNapoli MR, Lopez-Cepero M, Lopez DM. (1993) The impaired tumoricidal function of macrophages from tumor bearing mice is related to defective nitric oxide production. *FASEB Journal* 7(1): 58A.

Speransky AD. (1943) *A Basis for the Theory of Medicine.* New York: International Publishers.

Stark M, Mahler K, Gupta P, Epstein S, Cannon R, Leis J, Benjamin S. (1991) Visceral afferent blockade with ondansetron (Zofran) increases nociceptive thresholds in patients with chest pain of unknown etiology (CPUE). *Am J Gastroenterol* 86: 1305.

Steen KH, Reech PW, Anton J, Handworker HO. (1992) Protons selectively induce lasting excitation and sensitization to mechanical stimulation of nociceptors in rat skin in vitro. *J Neurosci* 12: 86-95.

Stefano GB, Smith EM, Cadet P, Hughes TK Jr. (1993) HIV gp120 alteration of DAMA and IL-1 alpha induced chemotactic responses in human and invertebrate monocytes. *J Neuroimmunol* 43: 177-184.

Stein MB, Miller TW, Larsen DK, Kreiger MH. (1995) Irregular breathing during sleep in patients with panic disorder. *Am J Psychiatry* 152(8): 1168-1173.

Stenfors C, Mathe AA, Theodorsson E. (1994) Repeated electroconvulsive stimuli: Changes in neuropeptide Y, neurotensin, and tachykinin concentrations in time. *Prog Neuropsychopharmacol Biol Psychiatry* 18(1): 201-209.

Steriade M. (1993) Central core modulation of spontaneous oscillations and sensory transmission in thalamocortical systems. *Curr Opin Neurobiol* 3(4): 619-625.

Steriade M. (1994) Sleep oscillations and their blockage by activating systems. *J Psychiatr Clin Neurosci* 19(5): 354-358.

Steriade M, McCarley RW. (1990) *Brainstem Control of Wakefulness During Sleep.* New York: Plenum.

Steriade M, Domich L, Oakson G. (1986) Reticularis thalami neurons revisited: activity changes during states of vigilance. *Brain Res Rev* 8: 1-63.

Steriade M, McCormick DA, Sejnowski TJ. (1993) Thalamocortical oscillations in the sleeping and aroused brain. *Science* 262(5134): 679-685.

Steriade M, Nunez A, Amzica F. (1993) A novel slow (<1Hz) oscillation of neocortical neurons in vivo: Depolarizing and hyperpolarizing components. *J Neurosci* 13(8): 3252-3265.

Steriade, M, Contreras D, Curro Dossi R, Nunez A. (1993) The slow (<1Hz) oscillation in reticular thalamic and thalamocortical neurons: Scenario of sleep rhythm generation in interacting thalamic and neocortical networks. *J Neurosci* 13(8): 3284-3299.

Steriade M, Deschenes M, Domich L, Mulle C. (1985) Abolition of spindle oscillations in thalamic neurons disconnected from nucleus reticularis thalami. *J Neurophysiol* 54: 1473-1497.

Steriade M, Pare D, Parent A, Smith Y. (1988) Projections of cholinergic and non-cholinergic brainstem reticular neurons to relay and associational thalamic nuclei in the cat and the monkey. *Neurosci* 25: 47-67.

Sterling P, Eyer J. (1981) Allostasis: A new paradigm to explain arousal pathology. In Fisher S, Reason HS (Eds.), *Handbook of Life Stress, Cognition and Health* (pp. 121-150). New York: John Wiley and Sons.

Stevens WR, McCarley RW, Greene RW. (1994) The mechanism of noradrenergic alpha-1 excitatory modulation of pontine reticular formation neurons. *J Neurosci* 14(1): 6481-6487.

Stojilkovic SS, Catt KJ. (1992) Neuroendocrine action of endothelins. *Trends Pharmacol Sci* 13(10): 385-391.

Stolarek I, Blacklaw J, Forrest G, Brodie MJ. (1994) Vigabatrin and lamotrigine in refractory epilepsy. *J Neurol Neurosurg Psychiatry* 57: 921-924.

Stoof JC, Drukovich B, Vermeulen RJ. (1993) Dopamine and glutamate receptor subtypes as (potential) targets for the pharmacotherapy of Parkinson's disease. In Wolters EC, Scheltens P (Eds.), *Mental Dysfunction in Parkinson's Disease* (pp. 19-34). Amsterdam: Vrije Universiteit.

Stout AK, Woodward JJ. (1994) Differential effects of nitric oxide gas and nitric oxide donors on depolarization- induced release of [^{3}H] norepinephrine from rat hippocampal slices. *Neuropharmacol* 33: 1367-1374.

Sukhov RR, Walker LC, Rance NE, Price DL, Young WS. (1993) Vasopressin and oxytocin gene expression in the human hypothalamus. *J Comp Neurol* 337(2): 295-306.

Susman VL, Katz JL. (1988) Weaning and depression: Another postpartum complication. *Am J Psychiatry* 145(4): 498-501.

Suzdak PD, Gianutsos G. (1985) Parallel changes in the sensitivity of gamma-aminobutyric acid and noradrenergic receptors following chronic administration of antidepressant and GABAergic drugs. *Neuropharmacol* 24: 217-222.

Suzuki T, Takamori K, Takahashi Y, Narita M, Misawa M, Onodera K. (1994) The differential effects of histamine receptor antagonists on morphine and U-50, 488H-induced antinociception in the mouse. *Life Sci* 54(3): 203-211.

Svensson A, Carlsson ML, Carlsson A. (1994) Glutamatergic neurons projecting to the nucleus accumbens can affect motor functions in opposite directions depending on the dopaminergic tone. *Prog Neuropsychopharmacol Biol Psychiat* 18: 1203-1218.

Svensson TH. (1994) Dysregulation of locus ceruleus: Significance for midbrain dopamine cell functioning. *Neuropsychopharmacol* 10(3S/Pt.1): 509S.

Svensson TH, Mathe JM, Andersson JL, Nomikos GG, Hildebrand BE, Marcus M. (1995) Mode of action of atypical neuroleptics in relation to the phencyclidine model of schizophrenia: Role of

5-HT$_2$ receptor and alpha$_1$-adrenoceptor antagonism. *J Clin Psychopharmacol* 15(suppl.1): 11S-18S.

Swanson LW. (1993) *Brain Maps: Structure of the Rat Brain.* New York: Elsevier.

Swanson LW, Sawchenko PE, Rivier J, Vale WW. (1983) Organization of ovine corticotropin-releasing factor immunoreactive cells and fibers in the rat brain, an immunohistochemical study. *Neuroendocrinol* 36: 165-186.

Swanson R. (1993) Introduction: Potassium channels. *Sem Neurosci* 5: 77-78.

Swerdlow NR, Koob GF. (1987) Lesions of the dorsomedial nucleus of the thalamus, medial prefrontal cortex, and pedunculopontine nucleus: Effects on locomotor activity mediated by nucleus accumbens-ventral pallidal circuitry. *Brain Res* 412 (2): 233-243.

Swerdlow NR, Wan FJ, Kodsi M, Hartston HJ, Caine SB. (1993a) Limbic cortico-striato-pallido-pontine (CSPP) substrates of startle gating. *Biol Psychiatry* 33: 93A.

Swerdlow NR, Auerbach P, Monroe SM, Hartston H, Geyer MA, Braff DL. (1993b) Men are more inhibited than women by weak prepulses. *Biol Psychiatry* 34: 253-260.

Swiergel AH, Takahashi LK, Kalin NH. (1993) Attenuation of stress-induced behavior by antagonism of corticotropin-releasing factor receptors in the central amygdala in the rat. *Brain Res* 623: 229-234.

Szymusiak R, McGinty D. (1986) Sleep related neuronal discharge in the basal forebrain of cats. *Brain Res* 370: 82.

Taal W, Holstege JC. (1994) GABA and glycine frequently colocalize in terminals on cat spinal motoneurons. *NeuroReport* 5: 2225-2228.

Taber AT, Fibiger HC (1993) Electrical stimulation of the medial prefrontal cortex increases dopamine release in the striatum. *Neuropsychopharmacol* 9: 271-275.

Takamatsu Y, Yamamoto H, Ogunremi OO, Matsuzaki I, Moroji T. (1991) The effects of corticotropin-releasing hormone on peptidergic neurons in the rat forebrain. *Neuropep* 20(4): 255-265.

Talley NJ. (1994) Why do functional gastrointestinal disorders come and go? *Dig Dis Sci* 39: 673-677.

Tanada G, Carboni E, Frau R, DiChiara G. (1994) Increase of extracellular dopamine in the prefrontal cortex: A trait of drugs with antidepressant potential? *Psychopharmacol* 115: 285-288.

Tang AC, Hasselmo ME. (1994) Selective suppression in intrinsic but not afferent fiber synaptic transmission by baclofen in the piriform (olfactory) cortex. *Brain Res* 659: 75-81.

Tang C-M, Shi QY, Katchman A, Lynch G. (1991) Modulation of the time course of fast EPSCs and glutamate channels by aniracetam. *Science* 254: 288-290.

Taniguchi K, Ichimata M, Matsumoto S. (1993) The effects of several calcium channel blockers on the pain threshold when administered by iontophoresis. *Abstract, 7th World Congress on Pain* (p. 46). Seattle: IASP Publications.

Tanum L, Malt UF. (1995) Sodium lactate infusion in fibromyalgia patients. *Biol Psychiatry* 38: 559-561.

Tasker RR, Dostrovsky JO. (1989) Deafferentation and chronic pain. In Wall PD, Melzack R (Eds.), *Textbook of Pain* (pp. 154-180). Edinburgh: Churchill Livingstone.

Tassorelli C, Joseph SA. (1995) NADPH-diaphorase activity and Fos expression in brain nuclei following nitroglycerin administration. *Brain Res* 695: 37-44.

Taylor AD, Cowell A-M, Flower J, Buckingham JC. (1993) Lipocortin 1 mediates an early inhibitory action of glucocorticoids on the secretion of ACTH by the rat anterior pituitary gland in vitro. *Neuroendocrinol* 56: 430-439.

Taylor CP. (1994) Emerging perspectives on the mechanism of action of gabapentin. *Neurol* 44 (suppl. 5): 510-516.

Teicher MH, Glod G, Surrey J, Swett C. (1993) Early childhood abuse and limbic system ratings in adult psychiatric outpatients. *J Neuropsychiatry Clin Neurosci* 5(3): 301-306.

Terao A, Oikawa M, Saito M. (1993) Cytokine-induced change in norepinephrine turnover: Involvement of corticotropin-releasing hormone and prostaglandins. *Brain Res* 622: 257-261.

Terrian DM. (1995) Persistent enhancement of sustained calcium-dependent glutamate release by phorbol esters: Requirement for localized calcium entry. *J Neurochem* 64: 172-180.

Terry AV, Gattu M, Buccafusco JJ, Sowell JW, Kosh JW. (1995) Enhanced spatial learning and recall in rats following administration of the novel ranitidine analog, JWS-USC-75-IX. *Abstracts, Soc for Neurosci* 21: 71.10, p. 166.

Tettenborn D, Fierus M. (1993) Clinical aspects of nimodipine treatment in brain ischemia. In Scriabine A, Janis RA, Triggle DJ (Eds.), *Drugs in Development* (vol. 2: Ca^{2+} Antagonists in the CNS, pp. 473-482). Brandford, Connecticut: Neva Press.

Thach WT, Goodkin HP, Keating JG. (1992) The cerebellum and adaptive coordination of movement. *Ann Rev Neurosci* 15: 403-422.

Thoenen H. (1995) Neurotrophins and neuronal plasticity. *Science* 270: 593-598.

Thorburn KK, Hough LB, Nalwalk JW, Mischler SA. (1994) Histamine-induced modulation of nociceptive responses. *Pain* 58(1): 29-37.

Thorson K. (1993) The limbic hypothesis. *Fibromyalgia Network* 3(27): 3.

Tolbert LC, Morris PE, Spollen JJ, Ashe SC. (1992) Stereospecific effects of ascorbic acid and analogues on D1 and D2 agonist binding. *Life Sci* 51: 921-930.

Tolbert LC, Thomas TN, Middaugh LO, Zemp JW. (1979) Effect of ascorbic acid on neurochemical, behavioral, and physiological systems mediated by catecholamines. *Life Sci* 25: 2189-2195.

Tomasch J. (1969) The numerical capacity of the human cortico-ponto-cerebellar system. *Brain Res* 13: 476-484.

Tonkonogy J, Goodglass H. (1981) Language function, foot of the third frontal gyrus, and rolandic operculum. *Arch Neurol* 38: 486-490.

Torack RM, Morris JC. (1988) The association of ventral tegmental area histopathology with adult dementia. *Arch Neurol* 45: 497-501.

Toselli N, Taglietti V. (1993) Baclofen inhibits high threshold calcium currents with two distinct modes in rat hippocampal neurons. *Neurosci Lett* 164: 134-136.

Traiffort E, Pollard H, Moreau J, Ruat M, Schwartz JC, Martinez-Mir MI, Palacios JM. (1992) Pharmacological characterization and autoradiographic localization of histamine H_2 receptors in human brain identified with [^{125}I]- iodoaminopotentidine. *J Neurochem* 59: 290-299.

Trautman PD, Meyer-Bahlburg HFL, Postelnek J, New MI. (1995) Effects of early prenatal dexamethasone on the cognitive and behavioral development of young children: Results of a pilot study. *Psychoneuroendocrin* 20: 439-449.

Travell J, Simon D. (1993) *Myofascial Pain and Dysfunction: The Trigger Point Manual* (vol. 2). Philadelphia: Williams and Wilkins.

Tucker DM, Williamson PA. (1984) Asymmetric neural control systems in human self-regulation. *Psychol Rev* 91: 185-215.

Uddman R, Goadsly PJ, Jansen I, Edvinsson L. (1993) PACAP, a VIP-like peptide: Immunohistochemical localization and effect upon cat pial arteries and cerebral blood flow. *J Cereb Blood Flow Metab* 13: 291-297.

Ueyama T, Nemoto K, Tone S, Senba E. (1995) Stress-induced unbalanced expression of neurotrophins and their receptors in the brain. *Abstracts, Soc for Neurosci* 21:L 126.2, p. 297.

Unger P, Berkenboom G, Fontaine J. (1993) Interaction between hydralazine and nitrovasodilators in vascular smooth muscle. *J Cardiovasc Pharmacol* 21: 478-483.

Uvnas-Moberg K. (1994) Role of efferent and afferent vagal nerve activity during reproduction: Integrating function of oxytocin on metabolism and behaviour. *Psychoneuroendocrinol* 19(5-7): 687-695.

Uvnas-Mohberg K, Alster P, Hillegaart V, Ahlenius S. (1992) Oxytocin reduces exploratory motor behavior and shifts the activity towards the centre of the arena in male rats. *Acta Physiol Scand* 145:429-430.

Uvnas-Moberg K, Bruzelius G, Alster P, Bileviciute L, Lundberg T. (1992) Oxytocin increases and a specific oxytocin antagonist decreases pain threshold in male rats. *Acta Physiol Scand* 144: 487-488.

Vaeroy H, Helle R, Forre O, Kass E, Terenius L. (1988) Elevated CSF levels of substance P and high incidence of Raynaud phenomenon in patients with fibromyalgia: New features for diagnosis. *Pain* 32(1): 21-26.

Valentino RJ, Page ME, Luppi P-H, Zhu Y, Bockstaele EV, Aston-Jones G. (1994) Evidence for widespread afferents to Barrington's nucleus, a brainstem region rich in corticotropin-releasing hormone neurons. *Neurosci* 62(1): 125-143.

Valtschanoff JG, Weinberg RJ, Kharazia VN, Nakane M, Schmidt HH. (1993) Neurons in rat hippocampus that synthesize nitric oxide. *J Comp Neurol* 331(1): 111-121.

Van Bockstaele EJ, Cestari DM, Pickel VM. (1994) Synaptic structure and connectivity of serotonin terminals in the ventral tegmental area: potential sites for modulation of mesolimbic dopamine neurons. *Brain Res* 647: 307-322.

Van de Kar LD, Rittenhouse PA, Li C, Levy AD, Brownfield MS. (1995) Hypothalamic paraventricular, but not supraoptic neurons, mediate the serotonergic stimulation of oxytocin secretion. *Brain Res Bull* 36(1): 45-50.

Van der Kooy D, Koda LY, McGinty JF, Gerfen CR, Bloom FE. (1984) The organization of projections from the cortex, amygdala and hypothalamus to the nucleus of the solitary tract in rats. *J Comp Neurol* 224:1.

Vasile RG. (1994) Increase in left frontal cerebral blood flow following electroconvulsive treatment for depression. *Neuropsychopharmacol* 10(3S/Pt.1): 147S.

Villablanca JR, Marcus RJ, Olmstead CE. (1976) Effects of caudate nuclei or frontal cortex ablations in cats, II: Sleep-wakefulness, EEG, and motor activity. *Exp Neurol* 53: 31.

Virsolvy-Vergine A, Bruck M, Dufour M, Caurin A, Lupo B, Bataille D. (1988) An endogenous ligand for the central sulfonylurea receptor. *FEBS Lett* 242: 65-69.

Vivas NM, Marmol F, Salles J, Badia A, Dierssen M. (1995) Action on noradrenergic transmission of an anticholinesterase: 9-amino-1,2,3,4-tetrahydroacridine. *Neuropharmacol* 34 : 367-375.

Vojdani A, Ghoneum M. (1993) In vivo effect of ascorbic acid on enhancement of natural killer cell activity. *Nutrition Res* 13: 753-764.

Vojdani A., Goldstein JA. (1992) One gram of oral ascorbic acid normalizes deficits in natural killer cell function in one day in patients with chronic fatigue syndrome (unpublished experiment).

Von Sattel J-P, Myers RH, Stevens TJ, Ferrante RJ, Bird ED, Richardson EP. (1985) Neuropathological classification of Huntington's disease. *J Neuropathol Exp Neurol* 44: 559-577.

Vorobjev VS, Sharanova IN. (1994) Tetrahydroaminoacridine blocks and prolongs NMDA receptor-mediated responses in a voltage-dependent manner. *Eur J Pharmacol* 253: 1-8.

Wafford KA, Bain CJ, Quirk K, McKernan RM, Wingrove PB, Whiting PJ, Kemp JA. (1994) A novel allosteric modulatory site on the GABA$_A$ receptor beta subunit. *Neuron* 12: 775-782.

Wallace D. (1995) Personal communication.

Wallace DJ, Silberman S, Goldstein J, Hughes D. (1995) Use of hyperbaric oxygen in rheumatic diseases: Case report and critical analysis. *Lupus* 4: 172-175.

Wang S-J, Huang C-C, Gean P-W. (1995) Tetrahydro-9-aminoacridine presynaptically inhibits glutamatergic transmission in the rat amygdala. *Brain Res Bull* 37(3): 325-327.

Watkins LR, Maier SF, Goehler LE. (1995a) Cytokine-to-brain communication: A review and analysis of alternative mechanisms. *Life Sci* 57(11): 1011-1026.

Watkins LR, Maier SF, Goehler LE. (1995b) Immune activation: The role of pro-inflammatory cytokines in inflammation, illness responses, and pathological pain states. *Pain* 63: 289-302.

Waylonis GW, Heck W. (1992) Fibromyalgia syndrome: New associations. *American J Phys Med Rehab* 71: 343-348.

Wayner MJ, Armstrong DL, Polan-Curtain JL, Denny JB. (1993) Role of angiotensin II and AT$_1$ receptors in hippocampal LTP. *Pharmacol Biochem Behav* 45: 455-464.

Webb DJ. (1991) Endothelin receptors cloned, endothelin converting enzyme characterized and pathophysiological roles for endothelin proposed. *Trends Pharmacol Sci* 12(2): 43-46.

Weber B. (1994) Quinoxalinedione-type antagonists at the glycine coagonist site of the NMDA receptor–in vitro and in vivo efficacy profiles. *Neuropsychopharmacol* 10(3S/Pt.1): 101S.

Weidenfeld J, Feldman S, Mechoulan R. (1994) Effect of the brain constituent anandamide, a cannabinoid receptor agonist, on the hypothalamo-pituitary-adrenal axis in the rat. *Neuroendocrinol* 59: 110-112.

Weinberger DR. (1993) A connectionist approach to the prefrontal cortex. *J Neuropsychiatry Clin Neurosci* 5: 241-253.

Weiser SD, Patrick SL, Mascarella SW, Downing-Park J, Bai X, Carol FI, Walker JM, Patrick RL. (1995) Stimulation of rat stria-

tal tyrosine hydroxylase activity following intranigral administration of sigma receptor ligands. *Eur J Pharmacol* 275: 1-7.

Weiss JM, Scott P. (1994) Stress-induced behavioral depression:
Update on the role of the locus ceruleus. *Neuropsychopharmacol*
10(35/Pt.1): 511S.

Weiss JM, Stout JC, Aaron MF, Quan N, Owens MJ, Butler PD,
Meneroff CB. (1994) Depression and anxiety: Role of locus coeruleus and corticotropin-releasing factor. *Brain Res Bull* 35:
561-572.

Welty DF, Schielke GP, Vartanian MG, Taylor CP. (1993) Gabapentin anticonvulsant action in rats: Disequilibrium with peak drug
concentrations in plasma and brain microdialysate. *Epilepsy Res*
16(3): 176-181.

Weston AH, Edwards G. (1992) Recent progress in potassium channel opener pharmacology. *Biochem Pharmacol* 43: 47-54.

Whitaker-Azmitia PM, Quartermain D, Shermer AV. (1990) Prenatal treatment with a selective D_1-receptor agonist, SKF 38393,
alters development of serotonin neurons: Behavioral and
biochemical studies. *Dev Brain Res* 57: 127-132.

White JM, Rumbhold GR. (1988) Behavioral effects of histamine
and its antagonists: A review. *Psychopharmacol* 95: 1-14.

Whitnall MH, Kiss A, Aguilera G. (1993) Contrasting effects of central alpha-1-adrenoceptor activation on stress-responsive and stress-
nonresponsive subpopulations of corticotropin-releasing hormone
neurosecretory cells in the rat. *Neuroendocrinol* 58: 42-48.

Wickramsinghe SN, Hasan R. (1994) In vivo effects of vitamin C
on the cytotoxicity of post-ethanol serum. *Biochem Pharmacol*
48(3): 621-624.

Williams CA, Gopalen R, Nichols PL, Brien PL. (1995) Fatiguing
isometric contraction of hind-limb muscles results in release of
immunoreactive neurokinins from sites in the rostral medulla in
the anesthetized cat. *Neuropep* 28: 209-218.

Williamson AM, Ohara PT, Ralston DD, Milroy AM, Ralston HJ.
(1994) Analysis of gamma-aminobutyric acid synaptic contacts
in the thalamic reticular nucleus of the monkey. *J Comp Neurol*
349: 182-189.

Wilson MA, McNaughton BL. (1994) Reactivation of hippocampal
ensemble memories during sleep. *Science* 265(5172): 676-679.

Wise TN, Mann LA. (1994) The relationship between somatosensory amplification, alexithymia, and neuroticism. *J Psychosom Res* 38(6): 515-521.

Witt DM, Insel TR. (1994) Increased fos expression in oxytocin neurons following masculine sexual behavior. *J Neuroendocrinol* 6: 13-18.

Won CK, Park MY, Park SH, Pyun KH, Park HJ, Shin HC. (1995) Interukin-1 beta facilitates afferent sensory transmission in the primary somatosensory cortex. *Abstracts, Soc for Neurosci* 21: 45.7, p. 98.

Wong M-l, Bongiorno PB, Gold PW, Licinio J. (1995) Localization of interleukin-1 beta converting enzyme mRNA in rat brain vasculature: Evidence that the genes encoding the interleukin-1 system are constitutively expressed in brain blood vessels. *Neuroimmunomod* 2: 141-148.

Wood JD. (1994) Efficacy of leuprolide in treatment of the irritable bowel syndrome. *Dig Dis Sci* 39(6): 1153-1154.

Woolf CJ, Thompson SWN. (1991) The induction and maintenance of central sensitization is dependent upon N-methyl-D-aspartic acid receptor activation: Implications for the treatment of post-injury hypersensitivity states. *Pain* 44: 293-300.

Wu C. (1993) NMDA receptor antagonist CPP inhibits ethanol-evoked ascorbate release in the brain of freely moving rats. *Neurosci Lett* 157: 111-114.

Wu C. (1994) Possible role of glutamatergic neurotransmission in regulating ethanol-evoked brain ascorbate release. *Neurosci Lett* 171: 105-108.

Wu L-G, Saggau P. (1994) Adenosine inhibits evoked synaptic transmission primarily by reducing presynaptic calcium influx in area CA1 of the hippocampus. *Neuron* 12: 1139-1148.

Wurpel JN. (1994) Baclofen prevents rapid amygdala kindling in adult rats. *Experientia* 50(5): 475-478.

Xu JY, Tseng LF. (1993) Increase of nitric oxide by L-arginine potentiates beta endorphin-but not mu-, gamma-, or kappa-opioid agonist-induced antinociception in the mouse. *Eur J Pharmacol* 336: 137-142.

Xu X-J, Wiesenfeld-Hallin Z, Hughes J, Horwell DC, Hokfelt T. (1992) CI988, a selective antagonist of cholecystokinin B receptors, prevents morphine tolerance in the rat. *Br J Pharmacol* 105: 591-596.

Yaksh TL, Malmberg AB. (1994) Central pharmacology of nociceptive transmission. In Wall PD, Melzack RM (Eds.), *Texbook of Pain* (3rd ed., pp. 165-200). Edinburgh: Churchill Livingstone.

Yamada KA. (1994) Personal communication.

Yamada KA, Tang C-M. (1993) Benzothiadiazides inhibit rapid glutamate receptor desensitization and enhance glutamatergic synaptic currents. *J Neurosci* 13(9): 3904-3915.

Yamamoto T, Yaksh TL. (1992) Spinal pharmacology of thermal hyperesthesia induced by constriction injury of the sciatic nerve: Excitatory amino acid antagonists. *Pain* 49: 121-128.

Yamamoto R, Bredt DS, Synder SH, Stone RA. (1993) The localization of nitric oxide synthase in the rat eye and related cranial ganglia. *Neurosci* 54(1): 189-200.

Yasin S, Costa A, Naverra P, Pozzoli G, Kostoglou-Athanassiou I, Forsling M, Grossman A. (1994) Endothelin-1 stimulates the in-vitro release of neurohypophyseal hormones, but not corticotropin-releasing hormone, via ET_A receptors. *Neuroendocrinol* 60: 553-558.

Yeomans DC, Proudfit HK. (1990) Projections of substance P immunoreactive neurons located in the ventromedial medulla to the A7 noradrenergic nucleus of the rat demonstrated using retrograde tracing comined with immunocytochemistry. *Brain Res* 532: 329-332.

Yoshida M, Yokoo H, Tanaka T, Emoto H, Tanaka M. (1994) Opposite changes in the mesolimbic dopamine metabolism in the nerve terminal and cell body sites induced by locally infused baclofen in the rat. *Brain Res* 636(1): 111-114.

Yunus MB. (1992) Towards a model of pathophysiology of fibromyalgia: Aberrant central pain mechanisms with peripheral modulation. *J Rheumatol* 19: 846-850.

Yunus MB. (1994) Psychological aspects of fibromyalgia syndrome: A component of the dysfunctional spectrum syndrome. In Masi A (Ed.), *Fibromyalgia and Myofascial Pain Syndromes*. London: Balliere.

Zavonik MK, Fichte CM. (1991) Trigeminal neuralgia relieved by ophthalmic anesthetic. *JAMA* 265: 2807.

Zhuo M, Small SA, Kandel ER, Hawkins RD. (1993) Nitric oxide and carbon monoxide produce activity-dependent long-term synaptic enhancement in hippocampus. *Science* 260: 1946-1949.

Ziegler MG, Ruiz-Ramon P, Shapiro MH. (1993) Abnormal stress responses in patients with diseases affecting the sympathetic nervous system. *Psychosom Med* 55 (4): 339-346.

Zorumski CF, Izumi Y. (1993) Nitric oxide and hippocampal synaptic plasticity. *Biochem Pharmacol* 46(5): 777-785.

Zuardi AW, Morais SL, Guimaraes FS, Mechoulam R. (1995) Antipsychotic effect of cannabidiol. *J Clin Psychiatry* 56: 485-486.

Zubenko GS, Nixon RA. (1984) Mood elevating effects of captopril in depressed patients. *Am J Psychiatry* 141: 110-111.

Index

Page numbers followed by the letter "t" indicate a table.